The Feds

The Feds

An Account of the Federated Dublin Voluntary Hospitals

1961–2005

Edited by
David FitzPatrick

A. & A. Farmar

British Library Cataloguing in Publication Data
A CIP catalogue record for this book is available from the British Library

ISBN 1-899047-37-9
First published in 2006
by
A. & A. Farmar Ltd
78 Ranelagh Village, Dublin 6, Ireland
Tel +353-1-496 3625 Fax +353-1-497 0107
Email afarmar@iol.ie

Printed and bound by GraphyCems
Typeset and designed by A. & A. Farmar
Indexed by Helen Litton
Cover designed by Kevin Gurry
Hospital drawings by Thomas Wilson

Dedication

This book is dedicated to those who had the vision to establish the Federated Hospital Group, to all who worked to maintain the Voluntary Hospital tradition in those hospitals and to those who continue today to maintain that tradition in both St James's and the Adelaide and Meath Hospital, Dublin Incorporating the National Children's Hospital.

Contents

The Feds in Pictures falls between pages 138 and 139

Part Three: The development of specialty units

Acknowledgements

It is customary in a volume such as this to thank the individual contributors but in this instance there are so many it has seemed appropriate to name and describe them in a separate section (see page x). There can be no doubt that without these contributions this book would never have been produced and I must sincerely thank all who have made it possible. From the outset the project has been greeted with great enthusiasm from all I asked to contribute and I appreciate the difficulties many have experienced in finding time to write during their busy schedules.

It is invidious to single out anyone in particular but for general advice I must especially thank Peter Gatenby, Desmond Dempsey, the former FDVH CEO, and the present administrator Tim Lyne. Miss Betty O'Dwyer has been a constant encourager and with Mary Cotter has provided names for some of the photographs. Other illustrations have been provided by Michael Butler, John Bonnar, Donald Weir, Colm O'Morain, Sibéal Carolan, Davis Coakley and the Adelaide Society but special thanks is extended to Bobby and David Coleman (Bobby Studios) for trawling through their archives and producing many fine photos relating to the Federated Hospitals. I must also make special mention of Thomas Wilson whose illustrations for the FDVH Annual Conference Brochure will be remembered by many. He has taken time to redraw many of these to make them suitable for reproduction here. Michael Pegum has been responsible for the recent photographs of the hospitals. The sources of the chapters on plastic surgery, physiotherapy and the Adelaide are attributed in the text. It is quite impossible to name all those who have advised, encouraged and generally helped in the creation of this volume. May I now acknowledge all those who are not mentioned above or in the list of contributors? Your help, advice and comments have always been greatly appreciated—I cannot think of any adverse criticism received during the production time!

For financial support I am most grateful to the Federated Dublin Voluntary Hospitals Central Council, and to the Meath Foundation. Without this assistance production would have been difficult if not impossible.

The volume has been published by A. & A. Farmar and Anna and Tony have been of immense support during the book's genesis. They took on the project I think with only an inkling of the amount of work the collation so many papers would involve. They have been tireless in their work, always approachable for advice and they have been a pleasure to work with. To merely thank them seems inadequate and my appreciation of their efforts is boundless.

I could not finish without thanking Felicity, my wife, for her encouragement over the past few years while work has been in progress, and for her tolerance of a house which from time to time has had the appearance of a record repository rather than a home.

David FitzPatrick
February 2006

Contributors

PROFESSOR JOHN BONNAR MB (Glas. 1958) MD (Glas. 1971) FRCOG
FRCPI. 1969–75 Reader in Obstetrics and Gynaecology University of
Oxford and consultant in John Radcliffe Hospital. 1975–9 Professor
and Head of Obstetrics and Gynaecology TCD. 1975–9 consultant in
Rotunda and Adelaide Hospitals. 1980–7 Dean of Faculty of Health
Sciences TCD. 1988–99 St James's and the Coombe Hospitals.

MR FRANK BRADY FFDRCSI MB BDS (UCD 1969) FRCSI FFDRCSI
FDSRCS (Eng.). Consultant maxillo-facial surgeon FDVH; assigned
to Dr Steevens' Hospital then transferred to St James's Hospital.

MR MICHAEL BUTLER MB BSc FRCSI FRCS FRCS (Edin. & Glas. (hc))
FAMS.Appointed FDVH 1974, assigned to GU Department Meath
and St James's Hospitals and National Rehabilitation Centre, transferred to Tallaght Hospital 1998. President RCSI 2003, 2004. Senior
Lecturer Urology TCD.

MS SIBÉAL CAROLAN Registered with An Bord Altranais: General, Child
Health and Tutor Divisions, SGN Meath Hospital 1984. Master's
Degree in Nursing (TCD 1999). Postgraduate Diploma in Clinical
Health Sciences Education. Currently Nurse Practice Development
Co-ordinator at AMNCH.

PROFESSOR DAVIS COAKLEY MB (Cork 1971) MD FRCPI FRCP (Lond.)
FRCP (Edin.). Consultant in geriatric medicine St James's Hospital,
sometime Dean of the Faculty of Health Sciences TCD. Medical
historian.

MS ANNA DOLAN SGN SCN. Trained in Dr Steevens' Hospital 1972-5,
A&E Certificate 1979. Appointments include St James's, St Vincent's
and Dr Steevens' Hospitals and CNM Trauma Arab Sultanates, then
CNM2 Meath Hospital, presently CNM2 AMNCH.

MR ERIC FENELON MA MB (TCD 1944) FRCSI. Consultant ENT
surgeon Adelaide, Dr Steevens' and Royal Victoria Eye and Ear Hospitals. Member of Adelaide Board and Central Council FDVH. Retired
1998. Died 2005.

Mr David FitzPatrick MA MB M.Ch FRCSI FRCS. Consultant orthopaedic surgeon FDVH 1971–2001, assigned initially to Dr Steevens', Adelaide and NCH, later to the Meath and finally (1998) to Tallaght . Sometime Lecturer in Surgery and in Orthopaedics TCD and orthopaedic surgeon to the Rotunda and Incorporated Orthopaedic Hospital of Ireland. Retired 2001.

Dr H. Joseph Galvin LRCP&SI (1955) LM Rotunda DA (Eng.) FFARCSI. Consultant anaesthetist FDVH 1961, assigned to the Meath 1961-92, Rotunda 1967–92, St James's 1974–85.

Professor Peter Gatenby MB (TCD 1946) MD FRCPI FRCP (Lond.) Hon. FRCP (Edin.) Hon. FACP Hon. FTCD. Consulting physician Dr Steevens' Hospital 1953–74, consulting physician Meath Hospital 1957–74, consulting physician Rotunda Hospital 1949–74. Professor of Clinical Medicine TCD 1961–74. Medical Director United Nations (New York) 1974–82. Chief Medical Officer FAO United Nations (Rome) 1982–7.

Dr Gerard F. Gearty MB (UCD 1953) ScD FRCPI. Consultant cardiologist FDVH, assigned to Royal City of Dublin Hospital, Baggot Street 1963. Member of Board of RCDH and of Central Council FDVH.

Professor Ian Graham MB (TCD) 1969 FRCPI FESC. Consultant cardiologist, Associate Professor of Medicine TCD and Professor of Public Health Medicine and Epidemiology RCSI. Appointed to FDVH 1982, assigned as cardiologist to Adelaide and Meath 1982, transferred to AMNCH 1998.

Professor Tom Hennessy MD MCh FRCS FRCSI, Regius Professor of Surgery TCD. Consultant surgeon St James's Hospital. Consultant surgeon FDVH—Royal City of Dublin Hospital Baggot Street and Dr Steevens' Hospital 1975–98. President of RCSI 1994 and 1995.

Professor Hilary M. C. V. Hoey MA MD (TCD) MB (UCD) DCH (UCD), DObsRCOG (Lond.) FRCPI FRCPCH FTCD MICGP. Head of Department of Paediatrics TCD and consultant paediatrician endocrinologist National Children's Hospital and Our Lady's Hospital for Sick Children 1991 to date.

PROFESSOR DERMOT HOURIHANE MD (NUI) FRCPI FRCPath FTCD (1976). Professor of Histology and Morbid Anatomy TCD. Principal Pathologist to FDVH.

PROFESSOR D. I. D. HOWIE MA BSc PhD LlD (h.c.) MIBiol FIBiolI FTCD. Formerly Registrar (1966–74) , Vice Provost (1974–81) and Senior Fellow TCD, Associate Professor of Zoology and Head of Department 1988–93. Chairman FDVH 1974–7. Chairman St James's board in alternate years 1973–84 and Chairman 1984–2002. Governor St Patrick's 1984–2004 and at various times a member of the boards of the Rotunda and National Childrens' Hospitals.

DR GERARD HURLEY LRCPI MRCSI (1967) FRCR FFRRCSI. Consultant radiologist Adelaide and Meath, transferred to AMNCH in 1998. Member of boards of Meath and AMNCH. Sometime Dean FAC-ULTY OF RADIOLOGISTS RCSI.

PROFESSOR CONOR KEANE MB (NUI 1961) MD FRCPath FRCPI FTCD FFPath RCSI. Consultant microbiologist FDVH 1971–82, assigned to the Adelaide Hospital; St James's 1982–2002 . Sometime Associate Professor of Clinical Microbiology TCD.

MS KAY KEATING MISCP MSCP DipTP. Taught at Mater Hospital, then Superintendent Physiotherapist at Central Remedial Clinic. President of the Irish Society of Chartered Physiotherapists 1983.

PROFESSOR BRIAN KEOGH MD FRCPI FFOM FFPHM FRCP (Edin.) FACP (Hon.). Consultant physician/nephrologist Tallaght Hospital, St Vincent's Hospital, Blackrock Clinic, the Coombe Hospital, Beaumont Hospital. Associate Professor of Renal Diseases, TCD. Past President and founder member Irish Nephrological Society. Member Renal Association of Great Britain and Ireland. Member American Society of Nephrology. Past President RCPI. Chairman National Immunisation Advisory Committee.

MR DENIS LAWLOR MB (NUI 1969) FRCSI (1973). 1980/81 Fellowship Melbourne Micro-vascular Surgery. Accredited Plastic Surgeon 1984. Appointed consultant FDVH 1985, assigned Dr Steevens', Mater and James Connolly Memorial, moved to St James's and Mater 1988. Currently senior plastic surgeon St James's and the Mater.

PROFESSOR J. B. LYONS MB (NUI 1945), MD (NUI 1949) MRCPI (1949) FRCPI (1959). Consultant physician St Michael's Hospital, Mercer's

Hospital and Sir Patrick Dun's Hospital. Professor of the History of Medicine RCSI.

Dr Edward A. Martin MD FRCPI. Retired neurologist Adelaide Hospital and St Vincent's Hospital.

Professor David McConnell BA PhD FTCD MRIA FZSI. Chairman of the Adelaide Hospital 1988–9. Played a leading role in the development of AMNCH and its Charter. Presently Professor of Genetics TCD and Chairman of The Irish Times Trust.

Dr W. J. McCormack, MA, DPhil, FRSA, is Librarian in Charge at the Worth Library (1733)—see www:edwardworthlibrary.ie. His most recent book is *Blood Kindred: W. B. Yeats, the Life, the Death, the Politics* (Pimlico, 2005). He is currently editing John Devoy's recollections of Michael Davitt for University College Dublin Press.

Dr David McInerney MB (UCD 1969) FFR RCSI. Studied in Dublin, Bristol, and Australia. Appointed consultant radiologist FDVH 1978, assigned to Dr Steevens' Hospital and in 1979 to the Adelaide and Meath Hospitals; transferred to AMNCH 1998.

Ms Mary T. Moore. Nurse Tutor Mercer's Hospital 1980-3.

Dr Fergus O'Ferrall MSc (Health Services Management TCD). Director of The Adelaide Hospital Society and member of the board of AMNCH, author *Citizenship and Public Service: Voluntary and Statutory Relationships in Irish Healthcare* (Dundalgan Press, Dundalk, 2000) and a number of works on Daniel O'Connell.

Ms Meadhbh O'Leary joined the NCH administrative staff in September 1966. Worked with House Governors Mr Donal O'Brien and Col. D. Graves. In 1969 joined the Department of Paediatrics TCD as secretary first to Professor Robert Steen and then Professors Eric Doyle, Niall Donohoe, and Hilary Hoey.

Professor Colm O'Morain MB (UCD 1972) MD MSc DSc FTCD FRCPI FRCP FEBG FACG. Consultant gastroenterologist FDVH, assigned initially to Adelaide and Meath Hospitals, then transferred to AMNCH 1998. Professor of Medicine TCD. Member of AMNCH Board.

Professor Desmond O'Neill MB TCD 1983 MD FRCPI. Consultant in geriatric medicine FDVH, assigned to Meath, Adelaide and St James's Hospitals, transferred to AMNCH in 1998. Associate Professor of Geriatric Medicine TCD.

Mr Michael Pegum MB (TCD 1962) MA MD FRCSI FRCS. Orthopaedic surgeon FDVH 1972-2003 (Meath Hospital 1972-98, Adelaide Hospital 1987-98, AMNCH 1998-2003). Lecturer in Orthopaedics TCD. Retired 2003.

Mr J. Brendan Prendiville LRCP&SI (1946) FRCSI (1949). Surgeon Dr Steevens' Hospital 1957-87. Consultant in charge, A&E Department Dr Steevens' Hospital 1971-87. Medical Director Plastic Surgery and Burns Unit FDVH , based at Dr Steevens'; also assigned to the GU Unit at the Meath Hospital.

Mr Desmond Rogan B.Comm. (NUI Galway) H Dip HSM. Secretary-manager NCH and Adelaide 1978-93. Project Director Tallaght Hospital Board 1994-2005. Director AMNCH 1998 to date.

Professor Gregor Shanik MB (TCD 1967) MD MCh FRCSI FRCS FACS. Consultant vascular surgeon St James's Hospital. Associate Professor of Surgery TCD.

Mr W. Salters Sterling MA Dip ED D Phil (h.c. DIT). Formerly Academic Secretary TCD. Chairman Board National Children's Hospital. Hon Sec. 1st Board AMNCH. Presently Member Tallaght Hospital Board. Chairman Central Council FDVH.

Dr Mervyn Taylor MA MD (TCD) PhD (Lond.) MRCP (Lond.) FRCPI FRCPCH FFPRCPI. Consultant paediatrician FDVH and Cherry Orchard Hospital and Senior Lecturer in Paediatrics TCD 1972–2005. Research Associate Department of Zoology TCD. Sometime Chairman of Paediatric Medical Advisory Committee National Children's Hospital and member of the boards of FDVH, National Children's Hospital and AMNCH.

Professor Ian Temperley MD FRCPI FRCPath. FTCD (Emeritus). Consultant haematologist FDVH 1966-95. Medical Director National Haemophilia Treatment Centre 1971–95. Consultant haematologist St James's Hospital 1977–95. Associate Professor of Haematology 1970–85. Professor of Haematology 1985–95. Dean Faculty of Health Sciences

TCD 1987–93. Full-time member of Trinity staff 1958–95.

PROFESSOR GERALD TOMKIN MB (TCD 1962) MD FRCP (Lond.) FRCP (Edin.) FRCPI FACP. Physician-endocrinology and diabetes FDVH 1975–2004, assigned initially to the Adelaide Hospital, then to the Adelaide and Meath Hospital, to AMNCH 1998–2004. Associate Professor of Medicine TCD. Past President Association of Physicians of Great Britain and Ireland. Past Vice President European Association for the Study of Diabetes.

MS SANDY WAGSTAFF Dip. Grad. Phys. (Lond.).MISCP (wife of late Paul Wagstaff, staff member DSP 1974–80, Director DSP 1980–89). Sessional physiotherapist, Adelaide Hospital 1977–97. Private practice 1988–93. Sessional physiotherapist TCD Student Health 1993–7. Senior Physiotherapist GP Service Baggot Street Community Hospital 1998 to date. Clinical supervisor and finals examiner for physiotherapy students TCD.

PROFESSOR DONALD G. WEIR MB (TCD 1958) MD FRCPI FRCP FACP FTCD. Undergraduate student and intern at Adelaide 1954–9. Lecturer Department of Clinical Medicine TCD 1964–7, Meath and Dr Steevens' Hospitals. Consultant physician St Patrick's Hospital 1969–81. Consultant gastroenterologist FDVH at Sir Patrick Dun's Hospital 1967–87, and St James's Hospital 1979–99. Regius Professor of Physic TCD 1977–99 and Head of Department of Clinical Medicine TCD.1982–99. Now retired.

DR MARJORIE YOUNG MD FRCP FRCPI. Consultant dermatologist. Appointed FDVH 1974, assigned initially to Adelaide Meath and National Children's Hospital, transferred to AMNCH 1998. Lecturer in dermatology TCD.

Foreword

W. Salters Sterling

David FitzPatrick's invitation to contribute a foreword to this book is indeed an honour. The work is an exercise of fundamental importance which will contribute significantly to the writing of the history of Dublin's health and medicine in the second half of the 20th century. It brings together in one volume the experiences and understandings of many of those who participated in the transformation of a major sector of hospital provision in the greater Dublin area. It adds to the work of others, notably Davis Coakley, Peter Gatenby, David Mitchell and J. B. Lyons, who have written histories of some of those hospitals that no longer exist in independent form—the Foundling Hospital, Dr Steevens', Sir Patrick Dun's, Mercer's, the Meath, the National Children's Hospital, the Adelaide and Baggot Street. The Central Council of the Federated Dublin Voluntary Hospitals is still enjoying an existence, albeit a somewhat attenuated one.

The origins of the first five of these hospitals are found in the 18th century and of the last three in the 19th century. They are the product of personal philanthropy, voluntary endeavour and medical enterprise. *Watson's Almanac* for each year from the sixth decade of the 18th century records just how creatively compassionate that time was. The same source discloses their contextual companions—the Dublin Society, the Rotunda Lying-in Hospital, the emergence of the banks, the insurance societies, the building of the canals, the elaboration of Dublin University, the College of Surgeons, the College of Physicians and much more. It was a time of exuberant enterprise and medicine and hospitals were at the heart of it. For them, the 19th century produced a future of enhanced patient care and crucial scientific discoveries leading to outstanding international reputations.

As the significance of other establishment institutions declined, the hospitals and the colleges associated with them flourished. Ireland in the 19th century, and Dublin in particular, became known worldwide for the excellence of its patient care and especially the patient-centred clinical care which grew from the nature and quality of the training and education which had been developed. Because of the religious loyalty and affiliation of most, if not all, of the hospitals which came together to form the Central Council of the Federated Dublin Voluntary Hospitals, it may be thought that this flourishing medical world was exclusively Protestant but this was not so; in the same historical context institutions of Catholic inspiration such as Jervis Street, the Mater Misericordiae and St Vincent's were equally dynamic. The sources of the time portray a society in which there was room for all and what competition there was, was of a 'seeking with' rather than a 'seeking against' variety. Those same sources reveal a Dublin of many institutions, some of which were the first of their kind in the world—like the Rotunda which still continues to function—but most of which have disappeared graciously into history.

How different was the 20th century! In the times of developing national aspirations, the Great War, the Easter Rising, the War of Independence, the Civil War, the Economic War, the Second World War, survival quickly became the name of the game. For the non-Catholic community, the matter was one not just of economic survival—the survival of identity was equally important. In companionship with parish and school, hospital played a central role in the maintenance of that identity. Parishes, schools and hospitals were nationwide, frequently small, and in the case of schools and hospitals, inhabited buildings which became increasingly inappropriate for the conduct of the particular enterprise. As far as schools and education were concerned, the new state acted as generously as it could in economic circumstances that were only intermittently prosperous until the mid-1990s. The non-Catholic churches were well organised, both separately and collectively, to make their case to government. Not so the hospitals which had never been under direct church control, as had most of the schools. In any case, the funding for health was not on the same basis as for education and the idea of Sweep money, as a source of capital funding for health projects, was anathema to certain sectors of the non-Catholic community.

By the middle of the 20th century the inheritance of 18th- and 19th-century medical distinction was almost exhausted: the increasing pace of medical technology development could not be accommodated in old buildings; small laboratories could not embrace the increasing specialisation of medical laboratory science; the buildings themselves were difficult and costly to maintain and this applied particularly to matters of hygiene. Small might be beautiful in the field of tender loving care but it was definitely not so in the value for money exercise driving most of the mushrooming areas of medical advance such as orthopaedics, cardiology, general and specialist surgery and oncology to name but a few. Here, units of a significant critical mass were essential in order to be economic as well as to provide sufficiently frequent opportunities for skills to be developed, maintained, expanded and taught. The Hospitals Federation and Amalgamation Act (1961) was the beginning of the process whereby new, purpose-built hospitals, designed and organised to recapture an international medical reputation for Dublin and Ireland, could emerge as partners with a new St Vincent's, a new Beaumont, an elaborated Mater and new regional hospitals throughout Ireland in that endeavour of teaching and practice.

This book, edited by David FitzPatrick, tells much of the story of the creation of the current St James's Hospital and of The Adelaide and Meath Hospital, Dublin Incorporating The National Children's Hospital, which embraces some of the work originally undertaken by St Loman's Psychiatric Hospital. These two hospitals are the abiding legacy of the Federated Dublin Voluntary Hospitals together with a much strengthened medical school—now the Faculty of Health Sciences—in Trinity College. Their creation required a deal of sweat and patience and the capacity, on occasion, to absorb insult without injury. The Central Council, far from being a forum for collaboration, often displayed destructive rivalries. Trying to understand that as a latecomer to the Federation scene, I sought insight from the Federation Act. Section 14 of the Act sets out the functions of the Council. It says:

> The following functions in relation to the participating hospitals . . . shall be performed by the Council:
> (a) during the period of four years beginning on the establishment day, the examination of annual estimates and supplementary estimates of expenditure on the running of hospitals, and suggesting of amendments to such estimates,
> (b) after the expiration of the said period, the approval of estimates and supplementary estimates of expenditure on the running of hospitals and the approval of any amendments of such estimates,
> (c) the submission of claims to the Hospitals Commission for payment on foot of deficits,
> (d) the control of capital expenditure . . . and of applications for funds for such expenditure,
> (e) the determination of the form of accounts to be kept by hospitals,
> (f) the appointment of visiting medical staff . . .
> (g) the assignment, subject to subsection (2) of this section, to individual hospitals of the visiting medical staff so appointed,
> (h) the determination of the hospitals in which particular clinical units shall be located,
> (i) the assignment of professorial units to particular hospitals,
> (j) the apportionment of beds among the visiting medical staff,
> (k) the co-ordination of activities in relation to medical education, the conduct

of negotiations in regard to such education with the appropriate university, college or other institution (including the making of suitable agreements with such bodies to ensure efficient clinical instruction for medical students) and the provision of facilities for post graduate instruction,

(l) subject to subsection (3) of this section, the co-ordination of activities in relation to nursing education and the conduct of negotiations in regard to such education with An Bord Altranais,

(m) any other functions which may be assigned to the Council by resolution passed by the boards of all the hospitals.

I have quoted the Act at length: what is envisaged is a comprehensive, developing, overseeing, integrative role for the Federation. In my experience this did not happen. Allowing for changed circumstances between the 1960s and the 1990s the Federation played no role in the financial affairs of the individual hospitals. Neither did it play any role in respect of nurse education in negotiations with An Bord Altranais. What it did, and did superbly well, was to organise the appointment of medical and surgical consultant staff; negotiate a teaching agreement with Trinity College; nurture the Dublin School of Physiotherapy until it was incorporated into Trinity College; provide shared computer facilities as they developed; provide a not always effective channel of communication between the Federated Hospitals and the Central Pathology Laboratory at St James's Hospital; support the research programmes of individual members of staff when so requested; act as a convening agent for formal and informal fora of discussion within and between the Federated Hospitals themselves and, on occasion, with St James's Hospital. It does not seem to have ever achieved the authoritative role envisaged in the Act. What space it had was what was permitted by the individual hospitals. When it came to the provision of the governing formula for the hospitals that transferred to Tallaght, it was excluded from the deliberations in spite of subsection (4) of section (14) of the Federation Act:

> On and after the transfer day, the Council shall perform the functions which, immediately before the transfer day, were performable by hospital boards.

In my search for an answer to the experience of rivalry, the Act could only provide a clue *via negativa*; the voluntary hospital principle was stronger than any Act of the Oireachtas. The roots of the saplings established in the 18th and 19th centuries had produced trees of vigorously independent growth and strength in their maturity.

Nevertheless, experiencing the rivalry one is left to ponder what the landscape might have been like today if collaboration had been a more central feature of relationships, particularly as between The Adelaide and

Meath Hospital, Dublin Incorporating The National Children's Hospital and St James's Hospital and between them and the University of Dublin, Trinity College. The vision of a smooth running partnership engaging all the talents, skills, creative energies and imagination of these three great institutions is tantalising; so tantalising that it allows the mind to engage with the idyllic images of enhanced patient care, major breakthroughs in the area of gene therapy, exciting programmes of preventive medicine and health promotion, a one-stop-shop for children becoming adults with chronic illnesses, a seamless service between community and acute hospital. The possibilities are legion.

I became involved in the affairs of the Federation as a representative of Trinity College at the behest of Provost Watts. I did so not only as a matter of professional duty but also as a matter of family service. Two hundred and fifty years after Edward Sterling and his brother Luke had immersed themselves in the affairs of Dublin medicine through the boards of the Rotunda and the Foundling Hospital, it is an enormous privilege to have been involved, to have been of service, and now to be associated with this exercise in telling the story of the Federation.

Introduction

David FitzPatrick

'The Dublin Voluntary Hospitals by their nature are proud of their independence and traditions which in themselves are excellent. However, when carried to extremes as sometimes happens these attributes can be counterproductive.' This was the view of the Hospitals Commission as stated in its *Annual Report* of 1935.[1]

Although these traditions and independence continued, as will be seen, a number of efforts were made to bring about amalgamation of at least some of these hospitals over the ensuing 25 years. First, discussions took place with a view to amalgamation of Sir Patrick Dun's, The Royal City of Dublin (Baggot Street) and Mercer's hospitals. Various sites for a new hospital were discussed including the site of Dun's itself, Mespil Road and Vergemount, Clonskeagh. Nothing came of these moves and it was not until 1961 that the Federation Act was passed enabling a potential merger of the seven hospitals which formed the nucleus of the Trinity teaching hospitals.

During the next 40 years plans were made to bring about formal amalgamation of these hospitals and initially the establishment of a single hospital to replace them. The end result, however, has been the closure of all seven hospitals and their replacement by the conversion and expansion of St Kevin's Hospital to establish St James's Hospital and the building of the new Adelaide and Meath Hospital, Dublin Incorporating the National Children's Hospital (NCH) at Tallaght. St Loman's Psychiatric Hospital also transferred some of its services to Tallaght, to a purpose-built unit.

This book is intended to provide a record of the negotiations which led up to the closure of the individual hospitals and the transfer first of Baggot Street, Dun's, Mercer's and Dr Steevens' to St James's and second, the establishment of the Adelaide-Meath complex. Subsequently, the remaining three hospitals, the Adelaide, Meath and NCH continued, becoming known as the 'MANCH' hospitals, until Tallaght opened in 1998. The first section of this volume therefore deals with the administrative arrangements and political negotiations which took place in the various hospitals individually and the formal discussions which preceded the final move to Tallaght.

Attention is also paid to the Tallaght Hospital Board which was responsible for planning and building the hospital and for the logistical arrangements for equipping and arranging the distribution of the various units. These arrangements involved hours of meetings and discussions between the board's staff, consultants in various specialties, and every group of staff in the base hospitals.

The second section sets out the relevant recent histories of the seven Federated Dublin Voluntary Hospitals—Dr Steevens', Mercer's, the Meath, Sir Patrick Dun's, Baggot Street, the National Children's Hospital and the Adelaide. The third section deals with the clinical developments which took place within the Federated Group and an attempt is made to detail how the small units in the individual hospitals came together to form the specialist units which are now active in the new hospitals. Finally, as an afterword, some thought is given to the future and possible developments.

Credit must be given to the staff, both medical and lay, of all the institutions involved in the transfers at one time or another and to the many members of the voluntary hospital boards who willingly gave of their time to ensure that the plans came successfully to fruition. Particular mention must be made of those who debated and negotiated the changes required in the original Adelaide Charter—not an easy task when one recalls the observations of the Hospitals Commission in 1935 which were as true in the 1980s as they were then.

It has not been possible to include details of all the specialties but the development of Accident and Emergency (A&E) services deserves special mention. When the Federation came into being each of the individual hospitals had its own 'accident room' where many of the patients were from the local area and would have declared a degree of 'ownership' of their local hospital. Each hospital also accepted patients from the ambulance service which brought accident victims to the nearest institution. In 1954, in the Meath Hospital, Derek Robinson, as well as having inpatient and operating duties, had been appointed consultant with responsibility for the accident department, but at that time in most of the other hospitals the clinical work was carried out by students in residence under the supervision of the junior medical staff. In the 1960s this changed with the appointment of casualty officers—junior doctors of SHO or registrar grade—who were responsible for the day-to-day organisation of the department.

After the publication of the FitzGerald Report in 1968 the system in Dublin was reviewed and in the early 1970s the smaller hospitals stopped taking ambulance cases. On the south side of the city four hospitals were designated as those taking A&E patients—St Vincent's, the Meath, Dr Steevens' and when it opened, St James's. In the Meath Mr Robinson remained responsible for the department, which was renovated and updated, until in 1989 he was succeeded by Geoff Keye, one of the first consultants appointed solely to an A&E department. Brendan Prendiville undertook responsibility for A&E in Dr Steevens' in 1971, and Patrick Plunkett was appointed to St James's as A&E consultant in 1988. Thus was the foundation for our present A&E service laid.

A new A&E department was constructed in Dr Steevens' a few years before its closure and abandoned when its services were transferred to St James's and the Meath. The department in St James's, where a second A&E consultant has now been appointed, continues to provide an invaluable service. The Meath department with Geoff Keye, single-handed until 2004, transferred to Tallaght where the excellent traditions of the Meath service have been maintained despite the difficulties arising from the bed shortage caused by the injudicious bed closures of the 1980s. These, of course, affect all the A&E departments in the city. In Tallaght the problems are compounded by the necessity now to take patients from Naas where there is no on-call orthopaedic trauma service. When Tallaght opened in 1998 the accident service from the National Children's Hospital was accommodated there in a purpose-built children's A&E department in whose development Dr Mary McKay, the A&E consultant in Harcourt Street, played no small part. This is but an outline of the development of A&E services, an account of which deserves a complete volume to itself.

Some of the logistical difficulties which had to be overcome in the transfers of the hospitals are outlined in the text. It must further be remembered that all the developments and negotiations took place in a period of economic and financial stringency. In addition, the pending moves cast a degree of 'planning blight' over the hospitals making rationalisation and development of units exceptionally difficult.

As I detailed in a paper in 1978,[2] the Federated Hospitals had never been particularly favoured when largesse was being distributed by the Department of Health. In this article I demonstrated that the Federated Hospitals attached to Trinity medical school were less favourably treated, in terms of financial allocation, than the teaching hospitals attached to the other medical schools in Dublin. This in itself made the day-to-day running of the hospitals difficult and when, in the 1980s, hospital closures and transfers were accompanied by considerable bed losses in the Federated Group the difficulties of maintaining a reasonable service, given the rate of rationalisation and development of units, were compounded.

Despite these difficulties the development of both St James's and Tallaght has progressed since the moves took place and each institution has now emerged as a major contributor to the Irish health service. In addition, both hospitals have retained the better aspects of the cultures of their predecessors and a separate identity has emerged for each. Fortunately, because of lessons learned from other hospital transfers, and good change management, the transition to a new institutional identity has not been accompanied by any significant rancour. This is especially true of the hospital at Tallaght where a smooth transition was achieved thanks to the planning team, led by Des Rogan, and the successful change and transfer process, overseen and implemented so effectively by the first CEO David McCutcheon.

This book is a tribute to all who over the years gave of their time and experience to form the Federated Hospitals Group in the first instance. Many of them were lay people contributing in a voluntary capacity typical of the voluntary hospital tradition. All those now working in the hospitals can be proud of those whose dedication has been so fruitful and of the fact that the voluntary tradition is healthily continued there today.

References

[1] Hospitals Commission *Annual Report* 1935.
[2] *Journal of the Irish Medical Organisation* 1978.

PART ONE:

THE GENESIS OF ST JAMES'S AND TALLAGHT

1. *From foundling hospital to university teaching hospital: the development of St James's Hospital*

Davis Coakley

Recurrent wars, famine, and virulent epidemics made 17th-century Ireland a harsh environment for its inhabitants. Many of them moved to Dublin hoping for a better life. For most it was a vain hope and instead they joined the throngs of beggars who roamed the streets seeking subsistence. Towards the end of the century Dublin Corporation came under increasing pressure to do something about the large number of vagrants in the city. They posed a threat to both the health and the safety of the affluent citizens and it was this consideration, rather than any altruistic motive, which stimulated the debate. The city assembly responded by deciding to build a workhouse outside the St James's Gate to the west of the city to house the vagrants.

The City Workhouse

An Act of Parliament in 1702 identified the 14-acre site on St James's Street as the location for the new building and the site was settled for ever for the use of the poor of the city. The governors of the workhouse were incorporated by this Act and numbered nearly 200 persons. They included the Lord Lieutenant, the Lord Mayor, the Lord Chancellor, the Archbishop of Dublin, Members of Parliament and other influential persons. They were assigned the following duties:

a) To assemble once a month to relieve, regulate, set to work, apprehend and inflict 'reasonable' punishment on all vagabonds and beggars.
b) To detain and keep in their service, until the age of 16 (this was afterwards reduced to 12) any poor child or children found, or taken up, 'above five years of age', and to apprentice them out afterwards to honest persons 'being Protestant'.

The foundation stone of the Dublin workhouse was laid on 12 October 1704 by Mary, Duchess of Ormonde. The stone has survived and can be seen in the Dublin Civic Museum in South William Street. The workhouse opened in January 1706 when 124 vagrants were apprehended in the streets of Dublin and brought to the new institution. The historian Edward McParland has identified Thomas Burgh as the architect of the workhouse. Burgh was also the architect of Dr Steevens' Hospital and of the Old Library in Trinity. The workhouse was modified later by the famous architect Francis Johnston.

The accommodation for the vagabonds was in the vaults underneath the hall of the workhouse. These vaults, or cellars, were 240 feet long and 17 feet wide with what was described as an 'airy' sunk along the outside of the building for the purpose of affording light and to drain the rain water. In these dark and damp vaults there were double rows of two-tiered bunks to accommodate 100 men and 60 women. These vaults were uncovered during the construction of the Trinity Centre buildings at St James's Hospital.

The Foundling Hospital

There was a tradition at the time that parishes should support children abandoned under the age of five. However, despite this tradition there was little enthusiasm for supporting these children. The practice of covertly moving abandoned infants from one parish to another in the dark, known as 'dropping', was very common. The Irish Parliament responded to the problem by passing legislation in 1730 which obliged the governors of the workhouse to admit all children irrespective of age abandoned in Dublin. The institution now became known as the Foundling Hospital and Workhouse. Archbishop Hugh Boulter ordered that a turning wheel be placed in the wall near the entrance to the hospital. A mother wishing to deposit a baby anonymously could place the infant in a basket attached to the wheel and ring a bell which would attract the attention of the porter inside. All infants admitted to the Foundling Hospital were assessed and those who appeared to be ill in any way were sent to the infirmary. The other children were given to nurses in the country as soon as this could be arranged. These children remained with their wet nurses until their eighth year. They were then re-admitted into the Foundling Hospital and Workhouse to be educated and given some skill. There were 265 infants admitted to the institution during the first year of the Foundling Hospital. The mortality rate was very high within the institution—as many as a third of the infants died.

The governors claimed that the death rate was so high because many of the children were moribund on admission. Children were brought long distances from all over the country in terrible conditions and often eight or nine would be carried in the same basket.

Shocking reports on the conditions within the Foundling Hospital in the late 1750s prompted one of the most influential women in the country, Lady Arabella Denny, to take a direct interest in the affairs of the hospital. She was the second daughter of Thomas Fitzmaurice, 21st Lord of Kerry. Lady Arabella enlarged and improved the buildings of the Foundling Hospital and she spent over £4,000 on the institution derived mainly from her own resources and those of her friends. She had a special clock made by Alexander Gordon of Temple Bar which she had placed in the nursery of the hospital to ensure that the infants in the institution were fed regularly. The clock was purchased by the Guinness family in 1829 and is still in their possession.

After Lady Arabella Denny's departure the mortality rate rose again and conditions deteriorated making it necessary to introduce further reforms in 1798. Gradually more children survived infancy but, ironically, this success for the governors presented them with yet another problem. They were supporting a large number of children, boys and girls, and they were unable to find employment for them. In 1829 the House of Commons in Westminster decided to stop all new admissions to the hospital. There were several reasons for this but there is no doubt that the financial cost of maintaining the foundling children was a major consideration.

During the course of the Foundling Hospital's existence several famous people were governors including Henry Grattan, Arthur Guinness and Jonathan Swift.

The South Dublin Union

The institution was now about to enter a new phase in its history. The Poor Relief Act was passed in July 1838. Under this Act the country was divided into unions and a board of guardians was elected in each union to supervise the Poor Law. The guardians were also responsible for the running of the workhouses. In 1839 the Poor Law Commissioners took over the buildings of the Foundling Hospital and began the process of converting them into a workhouse for the South Dublin Union. From the beginning the South Dublin Union was recognised as one of the principal workhouses in the country and staff were sent there from other unions for training.

The workhouses were hardly built before they came under enormous pressure because of the great famine of the 1840s. Starving, sick people thronged to the union desperately seeking help. The Temporary Relief Act 1847 empowered government agencies to use soup kitchens to feed the starving and one was set up in the South Dublin Union. The numbers of people being admitted to the union rose during the famine with 6,717 being admitted in 1848. The cost of running the institution also rose dramatically from £13,000 in 1844 to £45,000 in 1848. During the famine more accommodation to house 1,000 extra paupers was erected in the union.

The South Dublin Union, like all workhouses, had an infirmary and medical staff to treat sick inmates. Cathcart Lees was the first physician and Peter Shannon was the first surgeon. When Cathcart Lees retired he was succeeded by Dr Robert Mayne, a very able physician who published regularly in the medical literature of the period.

Following the expansion of the dispensary system in 1851 dispensary doctors began to admit their acutely ill patients to the workhouse infirmaries. The practice was recognised in 1854 when the Poor Law Commissioners opened the workhouse hospitals to the sick poor, and to the constabulary and domestic servants, and the policy was enshrined in law in the Poor Law Amendment Act of 1862. These developments signalled very clearly that the state was moving away from a policy of laissez-faire to direct involvement in the provision of health services. This was a very significant landmark in the country's social and medical history but it has received scant notice in most medical histories of the country as the authors tend to concentrate on the voluntary hospitals. In order to cope with the expanding workload a new infirmary (later known as Hospital 3) was built in 1876.

There were several complaints about the standard of care of patients in the infirmary of the South Dublin Union. As a consequence, the Board of Guardians decided to appoint Roman Catholic sisters to run the infirmary. In 1880, ten Sisters of Mercy were appointed as nurses at a salary of £30 per annum. They faced a daunting task. Patients slept in verminous straw beds covered by sheets. The walls and floors were filthy. These nuns became known as 'the invincibles' to sisters in other Dublin convents because of the problems that they constantly had to tackle. Gradually the community grew and there were over 30 nuns living in the infirmary convent by the beginning of the 20th century.

Most of the patients and inmates of the South Dublin Union were drawn from the lower rather than the upper or middle classes and they ended up in the union because of illness or hopeless destitution. In 1921 a small group of volunteers, encouraged by Frank Duff, a young civil servant at the time, formed themselves into a group to start regular visitations to the patients in the infirmary of the South Dublin Union. Elizabeth Kirwan, an office cleaner, was the first president of the group. This was the beginning of the Legion of Mary which went on to become the biggest lay organisation within the Catholic Church in the 20th century.

The South Dublin Union and the 1916 Rebellion

The early years of the 20th century were a time of great political turmoil in Ireland. The revolutionaries of the 1916 rebellion identified the South Dublin Union as of strategic importance. On Easter Monday 1916 the union was occupied by the 4th Battalion of the Irish Volunteers under the command of Eamonn Ceannt, Cathal Brugha and W. T. Cosgrave. They used the nurses' home as their headquarters.

Soon after the occupation, British soldiers approached the union through Mount Brown on their way to support the troops at Dublin Castle. The rebels opened fire on the soldiers, wounding one of their officers. After vicious fighting, with fatalities on both sides, the soldiers eventually gained access to the grounds. From then onwards the Volunteers concentrated on the defence of their headquarters in the nurses' home. On Thursday a very capable commander, Sir Francis Vane, arrived to lead the British assault. Later that week, in a letter to his wife from Portobello Barracks, Vane wrote a detailed account of his role in the action:

> Everything was bizarre on that day for we advanced through a convent where the nuns were all praying and expecting to be shot poor creatures, then through wards of imbeciles who were all shrieking—and through one of poor old women until we sapped our way right to the wall of the house occupied by the enemy. But when we got through the wall we were right up against a barricade and I lost 2 men killed and 1 wounded in the first moment of entry—and was jolly glad to get out of it alive. Then I sent another party to a place on the right which was near enough to throw bombs into the house and they had a most awful time poor fellows. I thought I would never see one of them alive again—2 were killed and 2 wounded.

During the fighting Nurse Margaret Kehoe and three inmates were killed and Sister M. Austin Frost, who worked in the cancer ward, received leg injuries from a bullet wound which left her with a permanent disability.

[11]

St Kevin's Hospital

After the War of Independence responsibility for the union passed from the Poor Law Guardians to the Dublin Board of Assistance. The institution was now to function along the lines of a county home and was renamed St Kevin's (The Union), the word 'Union' being maintained in the official title. St Kevin's was divided into six male hospitals and four female hospitals and the Rialto Hospital (now Hospital 7) was for patients with pulmonary tuberculosis.

The acute hospital service in Dublin was provided by the voluntary hospitals. However, they also admitted large numbers of patients from around the country. They were under no statutory obligation to accept all the sick poor of Dublin. On the other hand, the Dublin local authority had an obligation to provide hospital accommodation for the poor who needed it. Reports on the health services throughout the period began to hint that St Kevin's would be developed as a municipal hospital with a postgraduate medical school unless the major voluntary hospitals made a greater commitment to the sick elderly and poor of Dublin.

The Dublin Hospital Bed Bureau, which centralised hospital admissions, was opened in June 1941 and was operated by the Hospitals Commission. St Kevin's took part in the bureau from the very beginning. The bureau reports gave the government very valuable information with regard to the admitting policies of the Dublin hospitals. It soon became clear that the voluntary hospitals generally were reluctant to admit patients over 60 years of age who were suffering from medical or surgical conditions. In 1947 over 489 applications were made by the Bed Bureau on behalf of patients over the age of 60. Only 213 were admitted to the voluntary hospitals and St Kevin's on its own admitted 207.

In April 1942 the Dublin Board of Assistance was suspended for bad administration and corrupt practices and three commissioners, chaired by Mr Seamus Murphy, were appointed directly by the Minister for Local Government and Public Health to take over the administration of St Kevin's and to make recommendations for the future. It is quite clear from their report that St Kevin's still functioned largely as a workhouse. There was still an area for male and female casuals to sleep overnight. The old Foundling Hospital building was still standing and housing a large number of inmates. The commissioners recommended the demolition of the older buildings and the 'development of the present Acute

Hospital as a fully equipped hospital for the acutely sick poor and their children'.

The introduction of an ambulance service in 1947 for the emergency admission of poor patients also favoured the development of St Kevin's. Up to that time, patients had to make their own arrangements for admission and to fund the cost of a taxi or ambulance if it was needed. This created a problem for very poor patients. However, the Catholic Social Service Conference came to the rescue by funding a new scheme in March 1947. From that time onwards, if a doctor indicated to the Bed Bureau that a patient was too poor to secure transport, the bureau could order the ambulance and charge it to the Catholic Social Service Conference. This favoured the admission of more acutely ill poor patients to St Kevin's. The third *Dublin Hospital Bed Bureau Report*, published in 1949, acknowledged 'the importance of the part played by St Kevin's Hospital in meeting the demand on the Bureau for general and medical surgical cases'. In the first six years of the Bed Bureau's existence the voluntary hospitals had accepted 9,919 patients and St Kevin's alone had accepted 3,220. This brought rewards with the building of a new operating suite and the appointment of visiting medical and surgical consultants to the hospital.

The development of St Kevin's was now government policy despite strong opposition from Dublin's medical establishment who saw it as a major threat to the existing hospitals. Dr Noel Browne, when Minister for Health, gave strong support to the project. Throughout the 1950s funding was made available for a major programme of demolition and refurbishment. The work began in 1951 with the reconstruction and refurbishment of the building now known as Hospital 2. It was reopened in 1952 for acute geriatric cases making it one of the first acute units for elderly patients in Europe. Hospital 1 was refurbished for acute medical cases and Hospital 5 as an acute female medical unit. In September 1954 the 25-bed maternity unit was closed and replaced by a new well-equipped maternity unit with a bed complement of 89, built as an extension to Hospital 5. The delivery rate in 1954 was 118 and by 1959 it had risen to 1,216. Towards the end of 1957 a new surgical section was opened in the Rialto Hospital (now Hospital 7).

Miss Anne Young, matron of Jervis Street Hospital, was appointed matron of St Kevin's in 1950. She was appointed just before the major reconstruction of the hospital took place and she was matron for the whole period of development. She established a nurse training school at the hospital in 1967 and a midwifery training school in 1970. The Mercy nuns left St Kevin's on 4 July 1963 after an association with the South Dublin Union and St Kevin's of 124 years. In the 1950s advertisements were placed in the Dublin newspapers for full-time medical and surgical staff who would have no commitments to other hospitals. Two physicians, James Mahon and Patrick Blaney, and two surgeons, Charles Boland and Hugh McCarthy, and an obstetrician/gynaecologist, Dr Hanratty, were appointed. Another clinician, Jack Flanagan, joined the hospital staff as a geriatrician in 1968. When the refurbishment was completed at the end of the 1960s St Kevin's was the largest general hospital in Ireland and it was under the management of the Dublin Health Authority.

The Federated Hospitals

Several attempts were made to amalgamate the smaller Dublin voluntary hospitals throughout the first half of the 20th century without success. In the early 1950s a major player entered the field with a very determined purpose. This was Trinity College and its medical school. In 1953 a group from the American Medical Association assessed Irish medical education and presented a very negative report. As a result, for a time, no Irish medical qualification gave an entitlement to practice in the greater part of the United States. It was a major setback for Irish medical schools and urgent action was needed. The report criticised the lack of integration between the medical schools and the hospitals. Professor Jerry Jessop was appointed Dean of the Trinity medical school in 1959 and he set out on a major programme of reform. Jessop's vision and energy played a key role in developments during that period. He became very committed to the concept of amalgamating the smaller voluntary hospitals into a major teaching hospital on one site. Consultants in these hospitals also realised that federation of the voluntary hospitals was now urgently needed because of the rapid growth in expensive technology. Following detailed negotiations, the boards of the Adelaide, the National Children's Hospital, Baggot Street, Sir Patrick Dun's, the Meath, Mercer's and Dr Steevens' agreed to form an associated group and to consider a closer union later. The Hospitals Federation and Amalgamation Act became law on 8 July 1961. A Central Council was established to co-ordinate and eventually to administer the amalgamated hospitals.

St James's Hospital

Centralisation of its laboratory services was seen as a priority for the new federated group. The development also facilitated the emergence of specialised units in medicine and surgery in the seven hospitals and the creation by Dublin University of full time academic appointments in the major disciplines. The FitzGerald Report, published in June 1968, recommended that four major hospitals should be developed in Dublin. Under this plan the activities of the Federated Hospitals would be divided between new hospital developments at St Vincent's, Elm Park, and at St Kevin's, St James's Street. In 1970 a joint negotiating body was formed with representatives of the Federated Hospitals and the Dublin Health Authority to discuss the future administration of St Kevin's. Discussions between representatives of this group and the Department of Health finally led to an establishment order for a new board for the hospital which was to change its name from St Kevin's to St James's Hospital. In a symbolic gesture Erskine Childers signalled the new beginning by initiating the demolition of some of the original workhouse buildings in 1970. The new St James's board met for the first time on 2 July 1971 and it was composed of representatives of the Federated Hospitals and the Eastern Health Board in equal numbers. Mr Paddy Burke, representative of the EHB was elected chairman at the first meeting. Subsequently, Professor Ian Howie took over. Howie was a member of the zoology department in Trinity College but he was already respected as a very able college administrator. He held the post of registrar of the college when he was appointed to the board of St James's. He was to become deeply involved in the development of the hospital over the next 30 years.

The new board of St James's began negotiations with Trinity College, with the intention of developing the hospital as a major teaching hospital for that university. Comhairle na nÓspidéal presented proposals outlining a hospital strategy for south Dublin to the Minister for Health in 1973. These proposals suggested the establishment of three hospitals in south Dublin, one at St James's, one at St Vincent's and one in the Newlands Cross area. The boards of Sir Patrick Dun's, Mercer's and Baggot Street agreed that their institutions would transfer to the new hospital on the St James's site. Their representatives joined a development committee at St James's to prepare the planning of the new hospital. The Adelaide, Meath and National Children's Hospital would eventually move to the new hospital in Tallaght.

In 1974 Brendan Corish confirmed the government's intention to establish three major hospitals in south Dublin, priority being given to St James's. In the following year the project team for the new St James's Hospital was established. The team, under the chairmanship of Professor Ian Howie, immediately began the preparation of a brief. In June

1976 a design team was appointed and in November David A. Hutchinson of HLM Architects in Surrey and Mr Jim O'Beirne of Guy Moloney and Partners, Dublin, were selected as architects. In the same year the haematology/oncology unit transferred from the Meath to St James's.

The development control plan of the new hospital was published in 1978. Because of the complexities of building a new hospital on the site of an already existing, large, increasingly busy, general teaching hospital it was decided to build the new hospital in three overlapping phases.

The first phase was divided into three sub-sections:

phase 1(a) included the new entrance at the Rialto end of the hospital and a communication centre;
phase 1(b) the boiler house, engineering workshops and the Eastern Health Board's ambulance centre;
phase 1(c) a major part of the actual hospital building including a new outpatient department, accident and emergency department, x-ray department, intensive care unit, operating theatres and nine in-patient wards, a new psychiatry unit and the Robert Mayne Day Hospital.

Construction work began on phase 1(a) in November 1980 and the new Central Pathology Laboratory was handed over to the hospital in the same year.

Intensive negotiations on the closure of Mercer's and the transfer of its staff and services to St James's began in 1982. The hospital closed at the end of May 1983. The health care centre in Hospital 5 was built and commissioned in 1982 and came into full use in the following year. The department of gastroenterology moved from Sir Patrick Dun's in 1983. Also in the same year the governors of Sir Patrick Dun's and the board of Trinity College funded the construction of a new research laboratory attached to the Central Pathology Laboratory. Similarly, in 1988, Mercer's supported the Mercer's Institute for Research on Ageing and, in 1996, Baggot Street Hospital supported the Royal City of Dublin Hospital Research Laboratory. Funding from the sale of Dr Steevens' contributed to the construction of the teaching facility for Trinity students at St James's. The top floor of Hospital 1 was redeveloped to house oncology, haematology and the bone marrow transplantation unit. June 1984 saw the long awaited beginning of the construction of the clinical facilities of the new hospital (phase 1(c)).

Growing economic difficulties throughout the decade resulted in drastic cutbacks in health care, beginning in 1986. These cutbacks precipitated the closure and move of services from Sir Patrick Dun's, Dr Steevens' and Baggot Street to St James's, far sooner than was planned. Sir Patrick Dun's closed at the end of August 1986 and its services transferred to St James's. An unfortunate consequence of the whole process was the transfer of the maternity unit in St James's to the Coombe in September 1987. Immediate preparations were then made for the transfer of services from Baggot Street and some specialties from Dr Steevens'. Considerable progress was made in a short period of time and the staff and patients transferred on 1 December 1987 and on 1 January 1988 respectively. The transfer was completed without creating any major or lasting divisions within the hospital, an achievement that was in large part due to the skill of the chairman, Ian Howie, and his senior management team at the time. All this activity resulted in St James's attempting to provide the services of a major acute teaching hospital from a very limited number of beds situated in very old and inadequate buildings scattered over a large site.

On 30 June 1988 the contractors, G. & T. Crampton Ltd, formally handed the completed phase 1(c) over to the hospital board. In the design of the new hospital there was a deliberate attempt to build it on a human scale and to avoid the forbidding institutional appearance of many modern and older hospitals. The department of diagnostic imaging was opened in October 1988 and the outpatient and accident and emergency departments opened on 1 December 1989. However, the opening of the ward areas and other parts of the new building was delayed until January 1992, pending further capital investment. Meanwhile, work began on the Trinity Centre for students in the Faculty of Health Sciences and this was officially opened in 1994 by the Minister for Health, Brendan Howlin.

Two years later the 25th anniversary of the foundation of St James's was celebrated in a series of events over three days. The celebrations were inaugurated by President Mary Robinson, in her last week in office as President. There has been a whole series of major developments since then. These include the new hepatology centre, located at the Rialto entrance to the hospital, which was opened in 1998, and the new centre for hereditary coagulation disorders which was opened in the year 2000, the opening of the new cardiac surgery unit in February 2000 and the building of phase 1(h) of the hospital which includes a major day treatment centre, ward accommodation, and the concourse of the new hospital. There has also been a very significant expansion of teaching and research facilities in the hospital with the completion of a major development which houses academic departments from different schools and very significant research facilities which include the Durkan Institute for research on leukaemia and the new Institute of Molecular Medicine.

In 1998 Ian Howie oversaw a major reform of the hospital board. In planning its structure he was particularly careful to ensure that it would continue to reflect the unique mix of municipal and voluntary representation which has characterised St James's Hospital from the beginning and which has emerged from its unique history.

2. The beginning of the Federated Dublin Voluntary Hospitals

Peter Gatenby

Though amalgamation of certain of the small Dublin hospitals had been proposed in 1885 and again repeatedly throughout the 1920s and 1930s[1] and the amalgamation of Dun's, Baggot Street, and Mercer's had been especially discussed, all such proposals came to nothing in the adverse economic climate of the Second World War.

By 1950 there were still ten separate general teaching hospitals in Dublin. Though all these hospitals were open theoretically to all the medical students of the three Dublin medical schools, in fact, by tradition and historical factors, at that time each hospital was mainly associated with an individual school, as follows. The Mater Misericordiae (1861) and St Vincent's (1835) were allied to University College Dublin. The Charitable Infirmary, Jervis Street (1718) and the Richmond (1773) had strong connections with the Royal College of Surgeons and had begun a campaign to amalgamate in the 1960s which resulted in the construction of Beaumont Hospital in 1985.

The hospitals associated with Trinity College were all small. These were the Adelaide (1839), Dr Steevens' (1733), the Meath (1753), Mercer's (1734), the Royal City of Dublin, Baggot Street (1832), Sir Patrick Dun's (1810) and the National Children's Hospital (1821). These seven hospitals were all close together on the south side of Dublin and were housed in antiquated buildings. As medicine advanced in specialisation it was more than ever obvious that these hospitals should be amalgamated and replaced by modern facilities.

In the 1950s a series of inspections of the medical teaching in Ireland were made. These reported unfavourably on the organisation of medical teaching which in turn reflected on the out of date hospital buildings.

The first of these inspections resulted from an invitation from the Irish Medical Association to the American Medical Association to assess the 'comparability' of instruction in the Irish medical schools with those in the United States.

[19]

A very adverse report was issued as a result of this inspection, and for a period no medical qualification from the Irish Republic was accepted in the greater part of the USA. The report mainly criticised the poor laboratory facilities. A further inspection in 1955, jointly by the General Medical Council of the UK and the Medical Registration Council of Ireland, supported the American criticism and remarked specifically on the lack of integration between the medical schools and hospitals. These reports emphasised the need for reform, especially of the small hospital buildings founded in the 18th and beginning of the 19th centuries which were mainly associated with Trinity College.

In 1957 four junior clinical teachers in the Trinity medical school met informally and agreed that there was an urgent need to amalgamate the resources of the small old hospitals associated with Trinity, in order to develop laboratory facilities and facilitate specialisation. The four were George Fegan, surgeon at Dun's, Stanley McCollum and John Sugars, surgeons at the Adelaide, and myself, at that time physician at Steevens', and later the Meath.[2] We were aiming for a new large central hospital to replace some or all of the small hospitals.

In discussions with our colleagues there was little enthusiasm for change, especially from those who were senior and felt well established. There was one notable exception and that was Robert Woods, ENT surgeon at Dun's. We appointed him as our chairman and we met in the waiting room of his consulting rooms in Fitzwilliam Place on several occasions. Bobbie Woods was so enthusiastic that he constructed a board with a row of hooks fixed horizontally across the top, each designating one of the six adult hospitals, and a vertical row of hooks on the left marking the specialties. Then, with prepared labels marked cardiac, respiratory, orthopaedic, ENT, etc., he planned the placing of specialised departments across the six hospitals as if they were in one closely amalgamated group.

Of course, though showing his keenness on reform, this was quite unrealistic when dealing with completely independent hospitals each under a separate board of governors. Though it was a dream it was an inspiring demonstration. We decided to approach the lay members of the boards of governors, and to our surprise there was considerable support. These were voluntary people who had no vested pecuniary interest in the hospitals; sometimes coming from a business background they understood the need for reorganisation, and the business word 'merge' came into discussion. Those non-medical governors, who supported the idea of hospital amalgamation in the early days and were very active then or later, included Alex Bayne of Baggot Street, A. W. Masser of Dun's, Rex Dick of the Adelaide, Judge Kingsmill Moore of Baggot Street, Brigadier M. H. Clarke of Mercer's, R. E. Minchin Clarke of Steevens', and Mrs Kingsmill Moore of the National Children's Hospital, Harcourt Street.

Eventually the seven hospital boards agreed in principle to unite, and discussions were held with the Department of Health throughout 1960. The Minister for Health and his staff were supportive. A parliamentary Act was drawn up. It was entitled 'Hospitals Federation and Amalgamation Act'. It was introduced in Dáil Éireann, passed both houses of the Oireachtas and became law on 8 July 1961.

The Act established a federation of the seven hospitals and also presented a procedure for ultimate amalgamation of two or more hospitals as might later be agreed. The enactment established a Central Council to co-ordinate the activities of the hospitals and eventually to administer the amalgamated group. The Central Council had its first meeting on 6 November 1961 which was the day appointed by the Minister for Health as 'Establishment Day'. The first chairman was Arthur Chance, orthopaedic surgeon at Dr Steevens' Hospital. The government appointed C. F. Dowling, an ex-civil servant, as secretary to the Central Council thus ensuring an administrator independent of any of the individual hospitals. Much credit is due to Mr Dowling who was scrupulously fair in his dealings with the seven somewhat competitive hospitals. The Central Council met each month in the boardroom of one of the seven hospitals. These monthly meetings were held according to alphabetical order starting with the Adelaide and ending with Steevens', everything being done to avoid favouritism to any one hospital.

The Central Council was made up of five representatives from each hospital, three lay and two medical, and also five from the Dublin Health Authority which later became the Eastern Health Board. This gave a total of 40 members and in addition provision was made for two members representing medical schools.

The main legal powers given to the Central Council were the control of capital expenditure, and the appointment of all visiting medical staff throughout the Federation. Therefore, from 1961 all appointments were to the hospital group and the appointee was 'assigned' to work in one or more hospitals. At an early stage the Central Council ruled that all appointments should be subject to a retiring age of 65.

Arising from the legal agreement between the Federated Hospitals and Trinity College there evolved a very satisfactory procedure for appointments. Both the Central Council of the Federated Hospitals and Trinity College were represented on the selection committee for every appointment. When the post was for a hospital consultant the majority of the members of the committee were from the hospital, and when the post was primarily for the university, then university representatives were in the majority. An outside assessor acted in every case. This development proved successful in attracting good candidates, and it was clearly an advantage to be able to make appointments to the hospital group rather than to individual hospitals.

Prior to federation each hospital had its own small laboratory endeavouring to cover most aspects of pathology, and under the direction of a pathologist appointed to one or two hospitals. Though this system usually provided a satisfactory service and a close relationship between the clinicians and the laboratory workers in each hospital, it was obviously not possible to cater for the inevitable expansion of all branches of pathology on seven different sites simultaneously. Centralisation of the pathology services of the Federation was one of the dominant, not to say sometimes painful, activities of the Central Council in its first ten years. The gradual centralisation of histology, cytology, haematology, bio-chemistry, microbiology and immunology in certain hospital laboratories and Trinity College caused problems in communication between the clinicians and the pathologists. These were overcome to a large extent by improved communication services.

The development of specialised aspects of medicine and surgery in the seven hospitals was facilitated by the federated system. Since the 1961 Act the location of specialised units was decided or confirmed by the Central Council. This avoided duplication of staff and equipment, and consequently a balanced service evolved throughout the hospitals. Each hospital, except Harcourt Street which was paediatric, still catered for general medicine, general surgery, gynaecology and otorhinolaryngology.

Though these developments in co-ordination on different sites were useful and progressive, by far the most important long-term objective of the Central Council was the establishment of a new hospital. In 1962 a planning committee was formed to consider this problem and the Central Council finally decided in 1964 that 'five hospitals should be merged into one on the site of Sir Patrick Dun's, that Steevens' Hospital would be an orthopaedic centre and the Meath a centre for genito-urinary and gynaecological surgery'.[3] The Minister for Health backed this plan in principle and allowed £43,000 to be spent on acquiring property around

Dun's site. However, in 1965 it was revealed that a major road was planned which would run through the proposed site and it was decided with the Department of Health that there was no option but to abandon the project at Dun's. None of the other Federated Hospital sites being suitable for a major hospital development, other possible sites were considered. One of these was a six-acre site at Tullamaine, where the Burlington Hotel is now sited, but later the city manager suggested the 16-acre site of the fever hospital at Clonskeagh.

In September 1966 the Minister for Health, Donogh O'Malley, received a deputation from the Federation to discuss the problem. He disagreed with the choice of Clonskeagh and suggested the Cherry Orchard 60-acre site at Ballyfermot. There was considerable enthusiasm for this suggestion from the Federation, and, under the chairmanship of Dr David Mitchell, who had succeeded Mr Chance in 1964, it was agreed to retain the services of the hospital planning consultants Llewellyn Davies Weekes to report on the Cherry Orchard project. Their report was received in March 1967. It approved the site and gave an outline plan for a hospital of 1,244 beds. In June 1967 the Department of Health agreed to the appointment of a project team to proceed with more detailed planning. However, shortly after this, the Minister for Health requested that the project team not be appointed, as he was setting up a Consultative Council to report on hospital planning for the whole country. This was a great disappointment to the Central Council, which was not eased when the report of the Consultative Council was published in June 1968. This report, now usually known as the FitzGerald Report, recommended the development of four hospital centres for Dublin, two regional and two general. It recommended that the activities of the Federated Hospitals should be divided between the St Vincent's Hospital site at Elm Park, and the site of St Kevin's Hospital.

The then Minister for Health, Seán Flanagan, accepted the recommendations of the FitzGerald Report in principle and requested the hospital authorities concerned to meet and discuss their implementation. Accordingly, R. E. M. Clarke, who became chairman in 1967, led the Central Council in discussions with St Vincent's Hospital and the Dublin Health Authority. At the same time the minister agreed that Llewellyn Davies Weekes could again be consulted to advise the Central Council. They were asked to advise on the future siting of the Federated Hospitals in view of the FitzGerald Report. The sites now to be considered in turn were Elm Park, St Kevin's and Cherry Orchard. The hospital planning consultants issued a report favouring the Cherry Orchard site for the Federation and putting St Kevin's as a second choice. However, the Department of Health maintained the view that St Kevin's was preferable for development though Cherry Orchard would be an important hospital site for the more distant future.

In November 1969, at a special meeting, the Central Council passed a resolution accepting the proposal of the minister (now Erskine Childers) to provide beds between the St Kevin's and Elm Park sites but considered it important that the majority of the beds and priority in building should be given to St Kevin's. In 1970 a joint negotiating body was formed with equal representation from the Federated Hospitals and the Dublin Health Authority with a view to administering the entire institution at St Kevin's Hospital. Discussions between representatives of this group and the Department of Health finally led to the establishment order for the new board of St James's (formerly St Kevin's).

On 2 July 1971, the St James's Hospital Board met for the first time. The board was composed of representatives of the Federated Hospitals and the Eastern Health Board in equal proportions. The Minister for Health gave an undertaking that a new hospital of at least 350 beds would be constructed on the St James's site to replace some of the Federated Hospitals. So, after many years of countless meetings and discussions, the Federated Hospitals had at last a definite prospect of new hospital construction. The St James's site of 49 acres was well placed to serve a large population, and the synthesis of the local health authority services and of the voluntary hospital tradition promised a great development in patient care and medical teaching for the city of Dublin.

References

[1] T. G. Moorhead *A Short History of Sir Patrick Dun's Hospital* Dublin: Hodges and Figgis 1942, pp 62 and 202; J. B. Lyons *The Quality of Mercer's: the Story of Mercer's Hospital 1734–1991* Dublin: Glendale Publishing 1991, p 162.

[2] D. Mitchell *A 'Peculiar Place'; The Adelaide Hospital 1839–1989* Dublin: Blackwater Press 1989, p 210.

[3] P. B. B. Gatenby *History of the Federated Dublin Voluntary Hospitals (1961–1971)* Federated Dublin Voluntary Hospitals and St James's Hospital 10th Anniversary Celebration (commemorative publication), Dublin 1971.

3. The emergence of a hospital system to meet the challenges of 2000 and beyond

Ian Howie

Hospital amalgamation—a continuous thread

The objectives of what David Mitchell[1] describes as the 'young consultants' who sponsored the Hospitals Federation and Amalgamation Act (1961) were set out in a memorandum to the boards of the seven hospitals in 1957 as follows:

- ultimate amalgamation (of the hospitals) in one *or more buildings* (italics added)
- interim voluntary co-operation towards specialisation
- clinical units of 30 to 50 beds in the care of two consultants
- some professorial units with whole time staff
- co-ordinated complete laboratory service
- voluntary retirement for all staff at 65 years of age.

What was behind these objectives was the need to create a hospital large enough to justify investment in modern medical technology, staffing for a range of specialties and retention of teaching hospital status in the face of the threat of withdrawal of recognition of Trinity medical degrees from both British and American authorities (General Medical Council and American Medical Association). David Mitchell remarks somewhat insouciantly: 'without some form of combination, long term prospects seemed . . . to be poor, not so much in terms of standards of patient care [sic], as in regard to furthering medical research and education'.[2] There was also an unspoken concern, not referred to in the several texts on the history of the period, about the increasing dominance of the Mater and St Vincent's in service terms and the growing reputation of the much larger medical school of University College Dublin.

While Mitchell dismisses the Federation as a failure, in the decade

1961–71 there was progress on the clinical objectives listed above and despite many disappointments amalgamation in a new hospital was pursued with great persistence. Furthermore, the bond between the hospitals and the teaching authority was greatly strengthened. Ultimately, the Federation has participated in the formation and construction of two large hospitals, St James's and the Adelaide and Meath Hospital, Dublin Incorporating the National Children's Hospital (Tallaght), with the great range of regional and national specialties represented therein. They incorporate significant teaching and research facilities and are a force to be reckoned with in the knowledge-based medicine of the 21st century. The role played by the Federation (and Trinity) in the evolution of these new hospitals is unquestionably their chief contribution not only to Dublin but also to Irish medicine in the modern era. This chapter deals with the establishment of St James's Hospital and the part played by the Federation therein and in its subsequent development.

Public policy and the FitzGerald Report

It has long been recognised that the recommendations in the report of the Consultative Council on the General Hospital Services *Outline of the Future Hospital System* 1968 (the FitzGerald Report) had an important influence on subsequent hospital development including the future of the Federation. The Consultative Council did not believe that small is beautiful: 'There is a very strong case to be made in favour of larger hospitals, more specialisation and more recognition . . . that the relatively small population of this country must . . . restrict the number of specialised units'.[3] What was recommended was that the two regional centres which were proposed for Dublin 'should consist of groups or complexes rather than of single institutions'. On the south side of the city a separate hospital was to be built for the Federation on a 'site adjoining the new St Vincent's Hospital at Elm Park' with a total bed complement of at least 1000. The choice of the St Vincent's site was predicated upon the facts that a new hospital of 450 beds was already being built there and that it was situated close to 'the science department of University College, Dublin'. While intellectually there were those in the Federation who appreciated the need for concentration of resources to support specialisation and were attracted by the idea of a hospital of their own alongside St Vincent's, to others the concept of the two hospital managements operating on the same site, and remaining separate, was an unlikely proposition. An association with the campus of UCD also ran counter to the recent proposals of the Minister for Education, Donogh O'Malley, for a merger of the medical, dental and veterinary schools in Trinity. The Council's further proposal for the development of a 500-bed general hospital on the south side of the city was perceived to be similarly flawed, 'the general hospital to be sited at St Kevin's Hospital should be developed by transferring to some of the existing buildings the general services now provided by one or more of the Federated Hospitals . . . (which) would come under the day to day management of the Federated Hospitals' authorities'.[4] The remaining buildings were to remain under the management of St Kevin's (actually the Eastern Health Board). The grim history of St Kevin's[5] and a lack of appreciation, and possibly ignorance, of the work at the public hospital for the poorest sections of the community, made these proposals additionally unattractive to the Federation.

The teaching agreement between TCD and the Federation

Continuing uncertainty about the future of the Federated Hospitals coupled with the criticisms of its medical school by the AMA and the GMC was a matter of grave anxiety for Trinity College, which had been reliant upon access to these hospitals for general clinical teaching for approaching 200 years. The Dean, Professor W. J. E. (Jerry) Jessop, led Trinity's endeavours to respond to the criticisms of the licensing bodies with specific developments in, for example, pharmacology and pathology. Surprisingly, in the many texts relating to the history of the hospitals in this period there is no direct reference to the so-called 'teaching agreement' concluded between the college and the Federation's Central Council in 1970. The objective was to ensure efficient clinical instruction for students and the creation of 'professorial units' of 'not more than 50 and not less than 25 beds the patients in which shall be under the care of the relevant University Professor and his [sic] assistants'. This would ensure access to beds for the full time professors then being appointed by the college and in due course would ensure that beds would be available for their successors appointed in open competition. The nucleus of academic departments with teaching facilities and research space had already been established for medicine in the Meath and for surgery in Sir Patrick Dun's. The teaching agreement secured participation of hospital representatives on appointment committees for full time academic staff while the university was to be represented in appointing all hospital consultants upon whom the university was dependent for a

great deal of clinical teaching. The agreement therefore addressed one of
the chief criticisms of the AMA and GMC, the lack of integration between the medical school and the hospitals. It was also a formal mani-
festation of the bond between them which was to last through the subsequent difficult closure of the Federated Hospitals and continue into
the future teaching hospitals.

St James's Hospital—establishment

A significant meeting took place in September 1969 between the then
Minister for Health, Erskine Childers, and representatives of the Federated Hospitals. At that meeting he spoke favourably about the proposed
development of St Kevin's. In the following month Jessop and I presented a paper to the Central Council in which we argued that the state,
having just completed the new St Vincent's Hospital at Elm Park, would
only be able to sustain the development of one other hospital in the
foreseeable future on the south side of Dublin and that would be, or so
it appeared from the minister's statement, at St Kevin's. This was in part
a recognition of demographics and in part the need for hospital services
in an underprivileged sector of the city. Nevertheless, in November 1969
the Central Council still divided 15 to 4 in favour of a new hospital at
Cherry Orchard as had been recommended by their planning consultants, Llewellyn Davies Weekes. Apparently ignoring this decision a joint
negotiating body was set up shortly thereafter between the Central Council and the Dublin Health Authority (later the Eastern Health Board).
Through the efforts of this body and especially of the then chairman of
the Central Council, Minchin Clarke, the minister gave a written undertaking in February 1971 to build a new 350-bed hospital at St Kevin's
'with all the necessary support, services and teaching facilities'. After
that things moved swiftly. An establishment order under the Health
(Corporate Bodies) Act 1961 was signed by the minister setting up the
'St James's Hospital Board' and a lease of the former St Kevin's Hospital
site was granted by the Eastern Health Board, which owned the site, to
the new board. It was the minister who suggested the name 'St James's'
presumably recalling the proximity of the historic St James's Gate. The
establishment order provided that the board would be appointed by
the minister but made up of equal numbers of representatives nominated by the Central Council and the Eastern Health Board. The chairman was to be elected by the members, alternating annually between
the two groups. The first chairman (a nominee of the EHB) was Mr
Paddy Burke and I was the second (nominated by the Federated Hospi-

tals). It might be asked why the Eastern Health Board, which after all owned St Kevin's and its considerable site, acquiesced in these arrangements but it had been the intention of the Dublin Health Authority since the 1940s to upgrade the acute medical and surgical services at St Kevin's. Furthermore, J. J. Nolan (deputy CEO of the Eastern Health Board and subsequently a significant influence at St James's) personally was committed to the recognition of St James's as a teaching hospital. Despite the shared basis on which the St James's board had been established there was a continuing belief in the Central Council that the new hospital when built would be 'their' hospital, a belief no doubt sustained by the FitzGerald Report's recommendation of separate hospitals and separate managements on the same site. While these aspirations were unfulfilled the contribution made by a succession of lay and medical nominees of the Central Council to governance of the hospital up to a change in the establishment order in 1998 was substantial. They did much to form the ethic of the present corporate body.

Key influences on the development of St James's after establishment

(i) Comhairle and the Department of Health

In November 1973, six years after FitzGerald, Comhairle na nÓspidéal, led by its chairman, Professor Basil Chubb, who at that time was also the chairman of Sir Patrick Dun's Hospital, reported on the *Future development of general hospital services* in Dublin. So far as the south city is concerned the report modified the FitzGerald proposals by advocating a third hospital at 'Newlands', later to become Tallaght. While the report was brief and general in content it had an important impact on the development of St James's as a teaching hospital:

- it removed the distinction between regional and general hospitals;
- it recommended that regional and national specialties would 'tend to relate to (both) St Vincent's and St James's' (*loc. cit.*);
- it proposed a catchment area population for St James's of 250,000 and revised upwards the approximate scale of the new hospital to between 500 and 600 beds.

Inter alia the report noted that it was 'already agreed' that three of the Federated Hospitals, namely, Sir Patrick Dun's, Mercer's and the Royal City of Dublin, 'will amalgamate and move to St James's Hospital' (*loc. cit.* App.iii). Colloquially these hospitals were thereafter referred to as the 'designated hospitals'. Discussions on their amalgamation had been going on for some time (since 1969) but they ended without result. Nevertheless, the assumption of this agreement had a profound influence upon subsequent policy relating to St James's.

If the foregoing Comhairle report defined the scale and status of the new hospital then the subsequent publication of two reports of a joint working party of Comhairle and the Department of Health on the *Development of specialist services in Dublin hospitals* (1977, 1978) defined its clinical content. Having arrived at decisions on hospital rationalisation which were much less rigorous than those proposed by FitzGerald it became necessary instead to rationalise the distribution of 'regional' and 'national' specialties to ensure a sufficient concentration of expertise and resources to bring them up to international standards. The proposed allocation of specialties on the south side of the city was negotiated by Professors Gatenby and Beckett on behalf of St James's and the Federation with their colleagues from St Vincent's at the South City General Hospitals Council. This was the only useful function that this committee carried out. The allocation recognised where the specialty strengths of the existing hospitals lay and where the services of these hospitals were likely to transfer in the course of hospital rationalisation. While specialties have evolved and new ones have been added, the allocation, originally published in a scruffy cyclostyled document, has guided and informed the decisions of Comhairle and the Department of Health on consultant staffing in the south city for three decades.

(ii) The Establishment Order and the teaching agreement

Despite the fact that the second function of the new St James's board set out in the St James's order was 'to provide . . . facilities for the teaching of medical, nursing and paramedical students and for the conduct of medical research' there was no seat on the board for university representatives as there had been on the Central Council of the Federation. The Eastern Health Board was reluctant then, and later, to give up any of its seats, but whatever tensions might have existed from time to time between 'town and gown' in the Central Council/TCD relationship, the former maintained its commitment to the university and included, voluntarily, two representatives from Trinity among its nominees for membership of the St James's board. This practice continued until a revision of the statutory order in 1984 which granted direct representation to the university.

The university representatives lost no time in proposing a teaching agreement with St James's on the model of that between Trinity and the Federation. However, the Minister for Health, whose approval was required, was reluctant to sanction the draft agreement as it might be prejudicial to the future arrangements for medical education in Dublin which were contained in the Higher Education Authority's *Report on University Education* (1969) subsequent to Donogh O'Malley's proposed merger of TCD and UCD. Remarkably as it may now seem, the HEA had proposed that St James's should become the main centre in Dublin for the clinical teaching of medical undergraduates under the control of a joint medical school. Fortunately, the chairman of the HEA, in a letter to me, recognised the difficulties the TCD school was currently encountering with teaching scattered over seven hospitals and further that it was the Minister for Health's intention that units of the Federation should be transferred to St James's. In these circumstances the HEA saw the need for an 'appropriate agreement between the Board of St James's Hospital and Trinity College under which accommodation and facilities for medical teaching at that hospital may be provided.'[6]

Approval was given and an agreement was signed on 22 December 1972. Given the uncertainties of the political environment surrounding hospitals and universities at the time this outcome was both speedy and positive. The agreement was to give significant impetus to the evolution of clinical services at the hospital in the first decade after establishment. It was to lapse in the event that Trinity College ceased to be responsible for clinical medical education but this, fortunately, has not arisen.

The growth of clinical services during the 1970s

In 1971 the members of the staff of St James's were, naturally, health board employees and many remained so. Only nine consultants were covering about 1200 beds, the majority of which were long stay. They and the representatives of the EHB on the board, mainly local politicians, were, not surprisingly, committed to the socially orientated services given by St Kevin's—services for the elderly, the maternity and paediatric units as well as general medicine and surgery. Davis Coakley[7] has shown that at the time St Kevin's was the principal provider of these services for the most deprived sections of the community of Dublin. Nevertheless, after St James's was established a number of the consultants (led by Dr Blaney) were also committed to teaching and to the development of more comprehensive specialist services and this was strongly supported by Jim Nolan, then deputy CEO of the Eastern Health Board.

Up to the year 2000 three strategic development programmes characterised St James's:

- services development (allied to teaching and research)
- physical redevelopment, and
- organisation change.

The principal contribution of the Federation to St James's (and later to Tallaght) was to the first of these through the transfer of the specialties which had begun to emerge in the seven hospitals. Their main impact, however, was not felt in St James's until after the forced closure of the designated hospitals between 1983 and 1987; before that, however, a succession of academic appointments, which also originated in the Federation, spearheaded diversification of the clinical services. In February 1974 the St James's Board, the Federation and Trinity College sent a joint letter (signed by Lorcan Hogan, hospital administrator; Nevin Dowling, FDVH chief executive and planning officer, and Gerry Giltrap, secretary, Trinity College) to Comhairle stating that 'the St James's board is anxious to improve its consultant staffing structure, and is especially concerned to do this in the context of joint teaching appointments'. The letter went on to recall that in the previous year Comhairle na nÓspidéal had written indicating that it would look favourably on moves 'in the direction of the intended amalgamation of the services of St James's Hospital and the Federation'. The occasion of this letter was the retirement of the then professor of surgery, George Fegan, from Sir Patrick Dun's and the stated desire of the college to replace him with a whole time appointee. It was proposed that there would be a 30-bed professorial unit partly in St James's and partly in Dr Steevens', staffed by the professor and a whole time lecturer. The letter ended by advising that the application was to be viewed as part of an overall plan for the integration of consultancy services between the Federation and St James's. This application seems to have been the origin of the policy adopted by Comhairle na nÓspidéal that all new consultant appointments in the designated hospitals should be made jointly with St James's. It ensured that specialty development in one would be mirrored in the other and, crucially, reduced the contractual problems associated with the eventual closure of these hospitals as many of the consultants already held St James's appointments. Whatever doubts and uncertainties existed in the hospital community about what the future might hold the letter makes plain that the governing authorities and Comhairle were co-operating to ensure that the legacy represented by the specialties located in the designated hospitals would transfer successfully to St James's.

Other academic appointments followed. So long as consultants in the Federation were dependent for some of their income upon their share of the 'pool',[8] which related to the number of beds they held, not all the hospitals were comfortable with the commitment inherent in the teaching agreement between the Federation and Trinity to relinquish hospital beds for whole time professorial units. Professor Gatenby, the first full time professor of medicine, was attached to the Meath where he had both beds and modest research facilities. Subsequent to his resignation to take up an appointment at the United Nations, the dean and I, as vice provost, met representatives of the Meath consultants over dinner expecting that the vacant consultant post could be filled by open competition for a professor. Instead we were met with a request to remove the professorial unit from their hospital. Shortly afterwards there was pressure to move Professor Temperley from the Meath on the grounds that haematology was judged, correctly, to be too expensive. Fortunately it was now possible to appoint both Professor Graham Neale, who succeeded Gatenby in 1976, and Professor Temperley to St James's. The decisions to transfer the academic departments of surgery, medicine and clinical haematology to James's were the first practical steps in its conversion into a teaching hospital and a major contribution to the growth of its specialist services. Professor Neale and his successor Professor Weir developed both an active clinical service and research in gastroenterology. Professor Hennessy's specialisation in oesophageal surgery became a virtual national unit while out of Temperley's clinical haematology evolved the national units in coagulation disorders, leukaemia and bone marrow transplantation. Lest it be forgotten, as it often is, the chair of psychiatry, which was associated with the EHB catchment area service, had its inpatient accommodation on the St James's campus. Professor Peter Beckett was joined by Dr Webb in 1971; the latter succeeded to the chair in 1977. Thus the principal clinical chairs, with the exception of obstetrics and gynaecology (which came later), were quickly established on what by the late 1970s had become the principal teaching base for the Trinity medical school.

Hospital closures and clinical services in the 1980s

Further acceleration in the development of clinical services began with the opening of the Central Pathology Laboratory in 1980. This, the first new building at St James's, fulfilled the ambition of its chief architect, Professor Dermot Hourihane, to bring together, at one location, all the laboratory disciplines (immunology and histopathology from the pathology school building in Trinity, biochemistry from Dun's, haematology from the Meath and microbiology from the Adelaide) thereby creating a critical mass of staff and expertise which enabled effective participation in research and development. By 1991 the laboratory housed 240 staff including 15 consultants and, importantly, 20 trainee pathologists. This gave the hospitals served, which extended well beyond St James's and the remaining Federated Hospitals, the benefit of the early introduction of new diagnostic tests and technologies. It did not, of course, fulfil the ambition of many physicians in the Meath, Adelaide and National Children's Hospital, to have a complete laboratory service on their own doorsteps. Nor did the new central laboratory, as a structure, for long fulfil the ambition of the pathology staff to have an advanced laboratory building, based as it was on the already dated plans for laboratories in Cork and Gartnavel in Scotland.

The progressive increase during the 1980s in the number and range of clinical and diagnostic specialties and facilities at St James's was well documented by the late Professor John Pritchard, a respiratory physician with a rare talent for combining academic excellence, a caring clinical service and a commitment to the institutions to which he was attached. He produced a chart of new specialty developments year by year from 1980 to 1990 for the St James's Hospital *Annual Report 1988/9*. Most, but not all, of these new services, arose from the progressive closure of the designated hospitals beginning with Mercer's in 1983, followed by Dun's in 1986 and, accelerated by the worsening economic situation, by Baggot Street and Dr Steevens' in 1987/8. The present day regional cardiovascular specialties (now including cardiac surgery) had their origins mainly in Baggot Street, gastroenterology and ENT, again regional services, had most of their origins in Dun's, medical oncology originated in Mercer's, while plastics and reconstructive surgery, maxillofacial surgery and the burns unit all began in Steevens', and these too are national units. The closure of Steevens' and the opening of the A&E unit in the new hospital building in 1989 resulted in progressive increases in activity. The evolution of these services and expansion of associated research activity is the story of St James's. The St Kevin's tradition of providing services largely neglected by other institutions continued, notably the care of the elderly and genitourinary medicine, including STD and HIV, led by Fiona Mulcahy. The latter specialty might be said to have had an embryonic stage in the Federation in the service provided, in Dun's, by one of the most popular physicians in Dublin medicine, H. G. 'Bunny'

Ellerker, and in Dr Steevens' by Walter Verling.

Problems associated with the hospital closures

The chairman of St James's commented in his report for 1987 that the enforced hospital closures which had just taken place were 'probably the largest and swiftest closure and transfer of acute hospital services in the history of the voluntary hospital movement'. A controlled/planned amalgamation of institutions was one thing but no one had anticipated an event of this kind. The need to phase the construction of the new hospital and the inevitable withholding of building approvals by the Department of Health in a period of recession meant that while construction of the main clinical facilities had commenced none of these was commissioned when the closures took place. To accommodate the additional acute services the St James's maternity service was closed and transferred to the Coombe (ensuring that everyone in the system was suffering disruption) and an urgent programme of refurbishment was carried out in the former maternity and premature baby units to provide, among other things, a twin theatre suite and the specialised facilities needed for the burns unit and laboratories for maxillofacial surgery.

The move to the original St James's buildings, albeit with some refurbishment, the reduction in the overall number of beds and natural uncertainties about a change of employment and employer created natural disappointment and concern among staff required to transfer from the designated hospitals. The anxiety was probably greater among nurses and support staff. For some the situation was eased, if not assuaged, by the availability of options of early retirement and redundancy packages, so characteristic of periods of recession. Many, however, did transfer and made a valuable contribution to St James's. The last two closures resulted in the transfer of just over 170 staff. A remarkable aspect of the whole process was that at a time when industrial disputes were commonplace, all the closures took place without interruption of the service. Much credit is due to the forbearance of the staff and the skills of the personnel officers of the Federation and St James's, Pat Corcoran and Betty Coyle, both universally liked as individuals. The fact that the relatively new CEO of St James's, Liam Dunbar, had been group nursing administrator for the Federation and St James's helped, as did the realism of the then chairman of the Federation, Professor Bill Watts. The determination of Gerry MacCartney, who represented the Department of Health, ensured a swift result.

Most of the consultants already held a contract with St James's and their confidence in the future was somewhat increased by the amendments to the establishment order which had been signed by the then minister, Barry Desmond, in August 1984. The effect of the order was to reduce the representation of both the Eastern Health Board and the Central Council on the board and to introduce nominees of the Medical Board, Trinity College, the nursing staff and the unions. Subsequently there were always four senior consultants on the board, as either Medical Board, Central Council or Trinity nominees so that they were in a position of considerable influence. Ironically, it was commonly believed among consultant staff that Desmond was anti-consultant and bent on introducing a socialist national health service. The changes in the establishment order gradually transformed the perception of the board. Whereas previously the members were believed to be interested primarily in their nominating institutions, the new body was seen to be committed to the corporate interest of St James's.

Other development programmes

Organisation change has been an essential part of the transformation of St James's into a modern, stand-alone teaching hospital. The change process began uneasily. Liam Hogan, the hospital administrator, continued in charge of day-to-day operations but planning for the new hospital proceeded virtually separately under the supervision of a project team and planning officers. The appointment of Liam Dunbar as chief executive in 1985, at first in an acting capacity, effectively unified management of the hospital while his successor, John O'Brien, is the chief architect of the current management structure and organisation of the hospital. In all of this the Federation had little part to play except for the fact that at governance level the Central Council representatives lent strong support for the first chief executive appointments.

The aspiration to have a new hospital(s) was the incentive which drove the Federation throughout its existence and the cement which held the partnership of Federation, EHB and Trinity together in the early days of St James's. Despite the definition of the scale of the hospital in the 1973 Comhairle report, and the approval of the report by Mr Corish, Minister for Health, it was only in 1976 that a project team was set up, initially to write the brief. Its composition was inclusive of board members, consultant staff, nursing staff, the chief architect and other technical advisors and administrative officers from the Department of Health. Although it was not very fruitful in the long run, the chief architect of the Department of Education and the secretary of the Higher

Education Authority were also included. Plainly this was a major endeavour to involve and knit together all those who might contribute to planning and might also have a role in decision making for a teaching hospital. In the initial stages there was a tacit acceptance that Central Council staff would service the project team. Nevin Dowling, the chief executive of the Federation also held the title of planning officer and briefly served both Central Council and St James's in this capacity. When he resigned, in 1977, Padraig D'Alton who had been technical services manager for the Federated Hospitals became planning co-ordinator. Not long afterwards, however, he transferred to the employment of St James's as project and technical services manager and thereafter reported to the St James's board. D'Alton was the mainstay of the planning process. He wrote the briefs for the various stages of the new hospital and later supervised their planning and construction. A notable contribution to the functional success of the new building lies in the consultation groups (about 130 in all) he established to consider each draft brief and later plans, operational policies and commissioning. These groups were representative of all categories of staff who would occupy the department for which a brief or plan was being prepared. Prior to 1987 they included staff from both St James's and the designated hospitals. This gave many staff some 'ownership' of the new hospital although, of course, it was common to complain that there had been 'no consultation' when the plans were finally published.

The brief, completed in 1977, was for the 'St James's Teaching Hospital' and envisaged two main functional units, (a) the main teaching hospital complex of 750 beds, and (b) a clinical science facility; the latter was to provide for medical, dental and nursing education and a physiotherapy school. The acceptance of the brief by the then minister led to the appointment of a design team and a development control plan for the site was produced in 1978. Thereafter, progress was again painfully slow; detailed phasing was required to build on a complex site and the planning process involved numerous stages, most of which required sanction by the Department of Health which in turn was frequently delayed by the exigencies of the economic situation. None of the clinical facilities was open when the last of the Federated Hospitals closed in 1987, ten years after approval of the brief.

Despite the delays the prospect of excellent facilities was a major factor in recruitment and retention of well qualified staff from the outset and the fact that the main phase of clinical facilities (phase 1) was visibly under construction, if not open, gave some reassurance to staff required to transfer from the designated hospitals in 1987. The diagnostic imaging and outpatient departments were officially opened in January 1989 to be followed by the A&E department and the ward accommodation. At the time of writing most of the clinical facilities of the new hospital have been completed and there is a substantial clinical sciences complex (the Trinity Centre) which, although it does not include a dental hospital, has in its place a major research facility for molecular medicine.

The ultimate legacy

After 1987, and in the absence of revenue funding from the Department of Health, the designated hospitals could no longer deliver a service for patients. Nevertheless, each of these charities possessed valuable capital assets in the form of their property and various bequests and benefactions for which they acted as trustees. Upon closure they were not short of relatives hoping to inherit. The Department of Health made it clear that it expected that the remaining assets would be devoted first to clearing the operating deficits accumulated during the final difficult years of the hospitals' existence and then as a contribution to the capital cost of the new hospitals planned to replace them. Professor Watts, as chairman of Mercer's, articulated the opposition among the governors of the various charities to the surrender of the assets entrusted to them. If the original foundations were to close, the approval of the Commissioners for Charitable Donations and Bequests, and ultimately the courts, would be required for *cy près* schemes which would ensure that the assets would be applied to purposes close to the intentions of the original donors.

The first to draft a scheme was Mercer's. The governors prepared and received approval for a scheme which established a new charity, the Mercer's Hospital Foundation, to which the assets of the hospital, mainly arising from the sale of the hospital building, were transferred, and of which the governors effectively remained in control. The objectives were to provide 'public medical and hospital services, facilities, accommodation and care (such as are not already provided for out of public funds or other private sources) for diseased or infirm poor of Dublin', thus reflecting the intentions of the original donor and at the same time a policy of avoiding absorption into state funding. The scheme gave prominence to the 'provision and endowment of clinical research and training facilities'. In close pursuit of these objectives, the board of the new foundation established in 1988 the Mercer's Institute for Research in Ageing.

Research in this area had scarcely been the focus of attention in teaching hospitals or from the principal sources of research funding in previous times. The creation of this institute, for which St James's provided accommodation, resulted in a flow of publications and a growing reputation for Professor Coakley and the team of researchers supported by the institute. There is nothing like research for success breeding success and the Mercer's initiative led to further grants from the Health Research Board and from the Department of Health and Children for new services such as the dementia services information and development centre and a memory clinic.

Meanwhile, an affidavit sworn in 1989 by Donald Richardson, the last chairman of Sir Patrick Dun's, in support of a draft *cy près* scheme to determine the use and application of the assets of the hospital, set out in considerable detail the history of the charity. The primary objective of Sir Patrick Dun (the original donor) was to provide for a professor of physic in the College of Physicians. He left the college his house as a meeting place and a library for their use. Pursuant to the School of Physic Act of 1800, additional professorships were established and commissioners were appointed to construct, specifically, a teaching hospital. Thus Sir Patrick Dun's Hospital was built at Artichoke Road (later renamed Lower Grand Canal Street). Subsequently, professors were also appointed by Trinity College and all were finally assimilated by Trinity in 1941. Prior to the closure of Dun's both the professor of surgery, George Fegan, and the Regius Professor of Physic, Donald Weir, were prominent members of the staff. It was scarcely surprising in the light of this history that on the closure of the hospital the governors sought approval for a *cy près* scheme under which the assets of the hospital, mainly derived from the sale of the property (about £2.5 million), were to be divided as to two thirds to TCD and one third to the College of Physicians. To continue the provision of a teaching hospital the then provost had proposed that the moiety given to Trinity could 'be utilised through the development of TCD's medical school and ancillary activities at St James's Hospital'. The brief for the new St James's teaching hospital had included a clinical sciences complex with facilities for teaching medical, dental, nursing and paramedical students but up to 1987 no funds had been available to realise this ambition. In his affidavit Mr Richardson also recalled that a high proportion of the bequests made over the years to Dun's related to nursing education and that as a result one of the attractive features of Trinity's proposed development was to provide 'proper educational facilities for nurses in custom built accommodation'.

One of the more surprising aspects of the *cy près* scheme as finally approved was that the governors had persuaded the Department of Health to repay no less than £405,302 of uncovered net expenditure and this was included in the scheme as a direct transfer to St James's. The fact that this sum was actually handed over may have been due in part to constant reminders from the CEO and chairman of St James's that whereas the state had contributed to nursing schools elsewhere nothing had been provided at St James's. According to the terms of the *cy près* scheme this refund, along with the property fund, was to be 'applied to the construction, development, establishment and the activities of Trinity College Dublin's medical school and its ancillary activities at St James's Hospital which includes a nurse training school project'.

The *cy près* scheme was only the last of a number of benefactions given by the governors of Dun's to St James's and TCD. In 1969 they had entered into an agreement with Trinity to provide accommodation in Dun's for an integrated teaching centre and library, in fact, a nascent clinical sciences centre. Then, in August 1983, they entered into complicated agreements with St James's and Trinity whereby the former would construct a laboratory as an additional floor to the Central Pathology Laboratory which Dun's would pay for, lease and then licence to Trinity as the 'Sir Patrick Dun's Research Laboratory'. Dun's therefore has made major contributions to research and teaching facilities in the new teaching hospital to which its services and staff transferred.

The governors of Dun's took a different view of their own position from that adopted by Mercer's. They specifically rejected the idea of setting up a foundation under their control to administer their funds in perpetuity. They decided that once the hospital closed their role was complete and having defined the purposes for which their funds were to be applied they were content to allow Trinity and St James's to accept continuing responsibility for their application and administration.

The board of Dr Steeven's followed the example set by Dun's and their *cy près* scheme also devoted the assets of the hospital after its closure and sale (to the Eastern Health Board) to the Trinity teaching and research centre at St James's. Regrettably, in this case deficits which had mounted prior to the closure of the hospital were reclaimed by the Department of Health and the residual fund was relatively small.

As closure approached for Baggot Street, the board made a last minute attempt to promote a continuing future for their hospital through offering to deliver a general medical, surgical and casualty service for their area. This was rejected in 1987 by the Department of Health.[9] The acute

services were run down in November and December and the last patients and staff were transferred to St James's. There was a further surprising change of direction when the board agreed to lease the hospital
to the Eastern Health Board for badly needed long stay accommodation
for the elderly and as a base for various outpatient community services.
Thus, the Royal City of Dublin board remained the owners of their
valuable property in Baggot Street but they were not without other
disposable assets. The nurses' home was sold in 1988, the proceeds to be
administered by a new trust committed to supporting research and educational activities related to the hospital's former key specialties, cardiology, respiratory medicine and cardio-thoracic surgery. A research and
investigation unit was constructed and extended (in 1986) to form the
Royal City of Dublin Research Laboratory which is situated close to the
base of the CResT[10] directorate at St James's.

Conclusions

The closures of hospitals and with them the reduction in available beds
in the Dublin area in the 1980s has been blamed for the continuing lack
of capacity but the reduction in beds was not an inevitable ingredient of
hospital rationalisation. It resulted from the economic difficulties of the
time. Despite the reduction in bed numbers the concentration of expertise brought about by rationalisation has yielded improvements in the
quality and sophistication of the service. Many conditions are treated in
the new large hospitals by multidisciplinary teams with sophisticated
diagnostic capability and a substantial improvement in outcomes has
been achieved which would not have been possible without the up-
heaval of hospital rationalisation and closure. Also as a response to the
reduction in the number of beds St James's staff became pioneers of
endoscopy and day treatment in the Republic, thus making a virtue out
of necessity.

Almost unnoticed against the background of corporate and individual
trauma induced by the forced closures of the designated hospitals was
the fact that the original aspiration of the Federated Hospitals to 'own'
the new hospital had in effect been abandoned. In hindsight the reasons
are plain. There was at the crucial time no new hospital to 'own' and,
more fundamentally, since it was established St James's had acquired its
own corporate identity as a unique combination of municipal and voluntary hospital but belonging neither to the Health Board nor the Federation. The issue of separate managements was never discussed.

Although in a corporate sense St James's is very different from what the promoters of the 1961 Act expected their successors have a well equipped teaching hospital very much as envisaged in their original objectives with a high level of specialisation, professorial units and complete diagnostic services. The clinical sciences complex (the Trinity Centre) compares favourably with similar on-site teaching facilities in major UK centres. It has expanded to provide teaching for a large proportion of the health sciences and in very recent times major research institutes (the Molecular Medicine Institute and the Durkan Institute) have been added. In sum, the Federated Hospitals, through the specialisations they fostered, the teaching and research centres they have helped to fund and the young researchers they have supported, have made a continuing contribution to Irish medicine.

Depending on one's viewpoint the outcome is either a triumph of long term planning or a parable of the doctrine of unintended consequences.

References

[1] D. Mitchell *A 'Peculiar' Place: The Adelaide Hospital Dublin 1839–1989* Dublin: Blackwater Press, 1989.

[2] Mitchell *op. cit.* p 210.

[3] Consultative Council on the General Hospital Services *Outline of the Future Hospital System* (The FitzGerald Report) Dublin: 1968 p 25.

[4] *Ibid.* p 119.

[5] See Davis Coakley, Chapter 1 in this volume.

[6] Higher Education Authority correspondence, Ref. No. 198.

[7] See Chapter 1.

[8] *Editor's note*: 'Pool': a subvention was paid by the Department of Health for each occupied bed-day. Division of this was decided by consensual agreement between those consultants who held, or 'owned' beds. As may be imagined, 'consensual agreement' was not often reached without difficulty.

[9] Davis Coakley *Baggot Street: A Short History of the Royal City of Dublin Hospital* Dublin: The Board of Governors, Royal City of Dublin Hospital, 1995.

[10] Cardiology, respiratory medicine and cardiothoracic surgery

4. *The formation of The Adelaide and Meath Hospital, Dublin Incorporating The National Children's Hospital*

Fergus O'Ferrall

On 1 August 1996 three of Dublin's most famous hospitals became one. The Meath, founded in 1753, the National Children's Hospital, founded in 1821 and the Adelaide, founded in 1839, merged on that historic day to become The Adelaide and Meath Hospital, Dublin Incorporating The National Children's Hospital. Behind this unique merger lay years of complex negotiations. In 1988 discussions commenced in earnest as to how the proposed new hospital, which was to be built at Tallaght, would be governed and managed. The informal discussions and the subsequent formal negotiations were fraught and prolonged; they were characterised by high-minded vision and by an understandable vested interest within the three base hospitals as they sought to protect their heritage and future.

The leaders of the three hospitals succeeded eventually. They created a unique governance structure for the merged hospital and provided a new single corporate body for Ireland's most modern hospital campus at Tallaght. The merged hospital transferred to its new site on 21 June 1998 when the famous base hospital buildings were closed as all their patient services were continued from Tallaght. This brief account of how the three became one describes an important episode in Ireland's medical history.

The unique governance structure took legal effect through the Charter of The Adelaide and Meath Hospital, Dublin Incorporating The National Children's Hospital. This Charter was the result of extensive amendments to the Royal Charter of the Adelaide Hospital, Dublin (1920) which were approved by the Oireachtas in the Health Act, 1970

(Section 76) (Adelaide and Meath Hospital, Dublin Incorporating The National Children's Hospital) Order 1996. This order was facilitated by the Health (Amendment) (No 2) Act, 1996. These statutory measures received all party support in both Seanad Éireann (26 June 1996) and Dáil Éireann (3 July 1996).

The long and often controversial prelude to the approval of the amended Charter began in the 1980s and indeed earlier when the future of the Meath, Adelaide and National Children's Hospital (MANCH), as the last three hospitals in the Federated Dublin Voluntary Hospitals, had to be considered. Under the Central Council of the Federation a MANCH Council had been established to facilitate co-operation between the three surviving hospitals in the Federation: of the original seven hospitals four had already been effectively subsumed into St James's Hospital. It was intended that these three hospitals would provide the core services if and when the long-sought new hospital was built in Tallaght.

In 1980 the task of planning the new hospital at Tallaght was not given to the Central Council of the Federated Dublin Voluntary Hospitals but to a new Tallaght Hospital Board established by a Statutory Order under the Health (Corporate Bodies) Act, 1961. Though the new board had representation from the three base hospitals some at least felt that a clear signal had been given that the new hospital would be governed by a board appointed by the minister for health under the 1961 Act. The governance arrangements for St James's and for Beaumont, as they subsumed old voluntary hospitals in the 1970s and 1980s, had been made under this Act.

In the event the building of the new hospital was delayed for many years. Following a major architectural competition in 1985 architects were appointed.[1] It was not until October 1993 that the Minister for Health, Brendan Howlin, finally got the new building underway. In 1990, following intensive negotiations, a working party had been established by the then Minister for Health, Rory O'Hanlon, to agree upon a governance framework for the new hospital. It was chaired by David Kingston, chief executive of Irish Life, and Professor David Kennedy, a management consultant and former chief executive of Aer Lingus. The working party was composed of representatives of the three hospitals. Eventually, in May 1993, it produced 'heads of agreement' which were approved that month by the boards of the hospitals and subsequently by the government. The working party produced a draft text of the Charter based upon the heads of agreement and this was approved by the boards of the three hospitals in August 1995. The final text of the Charter, as expressed in the order as laid before the Oireachtas, was based upon this draft text as advised by the Attorney General and approved by government. It took legal effect on 1 August 1996 on which date a single board under the Charter took responsibility for the three hospitals as one hospital.

In retrospect, given the great success of the hospital at Tallaght, it may be difficult to understand why the process of agreeing the Charter was so long and complex. At the heart of the process was the issue of whether an agreed governance structure would be 'voluntary', that is have a board appointed by a voluntary body or bodies, or 'statutory', that is have a board appointed by the Minister for Health. The Adelaide, as represented by the Adelaide Hospital Society, expressed a deep commitment to an ethos and set of values which they believed required a voluntary board for the new hospital. The then chairman of the Meath, Councillor Gerry Brady, has observed that the Meath Hospital board did not see themselves as 'a voluntary hospital' in the same way as did the Adelaide: 'It wasn't a concept in the same way as I hear it now in the board of the new hospital. It was a hospital that provided a service dependent on the Department of Health for money . . . '[2]

The Adelaide by the late 1980s had come to hold a unique position within the remaining Dublin hospitals and the Protestant community in the Republic. Following the rapid sequence of closures in the 1980s of famous voluntary hospitals long associated with the Protestant community (such as Sir Patrick Dun's, Dr Steevens', Mercer's, Baggot Street, Monkstown and Barrington's, Limerick) the Adelaide by 1989 found itself the last remaining voluntary teaching hospital in the state under a largely (though not exclusively) Protestant lay board. It was governed by a Royal Charter, granted in 1920, which stated that the hospital was 'a religious and essentially Protestant institution' though, of course, its staff and patients were largely drawn from the Roman Catholic population. The famous Adelaide School of Nursing, founded in 1859, provided nurse education for students from the Protestant community.

The Meath was physically very close to the Adelaide and shared much of its history. More recently, consultant appointments and other services under the Federation Central Council were common to both yet the Meath represented quite a different ethos, one which was the product of its very different history. Founded in 1753 it had long been governed, under an 1815 local Act of Parliament, by a board of governors, or 'Joint Committee' as it was called, representing a Protestant ethos. The golden age of the hospital had occurred in the 19th century when a succession of famous doctors made it a great centre of teaching and research during the period of Dublin's international medical fame. The Meath had been constituted as the 'County Dublin Infirmary' under an Act of the Irish Parliament in 1774 and this Act conferred on the medical staff the privilege of appointing their successors. There was a long connection with local government in the Meath through grants received as the County Infirmary. In 1949 there was a concerted effort by the Knights of Columbanus, a Roman Catholic lay organisation, to oust the old, predominantly Protestant, Joint Committee. This led to major legal and political controversy which ultimately resulted in The Meath Hospital Act, 1951. This Act removed the power of the medical staff to appoint their successors and set out a very substantial proportion of public representation in the composition of the new Joint Committee (or Board) as follows: Dublin County Council 6; General Council of County Councils 2; Dublin Corporation 6; Medical Board 4; Hospital Corporation (Meath Society of Governors and Governesses) 4; and 2 co-options.[3]

From the late 1940s the Meath, while formally non-denominational in character, assumed a more overt Catholic tone and ethos than it had in its previous long history as a Protestant-led voluntary hospital. There was, therefore, a significant gap to be bridged in the values and perceptions of representatives of the Adelaide and the Meath as they negotiated in the working party from 1990.

The National Children's Hospital was founded in 1821 as the first teaching children's hospital in Ireland or Britain and it was governed by a lay voluntary board which took the legal form of a charitable company under the Companies Acts. The National Children's Hospital had a background and ethos similar to that of the Adelaide and it was perceived as a focus for Protestant participation in paediatric services as the other children's hospitals in Dublin were under Catholic auspices.

When in 1988 serious discussions commenced on the future management structures for the new hospital, the Adelaide proposed that it should be a 'public voluntary hospital' governed by an independent board with a continuing role in governance for the Adelaide Hospital Society, which governed the Adelaide Hospital under its Charter.[4] In 1988 the Department of Health proposed to amalgamate the management structures of the three base hospitals in such a way that the hospitals would have lost their voluntary status and would have become dissociated from Trinity College Dublin.[5]

The Department persisted in seeking a single management structure and a new chief officer for the MANCH group in preparation for the new hospital to be built in Tallaght. The Department wished through a 'single allocation' to ensure this occurred. The Adelaide refused unless such a structure had a 'non-profit' organisational base and was 'independent' of the state. It argued that such a structure would be publicly accountable so as to satisfy the state's requirements but it would facilitate a focus for the Protestant contribution to healthcare and maximise patient care which would benefit from on-going additional voluntary support. The Department's tactic was to withhold allocations to the three hospitals until they acceded to its demands.[6]

The impasse thus reached led to public controversy and the direct involvement of the leaders from the main Protestant Churches. At this stage the Adelaide board contemplated a minority role on the proposed new voluntary hospital board as sufficient to ensure a continuation of its tradition and ethos. However, as it became clear that the extinction of the Adelaide was intended, at least in some quarters, the stance of the Adelaide board hardened. Professor David McConnell, then chairman of the board, stated in 1992: 'Minority representation for the minority on the board of the new hospital came to look more like a prescription for slow extinction'.[7]

During 1989 there was considerable media coverage of the Adelaide issue and it was raised at the Church of Ireland Synod, the Presbyterian General Assembly and at the Methodist Conference in May and June of that year.[8] A meeting between the Protestant Church leaders and the Taoiseach, Mr Haughey, in September 1989 led to a positive response from Mr Haughey who stated that he would wish to see the ethos represented by the Adelaide maintained 'as an integral part of the hospital system'. He requested the church leaders to invite the board of the Adelaide 'to present to the Department of Health a detailed plan of what they would regard as the most advantageous future for the Adelaide Hospital'.[9]

The Adelaide board proposed that it play a significant and determining role in running a major teaching hospital and stated that it would welcome an invitation to run the new hospital at Tallaght and believed it could provide for appropriate participation by the Meath and the National Children's Hospital in the new institution. It felt that there should be one major voluntary hospital in the state governed with significant Protestant participation. There was no formal reply to this proposal. Neither did the financial pressure ease; the Anglican Archbishop of Dublin, Most Rev. Dr D. Caird, and the chairman of the hospital met with the Taoiseach, Mr Haughey, in January 1990 to discuss the crisis which as a result was partly relieved. A further financial crisis developed in 1991 and 1992. The board of the Adelaide interpreted the financial pressure as an attempt by the Department of Health to close the hospital as this had been the experience of the other hospitals which had been closed such as Dr Steevens' and Monkstown Hospital. Public controversy continued.[10]

It was against this vexed background that the working party established in 1990 worked to produce an agreement on the governance of the new hospital in Tallaght. Its terms of reference were 'to consider possible future management arrangements for the new public voluntary hospital with nursing school at Tallaght'. As set out by the minister, as a result of public pressure by the Adelaide, the terms of reference asked the working party to consider four management options:

(1) a management board established under the Health (Corporate Bodies) Act 1961;
(2) a management board established under primary legislation for the establishment of a new public voluntary hospital;
(3) a management board operating under an amended Adelaide Charter;
(4) a management board established under the Companies Act.

The proposals were to be based upon 'the premise that the traditions and emphases of the three hospitals are valuable and must be given expression in the management arrangements for Tallaght . . . In particular the position of the Adelaide as a focus for Protestant participation in the health services and its particular denominational focus must be continued in Tallaght'.[11]

The Department of Health, having been persuaded to concede these terms of reference by public and political pressure, chose not to participate in the working party. It was expected by many that the hospitals would find it impossible to agree and that a ministerially appointed board could be imposed in due course. However, as has been noted, after many detailed meetings held in the Irish Life building, where Mr Kingston had his office, agreement emerged by stages.

The working party submitted a report to the Minister for Health in November 1991 stating that the three hospitals had agreed that the legal instrument governing the new hospital at Tallaght should be by amendment of the existing Adelaide Charter under Section 76 of the Health Act 1970. The advantages of such a Charter outweighed those of the other legal options: a Charter would provide for the hospital the greatest degree of legal independence and it would maximise the opportunities for the participating hospitals to draft their own future governing instrument. Also, the hospitals would continue to hold the initiative in respect of any future changes to the Charter as such power resides in those bodies holding a Charter. It was noted that famous medical bodies such as the Royal College of Physicians and the Royal College of Surgeons rejoice in their status as chartered bodies and it was felt that it would be a great boon to the hospital, alone amongst Irish hospitals, to have such a status as a chartered body.

There were many complex and difficult issues in the working group still to be confronted. However, the skill and persistence of the chairmen of the group, as well as the leadership and indeed generous vision of the three hospital chairmen—Professor David McConnell of the Adelaide, Councillor Gerry Brady of the Meath and Mr Thomas McManus of the National Children's Hospital—were the key ingredients which were to lead to ultimate success in negotiations over almost 40 meetings of the working group.

In May 1991 the Meath Hospital Board had rejected the proposal by the working group in respect of the composition of the new board: 5 from the Adelaide, 4 from the Meath, 3 from the National Children's Hospital and 1 from Trinity College. As the largest of the base hospitals, the Meath naturally did not wish to be placed in a perceived 'minority' in any new structure; it was very concerned to protect its own staff's future interests and many on the Meath side resented the salience of the Adelaide's position in the context of the political need in a pluralist environment to recognise the contribution of the Protestant community to healthcare. Given the political developments on the island as a whole during the 1990s the project was always about much more than just merging three hospitals of varying sizes.

In 1992, during these long negotiations the then Minister for Health, Dr John O'Connell, invited the Adelaide to withdraw from Tallaght; however, at that stage the Adelaide was totally committed to the full Tallaght project. The Adelaide believed that a second major teaching hospital was essential to the future of the Faculty of Health Sciences in Trinity College so it rejected what it perceived as a ploy which would lead to a dead end for a small vulnerable hospital in respect of patient care, education and research. The Adelaide was also determined to secure the future of the National Children's Hospital as part of the new hospital. At that time the National Children's Hospital remained very vulnerable with respect to the development of paediatric services.

Eventually, vision and leadership paid off when the three hospital boards were able to approve a key agreement entitled 'Heads of Agreement' dated 25 May 1993. The government approved these Heads of Agreement and the critical breakthrough had been achieved.

Now a second detailed phase of negotiations commenced. The working party charged Dr John Barragry, on behalf of the Meath, and myself, on behalf of the Adelaide, to translate the Heads of Agreement into a draft text so as to produce a fully amended draft Charter. The working party approved our drafts which we produced working together with great cordiality and mutual respect. The draft text, after some final key help in respect of the merit basis for staff appointments from the Minister for Health, Michael Noonan, was approved by the boards of the three hospitals in August 1995. Within a year, as has been noted, this Charter became law and rapidly took effect on 1 August 1996. Prior to this, at the initiative of Mr Noonan, an interim board, composed as set out in the Charter, had been meeting from early 1996 in order to prepare for the formal responsibilities when the Charter took effect.

It was important in achieving this unique governance instrument and status to have each of the three hospitals understand that the newly amended Charter accorded exactly similar status to each of them. This parity of esteem has underpinned the success of the merger.

As a result of this long intensive negotiation the hospital which transferred to Tallaght on 21 June 1998 represented a fruitful hybrid of different traditions. These traditions were enabled to evolve under the Charter which provides for the name of the hospital, for a new president of the hospital (the Church of Ireland Archbishop of Dublin) and for a board of 23 (6 from the Adelaide, 6 from the Meath, 3 from the National Children's Hospital, 6 nominated by the hospital president, 1 from the Health Board and 1 from Trinity College). The voluntary bodies of the base hospitals (the Adelaide Hospital Society, the Meath Foundation and the National Children's Hospital Foundation) continue to make their appointments to the new board, appointed every three years, and to support the hospital through voluntary action and their voluntary funds.

The Charter provides that the focus for Protestant participation in the health services is to be maintained in the hospital and it has 'a multi-denominational and pluralist character'. The inclusiveness of the hospital is reflected in a Charter provision as to the confidential relationship between each patient and his or her consultant. This is crucial in respect of a medical ethic which allows all persons to be treated as they wish, taking into account their own beliefs and values. The Charter provides that spiritual welfare is essential to patient care and that freedom of conscience and of religious practice is to be honoured for both patients and staff. The key general principle that had been so strongly contested, that newly established public services might be run by voluntary agencies, was secured. In the Dáil debate on 3 July 1996, which proposed the Charter for approval, the Minister for Health, Mr Michael Noonan, said:

> I regard this as a time to place on record my appreciation of the invaluable contribution, made on a voluntary basis, by the members of the Boards of the three hospitals which are moving to Tallaght . . . The skills and commitment which these people, and their colleagues in many hospitals and organisations, bring to the health services, while always appreciated, are not enough acknowledged.[12]

The new board of The Adelaide and Meath Hospital, Dublin Incorporating The National Children's Hospital met for the first formal meeting in charge of the new hospital at 8 a.m. on Thursday 1 August 1996 in the National Children's Hospital boardroom. They were the inheritors of all those who had developed the three hospitals from the time when a voluntary charitable impulse in a house on the Upper Coombe near Meath Street in 1753 led to the establishment of the Meath Hospital. Now they had a governance framework fitted to serve a changing Irish society into the 21st century with the highest quality of patient care, health education and research. They were not to have an easy passage— the first board, led so ably by Mrs Rosemary French, chairperson of the Adelaide Hospital Society, had to overcome a major under-funding crisis.[13] The first board succeeded brilliantly with the new chief executive officer, Dr David McCutcheon, in transferring the services to Tallaght in June 1998, an achievement which reflected the outstanding *esprit de corps* amongst all the staff who ensured this very complex operation was completed without a hitch. The hospital, therefore, was enabled under the Charter to enter the new millennium utilising Ireland's most comprehensive hospital campus and with the exciting prospect of achieving the highest possibilities in respect of patient services, education and research beckoning during the 21st century.

References

[1] See Neil Steedman (ed.) *Tallaght Hospital Architectural Competition* Dublin: Tallaght Hospital Board n.d. (1986).

[2] Interview with Gerry Brady, 9 June 1999.

[3] This brief account is based upon Peter Gatenby's *Dublin's Meath Hospital 1753–1996* Dublin: Town House 1996, especially Ch. 13 'The Advance of the Knights 1949–50'.

[4] This was not a new position: in November 1977 when the board of the Adelaide first agreed to move with the Meath, it was 'on terms which would be acceptable to the Board with the constraint imposed on it by the Royal Charter of the Hospital'. See D. Mitchell *A 'Peculiar' Place: The Adelaide Hospital, Dublin 1839–1989* Dublin: Blackwater Press 1989 pp 227–8.

[5] In April, May and June 1988 there were confidential meetings between P. W. Flanagan, Secretary, Department of Health, and representatives of the board of the Adelaide; it is clear from the record of these discussions that Mr Flanagan very reluctantly considered the concept of a 'public voluntary hospital' as an option for the new hospital as proposed by the Adelaide. See minutes and transcripts of three meetings 11 April 1988, 12 May 1988 and 15 June 1988 in Adelaide Hospital Society papers.

[6] This was not the first occasion on which this technique had been used. *Ed.*

[7] See McConnell, p 68 in this volume.

[8] See editorial in *The Irish Times* 1 June 1989 and articles in the *Belfast Telegraph* 7 July 1989 entitled 'The Republic's "Mater"' for the flavour of the public debate.

[9] See McConnell, p 71 in this volume.

[10] See, for example, *The Irish Times* 19 May 1990 Seanad Éireann debate, 1 May 1990.

[11] Terms of reference for the Kingston Working Group from the Minister for Health, Dr O'Hanlon, July 1990; the group was asked to submit its report by 31 October 1990!

[12] Michael Noonan TD, Dáil Éireann Parliamentary Debates vol. 468, No. 1, Col. 18, 3 July 1996.

[13] See 'A Case Study: The Adelaide and Meath Hospital, Dublin Incorporating The National Children's Hospital 1996–1999' in *Citizenship and Public Service: Voluntary and Statutory Relationships in Irish Healthcare* Dundalk: The Adelaide Hospital Society, Dundalgan Press, 2000 pp 161–224.

5. The Tallaght Hospital Board and the building of the new hospital*

G. D. Rogan

The Tallaght Hospital project was the largest, the most exciting, and the most complex acute hospital project ever undertaken in Ireland. Until the end of the 1950s Tallaght, to the west of Templeogue in Dublin, was a small village. During the 1960s it became the fastest growing suburb of Dublin as, in a bid to replace the overcrowded tenements in the city centre, local authority housing augmented private development in the area. By the end of the 1970s Tallaght had a population approaching 60,000, which grew to over 100,000 by 2005.

In 1970 the Department of Health amended the proposals in the FitzGerald Report (1968) to include two more hospitals—one an expansion of the James Connolly Memorial Hospital in Blanchardstown and the other a new acute hospital in the Tallaght area where infrastructural development had been minimal. These were in addition to the two on each side of the river as suggested by FitzGerald.

By the early 1980s some of the FitzGerald proposals had been implemented. In particular, the services of three of the Federated Hospitals—Baggot Street, Dun's and Mercer's—had transferred to St Kevin's which was renamed St James's. Those of the others—the Meath, Adelaide and the National Children's Hospital (MANCH)—were to form the nucleus of the activity in the new hospital at Tallaght. Dr Steevens' services were to be divided between St James's and MANCH. With St James's well under way the Department of Health began in 1981 to put together the framework necessary to create the new hospital in Tallaght.

Tallaght Hospital Board

The Tallaght Hospital Board was established by ministerial order in February 1980 (SI No. 38 of 1980) by the Minister for Health, Dr Michael Woods. It was charged under the order, *inter alia*:

This article is based on the author's official report on the Tallaght Hospital Board.

(1) to plan, build, equip and furnish a general hospital in Tallaght

(2) when commissioned, to *conduct, maintain, manage and develop the hospital services* [emphasis added]

(3) to provide facilities for teaching and for the conduct of research.

The board held its first meeting on 8 May 1981 in Arus Mhic Diarmuida in Store Street. Having met at various venues it finally leased its own premises in Harcourt Street in December 1985. The first chairman of the board was Kevin Molloy, a Tallaght businessman, who was succeeded by Tony Enright, principal officer with the Department of Health. In 1987 he was followed by Professor Richard Conroy who continues to be chairman until the present time.

First steps

The board met formally each month and dealt with administrative matters. One of its first real tasks was to identify the bed requirements for the different specialties. The possibility of providing outpatient facilities prior to the opening of the hospital was considered as was the future role of Naas Hospital which was already providing acute hospital services in the catchment area. By September 1981 the Department of Health and the Eastern Health Board had agreed that Naas would be retained permanently. On the recommendation of Beaumont Hospital the board developed a planning sub-committee to progress planning, co-opting as necessary managers from the base hospitals and professional advisors from the Department of Health. The board itself concentrated on discussing with the department issues such as catchment area, a private hospital facility on site, and staffing requirements. The need to agree with TCD that the new hospital should be one of the two major teaching hospitals associated with the Trinity medical school was also high on the agenda.

Executive staffing

John Collins was appointed the first secretary to the board. He was seconded from the Department of Health in 1981. The board sought approval to employ a small executive staff to assist in planning but this was denied, the department suggesting that staff could be seconded from the base hospitals. In 1982 I became the board's part-time secretary as well as holding the posts of secretary-manager in both the Adelaide and the National Children's Hospital—a tricky balancing act. Carol McKay became my fulltime assistant in June 1983. In 1985 Catherine

McDaid, with the approval of the department, was appointed nurse planning officer.

During the following years the board experienced continuing difficulty in obtaining sanction to employ administrative staff. This resulted in great stress for all involved which could have been avoided by adequate human resources. The situation was compounded by a lack of management structure for the new hospital. At the same time it became clear that not all of the designated hospitals agreed that in time the Tallaght Hospital Board would become the governing body of the new hospital. The Department was reluctant to take any action which would jeopardise the negotiations on the integration of services taking place in the three transferring hospitals. This, of course, resulted in a delay in establishing a management structure under the auspices of the Tallaght Hospital Board.

Communication

By and large the board enjoyed good relations with the public and the staff of the transferring hospitals during the entire project. It also ensured that both the staff and public were kept informed of progress, the latter particularly at times when there appeared to be little tangible activity in relation to the new hospital.

The first formal report of the board to the Central Council of the Federated Hospitals was made in October 1983. Later, open information days were held for the staff of the transferring hospitals. A line of communication with the unions representing the staff was also established and the usual commitments regarding conditions of transfer were agreed with them.

A vision of the new hospital

The original objective of the Tallaght Hospital Board was to build a new acute teaching hospital with a total of 750–800 beds on a green field site in Tallaght. It was to provide services for a population of around 340,000 in the area of south Kildare and west Wicklow in addition to the expanding population of Tallaght itself. The development was to be phased, with a replacement for the existing services in the base hospitals being provided in the first phase. The second phase was to include the development of a 50-bed maternity unit, and 50 additional beds for medicine and surgery. In the third phase a 210-bed orthopaedic and trauma unit was to establish a key elective orthopaedic unit on the south side of the city. A final phase was to provide further beds for medicine and surgery, a 50-bed psychiatric unit, a 25-bed rehabilitation unit and 40 extended care beds for older patients. Overall, a significant expansion of the services of the transferring hospitals was to be provided.

In August 1981 the board was working on the basis that Tallaght Hospital should have 750–800 beds. In retrospect, this plan, while providing only the necessary services, was over ambitious but in January 1982 the Department of Health agreed to the plan, and indeed, in November 1983, sanctioned eight more paediatric beds. It took the view, however, that neither private nor semi-private accommodation should be provided from the public purse. In late 1983 the board did receive a letter from the Department granting permission for 100 beds for accommodation for student nurses. This plan was overtaken by developments in nurse training.

Federated Hospitals governance changes

Following the move of the three hospitals—Mercer's, Baggot Street and Sir Patrick Dun's—to St James's, and the dispersal of Dr Steevens' services, the Federation structure changed. The Central Council continued to function but in 1987, in terms of day to day management, many of its activities were taken over by the MANCH Council. Its purpose was to co-ordinate the services of its three members—the Meath, the Adelaide and the National Children's Hospital—and to develop a single management structure for the new hospital in Tallaght. The activities of the MANCH Council were, however, frustrated by the Department, which continued to deal with each of the constituent hospitals individually for funding purposes. The MANCH Council, however, did provide a unifying forum when it became clear that the hospitals involved in it did not wish Tallaght Hospital Board to become the corporate structure for the new hospital.

The site and architectural plans

In 1984 the Minister for Health secured a site for the new hospital at the Tallaght end of the Belgard Road and the board visited it for the first time in September that year. Site work was due to begin in May/June 1986 but fencing of the site was delayed and the initial access road was only completed in 1993.

The board initiated an architectural competition in September 1983 with a board of assessors consisting of Dr Tony Enright, who chaired the board, architects Paddy Bermingham, Frank Jackman and Moishe Zarhy (Union Internationale des Architectes), Drs Niall Tierney and Gerry

Hurley, and myself as registrar. By closure in November 1984 there were 65 applications of which 16 were short-listed for interview and 10 submitted plans. The winning design was submitted by Robinson Keefe Devane (RKD). All ten designs formed an exhibition in the Guinness Hop Store and the winning design was displayed in venues in the Tallaght area, where it was well received.

Formal plans were now drawn up by the design team headed by RKD, planning permission was applied for and a project team was established. A high degree of flexibility was built into the design. After various complications involving changes of design and planning details full planning permission was granted and in 1991 the board learned that the estimated cost of building and equipping the new hospital was £118 million. The board threw itself fully into the whole process and the level of detail reviewed by it is all the more remarkable because at that stage it was still not in a position to tell which services were to be provided at the hospital.

Work on whole hospital policies continued and pre-commissioning plans helped to maintain the interest of staff in the transferring hospitals from 1988 to 1992 when there was no clarity from the government as to when a date for commencement of construction would be set. This period was one of considerable uncertainty.

Complement reduction

In June 1990 the secretary of the Department of Health met Professor Conroy, chairman of the board; at that time the bed complement had been fixed at a maximum of 600, a reduction of 28 per cent. This was to have been confirmed in writing. In January 1991 the tendering process started, although the board was concerned that approval to go to tender had not been received and progress seemed to have slowed. This raised the concern that the MANCH hospitals would suffer because no new investment would be made in their infrastructure in anticipation of the move to Tallaght. In March 1991 news arrived that there would be no funding in 1991. The contractors were advised of the situation and tendering was put on hold.

About this time Professor David Kennedy was asked to chair the Dublin Hospitals Advisory Group (DHAG) which was considering, *inter alia*, emergency services in the Dublin acute hospitals. DHAG was later asked by the then Minister, Mary O'Rourke, to 'review and in the context of its report make recommendations on the function, scope and scale of the proposed Tallaght Hospital . . . and to consider and make recommendations on the possible methods of funding for it.'

The board was not unnaturally disappointed that its most professional work carried out over the previous eight years was to be reappraised by the Kennedy Committee. It was suspected that the exercise was calculated to downsize further the hospital which had originally been planned to contain 830 beds.

Dr John O'Connell became Minister for Health in February 1992 and asked DHAG to finalise its report. Some days later he met the Tallaght board suggesting that Tallaght would have only 300 beds and that the specialities at the transferring hospitals would be retained there. The board responded vigorously to this idea, pointing out the enormous problems such a system would cause.

In May 1992 DHAG reported to the minister recommending the downsizing of the hospital to 467 beds with a corresponding reduction in the support systems in the hospital thus sowing the seeds for many of the difficulties which continue to this day.

Decision to build

In November 1992 the Taoiseach, Albert Reynolds, announced that the new hospital would have 467 beds and that building would begin on 14 April 1993. In February 1993 the new minister for health, Brendan Howlin, announced that building would commence as soon as possible and later impressed upon the board the urgency of getting the project underway before the end of the year.

The board, while it was concerned that the minister had not addressed the provision of private accommodation at the hospital, and about the reduction in its physical size, nevertheless proceeded enthusiastically. It was elated that Tallaght would be an acute teaching hospital and immediately reappointed the project team. All the deadlines set by the minister were met by the design and project teams and a management control programme was produced which showed clearly that it was feasible to go to tender in June and start work on the site in November 1993. I was appointed project director and E. C. Harris, together with J. J. Balance, were appointed as the firm in charge of its management.

In May 1993 tenders were invited in accordance with EU protocols and in October 1993 an Irish/English partnership—Laing Paul Joint Ventures (Tallaght) Ltd—was appointed as the main contractor. They took possession of the site on 29 October 1993 and started work. The role of the project team henceforth was to ensure that agreed timetables were adhered to and that the construction programme remained within budget. The design team had the responsibility of ensuring that the quality of work achieved the required standard.

Progress was monitored by the use of site photographs provided by the main contractor every two weeks. It is significant that the percentage of on-site staff from the Tallaght area employed by the contractor rose from 19 per cent in May 1994 to 27 per cent by the end of that year.

New hospital board

In 1995, after considerable discussion, the structure of the new hospital board was agreed. A board-designate for the Adelaide and Meath Hospital, Dublin incorporating the National Children's Hospital (AMNCH) had been formed and in 1995 the chairman of the Tallaght Hospital Board, Professor Conroy, offered his congratulations to Mrs Rosemary French on her appointment as its chairperson, stressing the need for a good working relationship between the two boards.

To this end a joint liaison committee was formed. For a time the Tallaght Hospital Board was the only statutory body in existence and the situation required the closest co-operation between it and the board-designate. Although lines of responsibility were often blurred, this indeed resulted. The Tallaght Hospital Board concentrated on the completion and equipping of the new hospital while the AMNCH board seems to have been involved in the logistics of the transfer and the development of the additional buildings necessitated by the cutbacks imposed in 1992. These buildings included a 77-bed private facility, the expansion of the outpatient department, and a multi-storey car park.

In August 1996 the AMNCH board-designate became a statutory body and the Tallaght Hospital Board passed operational issues over to it.

Progress and problems

The topping-out ceremony took place in June 1995 and internal construction began. A problem arose when it became apparent that the size and shape of the theatres had been altered, perhaps at the time of the Kennedy Report revision. It was realised that this meant that they could not be used when modern equipment had been installed. The board was advised in July 1995 that correction of this would involve the additional expenditure of £770,000; the board agreed to access its contingency fund if the shortfall could not be covered by savings in other parts of the contract.

A further problem arose when the board, having assessed outstanding deficiencies in the new building in March and April 1996, submitted its findings to the Department of Health in May that year. It was finally agreed that works considered essential to the opening of the hospital should be undertaken. These included an extension to the outpatient department and alterations to the x-ray, theatre, ICU and recovery, and HSSD (hospital sterile services) departments.

In August 1996 the contractor estimated a delay of five weeks to completion which became seven weeks in September. In October the contractor presented a programme which would allow completion by April 1997. The Tallaght Hospital Board doubted that this would enable the hospital to open in August 1997. In December 1996 Michael Noonan, Minister for Health, admitted that August might not be possible but was adamant that opening in 1997 should be possible.

In November 1996 Dr David McCutcheon was appointed CEO by the AMNCH board and indicated that additional building works might be required to allow proper operation of the hospital. This comment was undoubtedly based on the reduction in facilities forced upon the hospital by the findings of the Kennedy Committee (the DHAG) in 1992. One of the CEO's first acts was to institute weekly meetings of a management advisory group comprising the secretary-managers of the transferring hospitals, the administrator of the Federated Hospitals and the project director.

AMNCH now established a commissioning team and a manpower committee, later to become the human resources committee, in preparation for the hospital opening on 21 June 1998. The schedule was extremely tight but the board considered that date sacrosanct and non-negotiable. The Medical Board reckoned that opening without completion of some areas would be less than safe and the CEO met the theatre manager and the senior surgeon at the beginning of May to discuss signing off issues which the Medical Board had raised. On 7 May the CEO said he would ensure that heads of departments signed off drawings or else he would sign them off himself!

Equipping

An equipping steering committee had been set up in 1994 and had started the enormous task of deciding how much equipment was required, how much could be transferred and how much additional new equipment would be needed. Eight to ten committees were established, composed of members of the Tallaght Hospital Board, MANCH staff members and representatives of the Department of Health, and they drew up equipment lists for each department before arranging tenders for purchase. The total budget was of the order of £23 million. It was a larger quantum of equipment than had been purchased previously for the Irish health service and under EU rules.

All the equipment was evaluated, ordered, and put into position in the appropriate department in time for the opening of the hospital. Inevitably one or two problems arose along the way. One of these was that the cost of theatre instrumentation far exceeded the original estimates. This was mainly because modern hospital sterile services departments require three times as many instruments as hospitals which do not use HSSD facilities; in addition EU regulations for such units had been revised and required much higher standards to reduce the risk of cross infection arising from operative procedures.

Trinity College teaching agreement

The Tallaght Hospital Board's view of the new hospital, and that of MANCH and the transferring medical staff, was that it would be a teaching hospital carrying on the traditions established over the years at the base institutions. At the end of 1986 TCD sent the Tallaght Board a copy of its draft teaching agreement with St James's. The board agreed to use this as a basis for discussion and some progress was made in January 1987. The Royal College of Surgeons also expressed an interest in education facilities at Tallaght but wanted an exclusivity clause. The board decided to explore the TCD option again before responding.

No real progress was made until March 1989 when the MANCH Medical Committee and the Central Council of FDVH agreed a draft teaching agreement with Trinity and this then went to the Tallaght Hospital Board for approval. In late 1989 Trinity was in the process of allocating £1 million to the project and the board decided not to pursue the RCSI proposal further.

It was not, however, until February 1993 that further progress was reported and in November the agreement was said to be in its final stages. It was ready for signing in January 1994 but was not actually signed until October 1995.

The Tallaght Board and Trinity established a project team for the required academic facilities. Planning was completed in September 1996 and construction finally got underway in February 1999. The building was first used in the academic year which began in September 2000.

Opening and afterwards

The enormous logistical exercise of shutting down the transferring hospitals and actually transferring equipment, furniture, files and records to Tallaght took place during the final two months while the last alterations were being carried out. Staff worked long hours with exemplary professionalism. The support of both boards was of paramount importance and it is a credit to all involved that the preparation and attention to detail during this final period culminated in the successful transfer of patients and the opening of the hospital on Sunday 21 June 1998.

After the hospital opened the relationship between the Tallaght Hospital Board, the board of AMNCH and the Central Council of Federation had first to be clearly defined and then the future of the Tallaght Board and the Federation had to be determined. The winding up of these two bodies whose work has been magnificently completed still remains to be done but I must conclude by emphasising that the task of building a new hospital on a green field site in a new catchment area, while replacing and enhancing the services provided by long-established hospitals in the centre of Dublin, was by any standards a major project successfully completed.

PART TWO:

THE FEDS—
THE LAST DECADES

6. The Adelaide Hospital—the last Protestant general teaching hospital in the Republic of Ireland

David McConnell

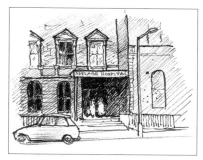

This paper was presented at a conference of The Cultures of Ireland Group in 1992 and published in Culture in Ireland—Regions, Identity and Power *(ed. P. O'Driscoll, Belfast: The Institute of Irish Studies, The Queen's University of Belfast, 1993). See also Editor's note p.77.*

Introduction

The Adelaide Hospital, Dublin, poses some important challenges and opportunities at a time when we are taking a more confident interest in the diversity of our culture. William Bateson, Balfour Professor of Genetics at Cambridge, and a leading exponent of Mendelism in the early quarter of this century, advised, 'treasure your exceptions'. The Adelaide Hospital is a particular exception in Ireland as I will explain, one among many others which may now find themselves threatened by a creeping, centralising, homogenising form of government. This is a story about a hospital but it may also be a story about the attitude of local and central governments of officials and politicians to minority interests of many kinds.

The questions are two: in what form will the Adelaide survive and will it be treasured? Putting it another way, will the Adelaide struggle on because it cannot or will not be destroyed, or will it prosper through a wholehearted belief by society that it must be sustained and enhanced precisely because it is an honourable exception?

With the recent closures of Sir Patrick Dun's, Dr Steevens', Mercer's, Baggot Street, Monkstown and Barrington's (in Limerick) hospitals, the Adelaide is the last voluntary Protestant general teaching hospital in Ireland. It has been apparently rather easy to close Protestant hospitals—the Adelaide has learned from the experience of the others and it may now be opportune to tell all other voluntary organisations what is in for them if they do not fit the mould of the mandarins of Hawkins House or for that matter of Marlborough Street. As John Hume implied, we may want unity but we must not ask for uniformity and that injunction applies equally north and south of the border.

The Adelaide Hospital, founded in 1839, is located in the Liberties in the historic centre of Dublin close to St Patrick's Cathedral, and it is a charitable institution. It is governed by a Royal Charter, given in 1921 and amended by the Oireachtas in 1981, which states that the hospital should be a religious and essentially Protestant institution. It is a public hospital, dedicated to the care of the poor and managed by a Board of Governors, drawn from the members of the Adelaide Society. It receives most of its monies from the Department of Health in Hawkins House and is answerable to the department for its expenditure, its services and in every other respect.

The hospital also receives substantial charitable support from every county of this island especially, but by no means only, from the Protestant community. It is widely regarded for its caring Christian ethics, and for its insistence on the privacy of the relationship between doctor and patient—the Adelaide has no ethics committee. In a country where public medicine is a religious matter these qualities distinguish the Adelaide from all other major general teaching hospitals in the Republic of Ireland. Happily there is widespread support for the hospital from people of all religious persuasions and none.

It is by modern standards a small teaching hospital, with an agreed bed complement of 190 and it is housed in very old buildings. It has for many years been closely associated with the medical school of Trinity College where the consultants have academic appointments. It has a well-known nursing school and it also teaches students of physiotherapy, dietetics and other paramedical subjects. The Adelaide, in association with the Meath and the National Children's Hospital, forms the MANCH Group, one of the six major acute hospital units in Dublin.

(The others are St Vincent's, the Mater, Beaumont, St James's and Blanchardstown.) About 8,000 inpatients are treated each year and 40,000 outpatients are seen in the Adelaide.

Plans for development of the small hospitals associated with the medical school of Trinity College

In 1955 the Trinity College medical school was primarily associated with seven small teaching hospitals, including the Adelaide, all more or less strongly associated with the Protestant community. Led partly by Adelaide consultants these hospitals formed an association, which was formalised under the 1961 Federation Act, with a view to amalgamating in one major modern hospital. Four of them (Baggot Street, Sir Patrick Dun's, Mercer's and Dr Steevens') eventually combined [with St Kevin's] to form St James's. Three others, the Adelaide, Meath and the National Children's Hospital, were not accommodated at St James's. Today these three are still run under the terms of the Federation Act and are co-ordinated to some extent by the Central Council of the Federation. Unlike all the other major hospitals in Dublin, they have not been developed, they have not been properly re-equipped and they are still housed in small, mainly Victorian, buildings.

Tallaght Hospital

Tallaght, the new suburb to the south west of Dublin, is larger than Limerick but has no hospital. The Department of Health proposed in 1977 to amalgamate the Adelaide, Meath and the National Children's hospital, which together would move to form the core of a new 750-bed hospital in Tallaght. The task of planning Tallaght was not given to the Central Council of the Federation but to a new Tallaght Hospital Board formed in 1980 with strong powers reserved for the Minister for Health. This was a clear and worrying signal that powerful interests intended that the new hospital would not be managed as a traditional 'voluntary hospital'.

The Adelaide was given representation on the Tallaght Board and looked forward to moving to Tallaght with enthusiasm. Tallaght should be a fine new hospital and it would be appropriate for a charitable foundation like the Adelaide to be involved in this, thus providing medical facilities in a rapidly growing part of the city.

The Adelaide could not make an absolute commitment to participate in Tallaght until many matters concerning its management became clear. Mr Barry Desmond, as Minister for Health, agreed that there would be a number of places reserved for Protestant trainee nurses in the new hospital which was helpful, but the Adelaide Board always recognised that this was not sufficient to ensure the continuation of the Adelaide tradition at Tallaght.

The planning of Tallaght was delayed for many years, but as soon as it was appropriate the Adelaide Board initiated discussions with the Department of Health, in March 1988, on the management structures of Tallaght, emphasising that the Adelaide wished to move to Tallaght. It believed that the Protestant community would be anxious to play a significant role in supporting and governing the Tallaght hospital. It introduced the idea that Tallaght should be a 'public voluntary hospital', governed by an independent Board, with a continuing role in management for the Adelaide. This was apparently acceptable to the Minister for Health in 1990 (see below). In 1988 the Adelaide believed that a minority role on the Tallaght Board would be sufficient to ensure a continuation of its tradition. However, it learned in the next two years that there was substantial opposition to the Adelaide tradition—minority representation for the minority on the Board of the new hospital came to look more like a prescription for slow extinction.

The design stages and specifications for tendering for the Tallaght project were completed by the Tallaght Board in 1990. However, the government did not include the Tallaght project in its budget for 1991 or 1992 due, it was said, to financial considerations. This was a severe blow to the Adelaide which had waited more than 30 years for the development of modern facilities. The delay led to suggestions that the government wanted to downgrade Tallaght or even to cancel it altogether. Doubts about the real reason for the delay intensified in late 1991 and early 1992 when the Adelaide came under strong pressure to withdraw totally from the Tallaght project. It seemed that government interest in Tallaght was waning in proportion to the insistence by the Adelaide that it should have a significant role in managing the new hospital. It would perhaps be more convenient, from the government point of view, to keep the Adelaide in Peter Street. From the Adelaide's point of view such an outcome would have amounted to the end of the hospital as a teaching institution—it would have withered away in its old and small premises.

Financial and political pressures in 1987–8

Atrophy seems to have been in the government mind for a number of years. In 1987–8 the Adelaide had been placed under severe financial and political pressure by the Minister for Health, Dr O'Hanlon, and his Department, to amalgamate with the Meath and the National Children's Hospital. The Adelaide, underfunded for many years, had accumulated a deficit of about £1 million by the end of 1988. This was not a promising position from which to start discussions about its future with its paymaster, the Minister for Health.

The Minister made it clear in 1988 directly, and indirectly through his Department, that unless the Adelaide, Meath and National Children's Hospitals amalgamated they would receive no budget for 1989. The Adelaide objected strongly to this proposal for amalgamation. The Minister also proposed, without consultation with the hospitals, to alter the structure of the Central Council of the Federation, which still had an important role in co-ordinating the activities of the three hospitals. He decided to replace the Chairman, Dr Watts, Provost of Trinity College, without consulting Dr Watts, and to remove the right of Trinity College to nominate members of the Council. The Adelaide Board believed that the combined financial and political pressures were intended to close the Adelaide as an independent institution and, of course, to separate the new hospital structure from Trinity College. It was suspected that Dr O'Hanlon intended to link the new hospital group to the College of Surgeons, a very fine institution in its own right but not appropriate for the Adelaide in the circumstances.

The pressures were somewhat crude, clumsy and they were certainly hurtful and worrying. They need, however, to be seen in the light of the political situation at the time. Two referenda had been held, on 'the right to life of the unborn' in 1983, and on divorce in 1986, and in each case the results had demonstrated, what Garret FitzGerald has noted in his autobiography, 'the sharp swing to the right in religious as well as political affairs'. Protestants in the Republic were gravely disturbed by the tone of both debates and most were dismayed by the outcomes. In this climate the Adelaide was very anxious indeed, being apparently bracketed by conservative politicians and nervous bankers.

Nevertheless, the Adelaide Board politely but firmly refused to accept the Minister's proposals to amalgamate with the Meath and the National Children's Hospital, and it objected, as did Trinity College, to his proposals for reorganisation of the Central Council (which in particular respects were believed to be *ultra vires*).

Although the hospital had no formal budget as of January 1989, it continued to function, somewhat anxiously making the assumption that the Department of Health would not or could not close it down. This turned out to be a correct reading of the situation. The Department paid the hospital monthly at the same rate as in 1988 but maintained the pressure on the Board by refusing to give any assurance that it would continue to do so. The Board was taking a considerable risk as it was continuing to enter into routine contracts without being sure that it could honour them. Members of the Board were informed by Senior Counsel that they might be personally liable for any failures to meet obligations.

The Board was, however, quite determined in its reaction to Dr O'Hanlon. Eventually, with important firm support from the three main Protestant Churches and, after vigorous public debate and private negotiation, a device was arranged which allowed the Department to agree a formal budget in the middle of 1989. The proposal to change Central Council was temporarily dropped, and further discussion of amalgamation of the Adelaide, Meath and the National Children's Hospital came to a halt.

Public debate 1989

There was considerable public discussion in the press, on radio and television and at the Church of Ireland Synod, the Presbyterian General Assembly and Methodist Conference in 1989. There was widespread support for the Adelaide. Indeed, very strong support came from the liberal centre of Irish society, possibly drawn from a coalition similar to the one which showed itself to be in the majority at the time of the election of President Robinson. An excellent editorial in *The Irish Times* (1 June 1989) and an article in the *Belfast Telegraph* (7 July 1989), give the flavour of the discussion.

Consultation with the Church leaders 1989

In January 1989 when the situation was most tense, the Adelaide sought advice jointly from the Archbishops of Dublin and Armagh, and from the Moderator of the Presbyterian Church and the President of the Methodist Church. The Adelaide explained the seriousness of the financial situation at a meeting in March 1989 and, being a small organisation, the Board asked whether the Protestant Churches considered the

Adelaide to be important; if so the hospital hoped for support from the churches in putting its case to the government. The Church leaders were extremely concerned, partly because of the closure of several other Protestant Dublin hospitals in recent years with very little consideration being given to the interests of the Protestant community but mainly because the Adelaide was in fact the last one which could possibly ensure that the Protestant community would *have* a distinctive and honourable role in a health system. The hospital was most grateful for the strong support of the leaders, and the Board was even more determined to stand its ground.

Discussions between the Church leaders and the Taoiseach 1989

The Church leaders believed that the situation was so serious that they arranged to meet Mr Haughey, the Taoiseach, in September 1989. He was most helpful as the record of that meeting shows. The minute notes that 'he would wish to see that the ethos represented by the Adelaide Hospital was maintained as an integral part of the hospital system'. He undertook that the Adelaide would not be placed under 'such financial pressure that its Board would be significantly reduced in its capacity to negotiate the future of the hospital' and he asked the Church leaders to ask the Board of the Adelaide 'to present to the Department of Health a detailed plan of what they would regard as the most advantageous future for the Adelaide Hospital'. The leaders met the Board and passed on this welcome encouragement and asked the Board to write its views to the Taoiseach.

Proposal by the Adelaide to the Taoiseach, September 1989

The Board wrote to the Taoiseach explaining the aspirations of the Adelaide to play a significant and determining role in running a major teaching hospital. It pointed out that it could not stay in the small and old premises of Peter Street. The Board stated that it would welcome an invitation to run the new Tallaght hospital which it had been involved in planning for several years. It believed that it could adapt to this larger role, and it believed it could provide for appropriate participation by the Meath and the National Children's Hospital in the new institution. After all, both of these hospitals had historical associations with the Protestant community, though the Meath, governed under the Meath Act of 1951, was by now strongly influenced by local politicians.

The Adelaide Board thought that the government might consider it highly desirable to respond to the growing if hesitant pluralism of the

Republic by agreeing that one of the more than 20 major hospitals in the Republic should be managed with significant Protestant participation. The memorandum of the meeting between the Church leaders and the Taoiseach, quoted above, seemed to indicate this would be possible.

The Adelaide received no written response to its letter to Mr Haughey. Nor did it receive any comfort from the Department of Health with regard to its financial difficulties which Mr Haughey had undertaken to deal with. Essentially nothing came from Mr Haughey's commitments in the next three months.

Public debate 1990

The Adelaide's position caused further public anxiety in early 1990. The financial situation was still desperate in spite of the Taoiseach's undertaking in September 1989. The Archbishop of Dublin and the Chairman of the Board met with the Taoiseach in January 1990 to discuss the financial crisis again. This time some action was taken and the crisis was partly relieved by monies paid in subsequent months—but the Adelaide is still in 1992 owed £182,000 for work carried out in 1989.

The miserable nature of the Adelaide situation led to public outcry and there were debates at the annual meetings of the Churches, and in the media. There was a second editorial carried by *The Irish Times* on 19 May 1990 which specifically referred to criticism of the Adelaide by Dr Newman, Roman Catholic Bishop of Limerick. Dr Newman was believed to have been influential in the closure of another Protestant foundation, Barrington's Hospital in Limerick, and now seemed to have the Adelaide in his sights. An interesting letter by Rev. G. B. G. McConnell (*The Irish Times* 4 June 1990) pointed out that the Anglo-Irish Agreement in Articles 2(b) and 5(a, b) might allow for consideration of the protection of human rights in the Republic.

The Adelaide was debated in the Senate on 1 May 1990 on foot of a special motion put down by Senator Norris. The Minister for Health, Dr O'Hanlon, reiterated the commitment made to the Church leaders by the Taoiseach and called the Adelaide to a meeting.

The Kingston Group 1990–91

Dr O'Hanlon set up a working group under Mr David Kingston, Chief Executive of the Irish Life Assurance Company, to 'consider possible future management arrangements for the new public voluntary hospital with nursing school at Tallaght'. The group had two members from each of the three hospitals (Adelaide, Meath, National Children's) and was given specific terms of reference by the Minister. These terms were clearly designed to take account of the national importance of the Adelaide. The Minister's terms stated that the management Board of the proposed hospital might operate 'under an adapted Adelaide Charter' and that the 'position of the Adelaide as a focus for Protestant participation in the health services and its particular denominational ethos must be continued in Tallaght.'

The Kingston Group met many times for several months and worked quite harmoniously. Eventually it agreed a scheme for amending the Adelaide Charter as the legal instrument for Tallaght. The new Board for Tallaght would be elected by three foundations (Adelaide, Meath and National Children's Hospital) and by Trinity. The foundations would also act as trustees for the assets of the old hospitals, using them for the benefit of the new hospital at Tallaght. The representatives on the new Board would be in the ratio of Adelaide: Meath: National Children's Hospital: Trinity = 5: 4: 3: 1 giving the Adelaide a significant though a minority position on the Board. The new hospital was to be called the Tallaght Adelaide. There were to be other safeguards for the Adelaide's interests in the mechanism for election of Chairman and President.

The Kingston plan was put to the Adelaide, Meath and the National Children's Hospital boards in May 1991. The Adelaide and National Children's Hospital agreed to it in a spirit of optimism and goodwill, but the Meath rejected four key provisions, all of which were well-known to be vital to the interests of the Adelaide. The Adelaide Board—knowing that the Meath representation in the Kingston Group had accepted it—was deeply shocked. More than that, the Meath Board had picked out items of critical importance to the Adelaide and dismissed them as 'minor'.

Many attempts in the summer of 1991, partly at the behest of Mr Kingston, failed to repair the breach between the Meath and the Adelaide. Indeed the situation actually worsened when the Meath appeared to misrepresent the proposals of the Kingston Group and repeated that the only differences between the Meath and the Adelaide were minor. The effect was to undermine the goodwill which had developed between the two hospitals, and to suggest that there was strong opposition to the Adelaide, especially among the local politicians who appeared to control the Meath Board.

This rejection shocked the Adelaide Board; it confirmed the views of a number of experienced members, which had been discounted for years by newer members of the Board, that the Adelaide ethos would not be safe without Protestant control. The newer members learned their lesson.

The crisis in December 1991—the end of the Adelaide?

The Department of Health had consistently underfunded the Adelaide; the allocation for 1991 had initially been less in money terms than the hospital spent in 1990—after strenuous negotiations it was improved somewhat. Nevertheless, the Adelaide had a budget overrun of £2–£300,000 for 1991 as it negotiated its allocation for 1992. Worse was to come.

For 1992 the Adelaide was given a quite derisory allocation. The Adelaide needed £11.5 million for 1992—it was allocated £9.13 million. The Secretary-Manager advised that the Board would have to lay off up to one quarter of the staff in 1992 and reduce services to patients, if it were to stay within this allocation. The capacity of the hospital to train nurses, continue undergraduate education and training of postgraduate doctors as well as paramedical students was seriously threatened. The Secretary-Manager advised the Board that the hospital would soon become suspect 'in terms of its ability to train', and 'therefore recognition for training in medicine, surgery, nursing, and paramedical disciplines would be re-examined and in some cases would inevitably be withdrawn'. The medical consultants advised the Board that the Adelaide would cease to be a teaching hospital.

In effect the 1992 allocation ensured that the Adelaide would be forced to close—a fact that was well-known to the Department of Health which had successfully used the technique of financial starvation to compel the closure of Dr Steevens' some years earlier. The Department had been told as much in meetings in the last quarter of 1991 during the negotiations for the 1992 allocation.

The Board decided to take the case once more, for the third time in three years, to the Minister for Health, and then if necessary to the public. Pending the Minister's reaction, the Board decided to run the hospital at the same level as 1991—staff would not be laid off while the case was made.

The determination of the Board to assert that the Adelaide had a future and to stand up to the Department was, of course, tested at each monthly Board meeting in early 1992 and at many sub-committees. The

Board is composed of more than 30 members who are seasoned businessmen, lawyers, engineers, some retired nurses and doctors, a few churchmen and other and thoughtful citizens. They were astonished at the way in which the hospital and especially its staff and patients were being treated by the Department of Health but they were by now also seasoned in the new brand of Irish politics. The Board was absolutely united and insisted that it would fight.

The Archbishop of Armagh, the Archbishop of Dublin, the Moderator of the Presbyterian Church and the President of the Methodist Church had been briefed at a meeting in Dublin by the Chairman and vice-Chairman of the Adelaide on 18 November 1991. The Chairman wrote to the new Minister for Health, Mrs O'Rourke, on 2 December 1991 to explain that the situation was very grave indeed. He sought an early and positive response.

The Minister was asked by the Chairman to proceed with the Tallaght project in 1992 and to announce that it would be completed and commissioned on a normal schedule. Her reply was non-committal and did not reveal any sense of urgency. She set up a committee, under Dr David Kennedy, to assess the Tallaght project. It was suspected that Dr Kennedy's committee was being asked to find reasons to downgrade Tallaght.

The appalling allocation to the Adelaide for 1992 was the subject of a further letter of 31 January to the Minister. It protested the clear indication that the Department of Health was intending to close the Adelaide. It was not possible to draw any other conclusion from an allocation which would have led to the laying off of one quarter of the staff. Difficult meetings followed and revealed that the Department indeed was not at all sympathetic to the Adelaide.

In the political turmoil which followed Mr Haughey's resignation, a new Minister for Health, Dr O'Connell, was appointed. A letter (24 February) to the Minister asked for assurances both on finance and on the Tallaght project. The Adelaide was invited at a more or less public discussion on 2 March 1992 to withdraw from the Tallaght project. The Adelaide quickly emphasised that Tallaght was the best solution to the Adelaide's future and it could not withdraw in the absence of an equivalent alternative development. The Adelaide believed that an alternative development was impossible unless Tallaght was reduced to a cottage hospital which was certainly not appropriate. In its submission to the Kennedy Committee (18 March 1992), the Adelaide gave strong support for the full Tallaght project, especially emphasising the large children's unit which was under specific threat. In April the Taoiseach Albert Reynolds also encouraged the Adelaide to withdraw.

Financial matters and the Tallaght project had by this time become so serious that the Adelaide called a press conference on 11 May. On 19 May the Archdeacon of Dublin, Rev. Gordon Linney, said at the Church of Ireland Synod that the Protestants were being edged out of the hospital system and the Archbishop of Armagh, Dr Eames, said, concerning the Adelaide, 'we are an angry people'. On the same day the Minister for Health met the Adelaide Board.

Finally in May, five months into the year and only after the Adelaide press conference, the Minister promised to be helpful on the financial problems of the hospital. He accepted that the hospital should not lay off staff and he undertook to seek ways of improving the basic funding for 1993. He appeared to accept that the long saga of underfunding should now be stopped and indeed reversed. He gave no useful undertaking about Tallaght. When approached by the Church leaders, the Taoiseach was unable to give any substantial help. The Minister for Health on 21 July expanded on his commitment to the funding of the Adelaide and he gave some cautious indications that Tallaght would be built essentially as planned. Once again he was evasive about the management, but the Adelaide emphasised the need to resolve the management question by government decision one way or another before Tallaght was announced. The Minister did, however, say in a letter of 28 July that he would meet with the Chairman 'in the coming weeks in regard to the other matters'. In the context of the discussions and correspondence this meant that the Adelaide would be consulted further about management before Tallaght was announced. In fact, the Minister did not meet with the Chairman of the Adelaide in the next three months in spite of many attempts by the Adelaide to obtain such a meeting. The next public information about Tallaght came from the Taoiseach's speech on 6 November 1992 in which he said that Tallaght would be built essentially as planned—management would be decided later 'with the necessary goodwill on all sides'. The Adelaide was delighted for the people of Tallaght and hugely disappointed that the Taoiseach and the Minister had ignored the interests of the Protestant community in the management of this great project.

The election November 1992

On the announcement of the election, the Adelaide immediately asked each of the political parties about the role of the Adelaide in the management of Tallaght. Mr Spring and Mr Desmond of the Labour Party, Mr O'Malley of the Progressive Democrats and Mr de Rossa of Democratic Left, wrote in strongly sympathetic terms. Fine Gael wrote briefly in more general terms. Fianna Fail repeated its commitment to the Adelaide which amounted to 'trust us'. The Adelaide, in a message to the people of Tallaght, said: 'We now need to make sure that the promises made in the heat of an election are fulfilled. With you we want to make Tallaght one of the best teaching hospitals in Europe.'

Conclusion

The Adelaide was determined throughout this period of its history that its traditions and ethos should be maintained in an identifiable and secure way. In later years it will perhaps be recognised that this time was one in which a fundamental and permanent sea change in the attitude of some reluctant fully to embrace a pluralist society occurred. It may also become apparent that at the same time from the 'Protestant' of the Adelaide a similar 'liberal' ethic developed to which all sections of Irish society could subscribe. The voluntary hospital tradition for the time being had survived and indeed strengthened its position. It may well be suspected that the way the Adelaide was treated at that time was but part of a much wider question which affected and may still affect the future of all voluntary elements of the health service and other social activities. This is the question of government against the people.

The Adelaide in this instance was but one of many excellent religious and non-religious voluntary foundations contributing to the well-being of our society. In its own way the hospital and its Board made a case for all such institutions to be allowed to develop and continue to play a part. These are the exceptions, each in its own way, which would be treasured in a truly pluralist state.

Editor's note

This article was written and published before the discussions relating to the Charter were completed and before the new hospital in Tallaght was finally opened. Details of the further events leading up to the Charter agreement and hospital opening are to be found in other contributions to this book. The three hospitals agreed to combine in August 1995 and to be governed by the Charter of the Adelaide and Meath Hospital, Dublin Incorporating the National Children's Hospital. This Charter is derived by amendment of the Charter of the Adelaide Hospital as approved by Seanad Éireann (26 June 1996) and Dáil Éireann (3 July 1996) with all-party support. The new hospital in Tallaght opened to patients in 1998.

The importance of Dr McConnell's article, however, lies in its account of the difficulties experienced in maintaining the voluntary tradition for the new hospital and indeed for medical services in Ireland generally. It would now seem that had the Board of the Adelaide and the Adelaide Society not been prepared to take such a firm stand on this as a matter of principle that tradition might well have been lost.

It is also apparent from the above account that there were indeed quite serious differences for a time between the negotiating parties, in particular the Meath and the Adelaide. It cannot be emphasised too strongly that these were overcome long before the hospitals moved to Tallaght and are now part of history. In fact, it may be said that one of the successes of the amalgamation has been the manner in which three institutions with distinct cultures have maintained in the new organisation the better parts of these. This has enabled the new hospital to develop a culture of its own, fitting for the 21st century, which perpetuates the voluntary hospital tradition in a medical service which today is very different from that which was extant when the hospitals were founded.

7. Dr Steevens' Hospital

David FitzPatrick

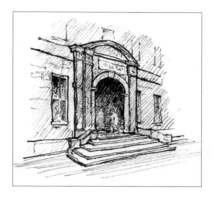

'He passed under the ancient archway, with its ponderous nail-studded door and the enormous scroll-work hinges, into the dim-lit square beyond. All was very quiet; and his footsteps in the stone-flagged colonnade that ran around the square echoed cavernous, ghostly. The hospital seemed dead as the dodo. Even the lights shining through the windows above, looking into the square, were shrouded, dim. At one corner of his path, however, as if to accentuate the gloom, a broad strip of light fell across the flagstones and drew him moth-like to the open door of the accident room. . . . Overhead in the clock tower the bell slowly clanged the hour of seven.'[1]

Thus did Johnson Abraham, a former resident, describe Dr Steevens' Hospital in 1913 and the atmosphere he evokes had changed little by 1961 when the Federated Hospitals were established by Act of the Oireachteas; indeed much of what has been quoted above will bring back memories to most of those who worked in Dr Steevens' up to its closure in 1987. That Abraham's own memories lived on is evidenced by his description of a visit he paid to the hospital with his daughter in 1946.[2]

There can be no doubt that being one of the oldest hospitals in Dublin was something of which all the staff were extremely conscious and proud. Most would be aware of its history and the associations with Dr Richard Steevens, his sister Grizell (apocryphally reputed to have been born with the face of a pig), Dean Swift, and Stella who endowed the hospital with funds to provide a chaplain. This chaplain was to be Irish and educated in Trinity College. He was to be unmarried and was not to sleep outside his lodgings in or near the hospital more than once a week. Should he marry he was to be immediately removed from office. These provisions gave rise to many anomalous situations over the years and discussions of them occupied a considerable amount of the time of the Board.[3]

Stella also stipulated that on disestablishment of the Church of Ireland her bequest should become null and void. In fact, although the possibility that a claim would be made on disestablishment in 1869 was considered and legal advice sought, no further action was taken.

Many were the famous names associated with the hospital—Colles, Crampton, Cusack from the older generation and more recently the medical historian Kirkpatrick, Thomas Wilson, President of the Royal College of Surgeons in Ireland and Brian Pringle, President of the Royal College of Physicians of Ireland. Thus the oldest of the hospitals to federate in 1961 brought with it a proud tradition of service to the community and of being at the forefront of medical advances.

Perhaps in 1961 some of the hospital's better days were behind it and the atmosphere as described above was somewhat anachronistic though continuing. However, with the coming together of the seven hospitals as the Federation's considerable development was to take place in Dr Steevens' before its somewhat abrupt closure in 1987.

The main specialties practised in Dr Steevens' at the beginning of the 1960s were general medicine and surgery, orthopaedics and small commitments to ENT, gynaecology and paediatrics. The three general surgeons, Chance, Cherry and Dunlop, were responsible for the management of trauma coming to the hospital and each had a major interest in elective and paediatric orthopaedics. Brian Pringle, who had an appointment to Arthur Guinness & Son, was one of the first to develop occupational medicine. Douglas Mellon, a general physician, was also in charge of the laboratory in the Rotunda, and Peter Gatenby, recently appointed as Professor of Medicine in Trinity, apart from his clinical expertise was renowned throughout the city for his teaching and his morning clinics were always packed.

In the early 1960s the three surgeons were joined by Brendan Prendiville, also appointed as a general surgeon but one who had been trained in Chepstow in the UK as a plastic surgeon. After his appointment he was also placed in charge of the accident room as the A&E department was then called. He was joined by Niall Hogan whose area of expertise was maxillo-facial surgery which complemented Prendiville's plastic work as he soon developed a national service providing repair of cleft palate.

While the orthopaedic and general surgical services continued Prendiville started the development of a plastic unit proper. In addition to his work with children he rapidly established the first plastic surgery unit in Ireland. He started a training programme from which emerged first Gearóid Lynch and then Gerard Edwards; with Seamus Ó Riain they formed a three-man unit to match that in orthopaedics.

In 1968 Nigel Kinnear was appointed Regius Professor of Surgery and his appointment included sessions in Dr Steevens'. I was appointed Lecturer in Surgery and, having training and an interest in orthopaedics, was also attached to Mr Dunlop. Following the retirement of Chance, I was appointed as orthopaedic surgeon and was joined later in the 1970s by Frank Dowling and E. Fogarty, both of whom had attachments to Our Lady's Hospital in Crumlin.

On the medical side Peter Gatenby retired to lead the United Nations medical service in New York. He was replaced by Professor Neale and by Eoin Casey, a rheumatologist. At the same time Victoria Beckett, wife of the Professor of Psychiatry and Dean of the Trinity medical school, Peter Beckett, took up a clinical teaching and research attachment at the hospital.

Obviously, with the development of specialised units and the increase in personnel, changes in the facilities in the hospital were essential. At the time, much responsibility for the running of the hospital still rested with the Medical Board who advised the hospital Board as to which developments were desirable. The Medical Board met outside the hospital, as had been the practice in many of the voluntary hospitals. The Steevens' Board met in 25 Fitzwilliam Place where Boyd Dunlop had his rooms. Minutes were still kept handwritten in a ledger, not circulated but read at the commencement of the meeting—provided the secretary, or someone who could read his writing, was present. There was no secretarial assistance provided by the hospital. The meetings were well attended; discussions could be heated and sometimes prolonged. Perhaps one of the faults of the system was, as is still often the case, that sectional interests could become an obstacle to progress.

Some apparently unimportant items caused considerable debate. It had been the practice in the hospital that when a consultant arrived in the morning the porter at the main entrance would ring a bell situated in the clock tower. As the number of consultants increased the time spent ringing the bell did so too. This gave rise to an agenda item listed by the then secretary Nick Jaswon, the pathologist to the hospital, as 'For whom the bell tolls?' Positions being jealously guarded there was considerable discussion before it was concluded that only those who had been appointed as physicians or surgeons 'to the Hospital' should be greeted in this manner. This established a slight divide between those who had been appointed to Steevens' before the Federation Act and those assigned to Steevens' after the Act, following their appointment to Federation. Such division was not significant really because enough rivalry already existed between the different specialist groups, each hoping to develop their services further.

Developments of the major specialties in the hospital, namely orthopaedics and plastic surgery, were to take place in the latter part of the 1970s and the early 1980s. These developments were made more necessary by rationalisation of the services in the Federated Hospitals. The first requirement was renovation of some of the old wards. Upgrading of these was carried out between 1976 and 1979 and included the replacement of one of the main staircases in the hospital. The cost was in the region of £500,000.

After considerable debate an agreement in principle was reached to establish the Federated Hospitals' orthopaedic unit solely in Dr Steevens' and to make room for this by moving the gynaecology and ENT services to the Adelaide and the Meath. The location of elective orthopaedic services in Dr Steevens' was in keeping with a 1977 report from Comhairle na nÓspidéal[4] which approved the concentration of elective work there. After a great deal of discussion with the Federation orthopaedic surgeons this plan was agreed. This development in Dr Steevens' was in keeping with Comhairle's plan to establish two elective orthopaedic units in Dublin, one on the north side—Cappagh—and one on the south. The Federation's surgeons regarded their brief as being to develop as far as possible the unit in Dr Steevens' so that it could become either a standalone unit there or the nucleus of one to transfer to St James's or Tallaght.

This plan was dependent on the movement of ENT and gynaecology to the Adelaide and the Meath—anticipating the findings of another Comhairle report on ENT services.[5]

The children's unit in Harcourt Street, under the Comhairle plan, would move with the Adelaide and Meath units to Tallaght.

The reorganisation required to implement these changes necessitated further capital expenditure. It was proposed that the two existing operating theatres be replaced by four, but in the event the Department of Health would only sanction three. However, two of these were equipped with sterile air systems ensuring that up to date facilities were available for modern orthopaedic practice.

A new accident and emergency department was built in the hospital grounds with an entrance opposite Heuston Station. Easy access for ambulances was thus provided. Previously they had to pull up at the Steevens' Lane entrance and trolleys had to negotiate steps and turns to reach the accident unit which over the years had become inadequate for the volume of patients. The new unit contained a large, cubicled reception area, separate x-ray room, a resuscitation room and minor theatre.

The old accident department was then converted into a separate burns unit. This ensured that burns patients were given specialised care and no longer occupied beds in general or orthopaedic wards. The consequent diminution of the risk of cross infection was welcomed, not least by the infection control committee which had battled with this problem for some years.

A new and enlarged physiotherapy unit was built under the theatre extension, an intensive care unit was designed and replaced one of the wards adjacent to the theatre suite, and some of the wards on the ground floor were renovated.

The capital cost of these alterations and buildings was: A&E development £300,000, operating theatres £1.25 million, ward renovations £500,000, new physiotherapy £200,000, burns unit £150,000, and intensive care unit £100,000, a total of some £2.5 million in addition to the monies already spent on ward renovation. These developments were funded by the Department of Health.

After all these changes had been completed the plan was implemented and in 1984 the ENT and gynaecology units moved to the Meath and the Adelaide. The plastic/maxillo-facial and orthopaedic units established themselves in Dr Steevens' and, within the constraints of finance and bed numbers, continued their development over the next few years. In the case of orthopaedics the number of elective outpatient attendances rose from 4,282 in 1984 to 5,327 in 1986 and inpatient numbers from 2,150 to 2,497 in the same period. All seemed well but 1987 was to prove a remarkably unpleasant year. The plan at this stage was that in due course the plastic surgery unit would move to St James's and orthopaedics would be further developed in Dr Steevens'.

A meeting between the Board and officials of the Department of Health had been planned for November 1986 to discuss the future of the hospital. This did not in fact take place until 19 January 1987. A summary of the meeting was sent from the Assistant Secretary, J. Dwyer, to the Chairman of the Board, Brian Campbell, a week later, 26 January. This included the following:

As agreed, the following would appear to be necessary at this stage:—

(a) *The role of Dr Steevens' as the nucleus of a regional orthopaedic unit pending transfer to Tallaght (including clarification of the number of beds in the medium and long-term) should be determined as soon as possible* [emphasis added]. A small team representative of the hospital and the Department should assess the implications and develop an outline plan for implementation once the role has been clarified. We will take the initiative on this matter.

(b) Certain aspects of the proposed later phases of the development of Tallaght Hospital should now be reviewed, so that the position regarding the provision of orthopaedic beds on that site is agreed. *Planning of facilities for the nucleus of the regional orthopaedic unit at Dr Steevens' (or one of the hospitals to be vacated circa 1993) might proceed on the basis that it will remain in service for about twenty years.* [emphasis added]

(c) *Planning towards the move of facilities[6] to St. James's needs to start soon in anticipation of the transfer taking place during 1989.[7]* [emphasis added] Mr Phelan, who is a member of St James's Board, will facilitate early discussions between both hospitals.

(d) Dr Steevens' future role in the A&E scheme will need to be considered soon in view of the timescale for the move to St James's.

(e) The Board of Dr Steevens' will consider developing closer links with the Tallaght Hospital Board. Consideration will be given to the desirability of integrating the management of the orthopaedic unit under the Tallaght Hospital Board, when the other services have been transferred from Dr Steevens' to St James's. The membership of the Board would be adjusted accordingly.

(f) In relation to the hospital's immediate and pressing requirements Messrs. Phelan and Synnott and Dr Tierney will visit you in three to four weeks time to examine the situation and report on requirements. These officers would also, most likely, be the representatives on the group proposed at (a) above.

(g) The potential for improvements in patient admissions and financial analysis systems will also be examined.

(h) Certain problems which have arisen in relation to the provision of patient services (and which were outlined at our meeting) will be considered by you and your colleagues. Additional information in relation to complaints about quality of service are being forwarded under separate cover to Mr Hope [Hospital Secretary].

I hope that this represents a full and accurate summary of the points we covered. If there are any items which you feel have not been properly reflected, perhaps you would let me know, so that we are in complete agreement about the understandings which were reached. May I take this opportunity of thanking you and other members of the Board for the work which you *are undertaking in seeking to maintain the services at your hospital under quite difficult circumstances. My colleagues and I look forward to working with you in the implementation of what must now be done.* [emphasis added]

The proposed move of the plastic unit was not generally approved, but it became generally accepted. Some renovation work remained to be done and approval was given for this in February 1987. A letter from the hospital secretary to the architect Peter Stevens indicates this:

Mr D. P. Stevens MRIAI
Peter Stevens & Associates, Architects
2B Sandymount Green
Dublin 4   20 February 1987

Dear Mr Stevens,
I am enclosing a copy of a letter I have received from the Department of Health through *Federation as regards renovation work to Wards 5, 5A, 6 and the staircase replacement.*
It would seem from the letter that the hospital may now proceed to compile the bill of quantities in accordance with Hospitals' Planning Office Stage 5 procedure. [emphasis added]
As regards the form of contract, from the letter it would seem that the government contract conditions will apply when quantities do not form part of the contract. The specification requires to be full and detailed and to include preliminaries, P.C. sums, provisional amounts etc.
I believe, too, that in fact the letter conveys approval for the preparation of tender documentation.
I have little doubt that when you receive it you will be in touch with me.
Yours sincerely
D. S. Hope
Secretary-Manager

At a hospital Board meeting on 25 February it was generally felt that the meeting with the Department officials (19 January) had been satisfactory.[8] A general discussion took place during which plans for the renovations which had been approved and other items arising from the meeting were considered.

Despite the general optimism about the future a further letter from the Department received on 9 April caused some consternation.[9] This was the usual annual letter detailing the non-capital allocation for the hospital for 1987. That year almost all the voluntary hospitals experienced a reduction in their allocations. That for Dr Steevens' was £5.475 million. Of this the Department reckoned that, having paid off monies due for unmet approved balances for previous years, the total expended up to the end of March 1987 was £2.3 million leaving a grant of £3.175

million to maintain the hospital for the remaining nine months of the year.

The Secretary concluded his letter by emphasising that 'in no circumstances should the hospital anticipate that the grant available on the approved expenditure level as set out above will be increased.'

The hospital governors, when they considered this letter, came to the conclusion that in order to maintain the plastic and orthopaedic services, which had figured prominently at the meeting in January, it should propose to the Department that the only way to contain expenditure within the allocation provided for 1987 would be to close the A&E department. A letter expressing the concern of the governors regarding the financial constraints and outlining a plan which would enable the hospital to stay within budget was sent to Mr Flanagan on 6 May. This invited a response from the Department but none was forthcoming.

The A&E department was closed as from 31 May 1987 in accordance with the plan notified to the Department. On 4 June the Chairman of the Board and the hospital Secretary were invited to the Department of Health to meet the Department Secretary. They reported to the Board at its next meeting that they had been told that it was expected that the hospital would be closed by 30 September.

This was confirmed, although not as explicitly stated, in a further letter sent on 8 June:

> Mr Brian Campbell
> Chairman
> Dr Steevens' Hospital
> Dublin 8
>
> Dear Mr Campbell,
> I wish to refer to my discussions with you and your colleagues on 4 June and to your earlier meeting with Mr J. O'Dwyer on 27 May 1987 regarding the future role of Dr Steevens' Hospital.
>
> As was explained during these discussions, it is necessary for the Department, as part of the current review of acute hospital services, to consider with hospital and health boards the steps necessary to maintain essential acute hospital services and to ensure that the decisions made in this regard fit in with the long-term plans for the development of hospitals, particularly in the Dublin area.
>
> In the discussions which have been held with the representatives of St James's, Dr Steevens', Baggot Street, Harcourt Street, Meath and Adelaide hospitals there was general agreement that to make the best use of the resources available *the following services should, as quickly as possible, transfer from Dr Steevens' to St James's*:

Plastics
Burns
Maxillo-facial

and that the accident and emergency and <u>orthopaedic</u> services at present provided at Dr Steevens' should transfer to the MANCH group.

In the course of the discussions with me on 4 June it was evident that the representatives of your Board accepted the logic of the conclusion that Dr Steevens' Hospital should close.[emphasis added] A very early decision by your Board to cooperate with the Department and the other hospitals concerned in bringing about these changes would be most appreciated. Should your *Board agree to proceed as suggested,* [emphasis added] immediate arrangements will be made to establish a small group representative of the Department and the hospitals involved to deal with the various matters which arise, including the transfer of services and consultation with staff. On receipt of your Board's decision Mr J. A. Enright will convene a meeting of the group.

The Department fully appreciates the concerns which your Board have to ensure that essential services continue to be maintained and that the best interests of the staff employed in your hospital are fully protected.

Please accept my appreciation of the courteous and constructive manner in which you have dealt with me on this very difficult issue.

Yours sincerely,
P. W. Flanagan
Secretary

This really was the beginning of the end for Dr Steevens' as an acute hospital. Discussions and resistance to closure continued for some time. The allocation was reduced further by £600,000 in July to pay for increased A&E services in the Meath necessitated by the closure of Dr Steevens' A&E. On 13 August the Board wrote to the Secretary having reconsidered their position and acceding to the Minister's request to transfer all services out of the hospital.

Mr Hope, the Secretary Manager, wrote:

. . . I am also conveying that in acceding to the request of the Minister for Health the governors decided that the hospital will close on 30 September.

Their decision was reached on the basis that funding will not be adequate for the hospital to maintain its services after 30th September and as services cannot now be provided adequately it was felt preferable that all of the hospital's services should be transferred to appropriate alternative sites.

The decision was taken with reluctance and deep regret . . .

There were two further twists to the tale.

On 9 September the Board wrote asking Mr Flanagan for details of arrangements after the closure on 30 September and indicating that unless definitive plans were provided the Board would be forced to issue protective notices to all staff.

The reply after further discussions was sent on 22 September:

Dear Mr Campbell,

Further to recent correspondence and discussions concerning the transfer of facilities and services from Dr Steevens' Hospital to St James's Hospital and the Meath/Adelaide Hospitals I wish to outline the temporary arrangements which the Minister would wish to see put in place to ensure that adequate provision is made for these services in the immediate future.

It is now clear that the capital works needed to receive the services at St James's and the Meath/Adelaide will not be completed until late November/early December. [emphasis added] Clearly some further time will be needed to transfer equipment, records etc. and to allow staff to become familiar with the new facilities. Accordingly *the Minister would appreciate it if the Board of Dr Steevens' Hospital would agree to allow the services to remain in their present location until the new facilities are available.* [emphasis added] It is anticipated that this arrangement would be needed until the end of December, 1987.

Officers of the Department will be available to discuss the details of this arrangement with you and your staff. It would be appreciated if agreement in principle could be communicated as soon as possible. To facilitate this process I can outline the general principles which we would adhere to.

1) The services would be managed by the Board of Dr Steevens' Hospital on behalf of St James's and the Meath/Adelaide.
2) It is the intention to provide funding for the maintenance of the services through the Federated Dublin Voluntary Hospitals.
3) The staff employed by Dr Steevens' Hospital would continue to be employed by the hospital until such time as they are redeployed to other hospitals or accept early retirement or redundancy as appropriate.
4) The Board of Dr Steevens' Hospital would continue to insure itself against the normal risks.
5) The Department of Health and representatives of all the hospitals concerned would agree on the level of service to be provided at Dr Steevens' Hospital under this arrangement.

The hospital did remain open until the end of December when the plastics and maxillo-facial units transferred to St James's and the orthopaedic and trauma units transferred to the Adelaide and the Meath respectively.

Of course there were some demonstrations and considerable criticism of the Department of Health who steadfastly proclaimed that the Board had decided upon and were responsible for the closure of the hospital. Hospital closure was not part of the Department's agenda and of course the Department would *never* interfere with the governance of any voluntary hospital. It was, however, crystal clear to anyone who had been involved in the negotiations leading up to the closure that, although in February 1987 the Department of Health seemed willing to fund further renovations in the hospital, the reduction in allocation in April and further subsequent discussions meant that the Board was to be forced to close the hospital because of lack of finance.

It is often forgotten that in 1987 virtually every voluntary hospital had its allocation reduced. With the closure of Dr Steevens' the Department now intended and did indeed spend in the region of £4 million building new theatres in the Adelaide and renovating those in the Meath. This expenditure was necessary to accommodate on a temporary basis specialties moved from Dr Steevens'. The fact that in the previous seven to ten years about £2.5 million had already been spent on new theatres, physiotherapy and a new A&E department in Dr Steevens' was conveniently ignored by the Department of Health.

Following the closure the hospital was purchased by the Eastern Health Board and completely renovated. The resulting refurbishment of the hospital was an architectural success; the plans for this were based on ones drawn up by the hospital architect, the late Peter Stevens.

Dr Edward Worth, who died in 1733 just before Dr Steevens' opened, bequeathed to the hospital £1,000 together with all his books. The books were to be for the 'use, benefit, and behoof of the Physician and Surgeon for the time being';[10] they were not to be removed from the room in which they were appointed to be kept. This was and is an important library in terms both of the books themselves and of their bindings. (A full description was provided by the then curator, Dr Muriel McCarthy.[11]) In 1987 they were still housed in the boardroom in the glass cases which had been provided by Worth's son after his death. When the decision was taken that the hospital should close the then Provost of Trinity College, Professor Bill Watts, suggested that because the library would be at risk after the closure the books should be given into the care of Trinity College where they would be meticulously cared for. He intimated that a replica room could be provided for them.

The Board agreed and one week later the whole library, together with portraits and other artefacts, had been removed to Trinity.

Following the sale of the hospital to the Eastern Health Board the question of the library arose. The EHB were anxious to restore the books to the room in which they had been since Dr Worth's demise and promised to arrange that the boardroom be made fully secure against theft, fire and damp. Trinity, however, was reluctant to return the library and the matter finally was decided by the court. Brendan Prendiville, who was one of the 'surgeons for the time being' at the close of the hospital, was instrumental in providing the EHB with details of the bequest. Judgement was found in his and the EHB's favour, each side paying their own costs.

The library today still resides in the hospital and a museum has also been established so that the memory of the munificence of Richard and Grizell Steevens, Edward Worth, and the influence of Swift and Stella will be perpetuated.

References

[1] Anon. (J. Johnson Abraham) *The Night Nurse* Modern Library 1936 (1st ed. London: Chapman and Hall 1913) pp 11–12.

[2] J. Johnson Abraham *Surgeon's Journey* London: William Heinemann 1957 p 370.

[3] T. Percy C. Kirkpatrick *The History of Dr Steevens' Hospital* Dublin: Dublin University Press 1924.

[4] *Development of Orthopaedic Services—A Discussion Document* Dublin: Comhairle na nÓspidéal 1977.

[5] *Development of Ear Nose and Throat Services—A Discussion Document* Dublin: Comhairle na nÓspidéal Nov. 1983.

[6] The plastic and maxillo-facial units.

[7] This referred to the proposal to move the plastic unit to St James's and allow expansion of the orthopaedic unit in Steevens'.

[8] Hospital Board Minutes 25 February 1987.

[9] P. W. Flanagan, Secretary, Department of Health, to Secretary-Manager, Dr Steevens' Hospital, 8 April 1987.

[10] T. Percy Kirkpatrick MD 'The foundation of a great hospital, Steevens' in the XVIIIth century' *Irish Journal of Medical Science* July 1933.

[11] Muriel McCarthy *Journal of the Irish Colleges of Physicians and Surgeons* Vol. 6 No. 4 April 1977.

8. The Meath Hospital

Gerard Hurley

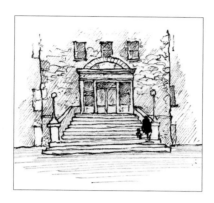

In the late 1970s the Meath was one of the oldest of the Federated Hospitals all of which had, in previous centuries, been set up by the munificence and voluntary efforts of concerned physicians and benefactors, mainly of the Protestant faith, to alleviate the suffering of the citizens of Dublin and surrounding counties. The Meath had a deservedly high reputation as a teaching hospital. Meath physicians had developed and promoted bedside teaching of medical students and postgraduates. It was an independent institution up to 1950 when, following an attempt to oust the Medical Board, which had previously strongly influenced the recruitment of physicians and surgeons to the hospital, matters became so acrimonious and of such public concern that an Act of the Dáil was required to resolve the situation—the Meath Hospital Act of 1951. This, along with the legislation setting up the Federated Dublin Voluntary Hospitals (1961), determined the structures which governed the Meath until its transfer to the new hospital at Tallaght in 1998. In the 1970s, 1980s and 1990s the Meath provided general adult medical and surgical services, had a busy accident and emergency department and a specialist genitourinary surgical department which had been set up by the farseeing urologist T. J. D. Lane in the 1950s.

The Federated Hospitals were all relatively small in size—the Meath, one of the larger, had just under 300 beds—and because of poor infrastructure were felt to be inappropriately equipped to become involved in the long term development of acute hospital services following the re-organisation of the health services arising out of the 1970 Health Act. The blueprint for acute hospital development in the country was the FitzGerald Report (1968). After the other hospitals in the Federated Group had transferred to the newly named St James's Hospital it was agreed in principle that along with the Adelaide, the Meath would form the core of a new hospital to be built on the expanding west side of Dublin city in the region of Newlands Cross. Later the National Children's Hospital also committed its future to this proposed new development at Tallaght and, following its closure in 1987, some of the services of Dr Steevens' were transferred to the Meath and the Adelaide. Later still the acute services from St Loman's Psychiatric Hospital were also included in the Tallaght development which would become one of six acute teaching hospitals serving the greater Dublin area.

The Tallaght Hospital Board was set up by Ministerial Order under the Health (Corporate Bodies Act) (1961) in February 1980 and was comprised of representatives of the Meath and Adelaide hospitals, the Eastern Health Board, Dublin University and some nominees of the Minister for Health. The Board held its first meeting at Aras Mhic Diarmuida on 8 May 1981 under the chairmanship of Mr Kevin Molloy, a local Tallaght businessman. In 1985 the Board leased its own premises in Harcourt Street and meanwhile had been expanded by the addition of representatives from the National Children's Hospital and Dr Steevens' and by increase in the representation of the Meath and the Adelaide and of the EHB and the Minister for Health. In 1987 Professor Richard Conroy was appointed Chairman and continues in office to the present day. It is clear from the Establishment Order that it was the intention, at that time, that this Tallaght Hospital Board would, following commissioning, become the governing board of the hospital.

A green field site was chosen on lands then in the hands of Bord na gCapaill to the west of Tallaght village and the Priory. The brief for the hospital envisaged a total bed complement of 835 beds with comprehensive support services in radiology, pathology, theatre suites etc. The size of the operating theatres was based on the British Standards prevailing at the time of the original brief. Subsequently, when the building was shelled out, it became apparent that the theatres were too small for modern surgical techniques. There was much debate about the provision of a nurses' home. This was strongly supported by the hospital representatives but resolutely opposed by those from the Department of Health on the grounds that student nurses were no different from other students and were also in receipt of some pay. The provision of adequate parking space was another bone of contention. As car owner-ship increased over the development years and the public transport sys-tem was based on buses, until Luas opened in 2004, additional parking space had to be provided at the time of the hospital opening in 1998. While there was steady progress in the planning of the hospital the financial climate was unfavourable to a major hospital development. In fact there were severe cutbacks in the health service particularly follow-ing the economic downturn in the mid-1980s. The base hospitals strug-gled to maintain existing services and the development of new services required fund-raising activities and endless negotiations. It was difficult to maintain staff morale and many staff felt that the Tallaght hospital project would never go ahead.

However, an architectural competition for the design of the hospital was set in train in September 1993 with the approval of the Minister for Health, Barry Desmond, who also indicated his disapproval of the set-ting aside of part of the site for a private hospital. The successful entry was that submitted by the Dublin firm Robinson Keefe Devane who were appointed as the design team. In 1987 Health Minister Barry Desmond turned the first sod on the site which then was cleared down to black boulder clay. Surrounding banks were formed giving the site the appearance of a giant arena. This was an irrevocable step in the development for although the severe financial cutbacks of the late 1980s and early 1990s had delayed the start there was no turning back and plans for detailed operational policies got underway.

Meanwhile, the activities of the three hospitals remained largely un-coordinated. The Adelaide Society did not want the Tallaght Hospital Board to be established as the governing body of the new hospital. They were adamant that, as all of the other Protestant hospitals had closed, it should be a focus for Protestant participation in the health services. In 1988, the Minister for Health, Rory O'Hanlon, proposed an interim arrangement which would co-ordinate the management of the three hospitals. This would involve re-constitution of the Central Council of the Federated Hospitals which would have two representatives from each of the three hospitals under the chairmanship of Professor Richard Conroy, Chairman of the Tallaght Hospital Board.[1] The Meath Board generally supported the proposal, but as the largest hospital and the hospital providing frontline A&E services they wished to have greater representation. The Meath Chairman, the late Austin Groome, also sought clarification on the relationships, roles and functions of the individual hospital boards, Central Council and the CEO in the proposals. He also sought further details of the proposed service plan and joint budget for the suggested group. In any event these proposals were unacceptable to the Adelaide and they refused to amalgamate. The Adelaide sought and received the support of the leaders of the Protestant community. This culminated in a meeting between Church leaders and the then Taoiseach Charles Haughey who stated that 'he would wish to see that the ethos of the Adelaide Hospital was maintained as an integral part of the hospital system'. He furthermore asked that the Board of the Adelaide present to the Department of Health a detailed plan of what they would regard as being most advantageous for the future of the Adelaide Hospital. The Board stated that they could adapt to the role of running a larger hospital, provide for appropriate participation by the Meath and NCH, and would welcome an invitation to run the new hospital at Tallaght. The Adelaide received no written response to its letter to Mr Haughey.

In 1990 a working party was set up by the Minister for Health Dr Rory O'Hanlon under the chairmanship of Irish Life CEO David Kingston with two representatives from each of the three hospitals. The working party was asked 'to consider the possible future management arrangements for the new public teaching hospital and nursing school at Tallaght'. They agreed that the hospital would be a public voluntary hospital with a multi-denominational and pluralist character and that it would develop medical research and education at both undergraduate and postgraduate level. Initially they were offered four choices of possible governance structure but concentrated on two of these—the Adelaide Charter, and a management board under the Companies Act—as the most appropriate vehicles for a voluntary hospital. By this time there had of course been a complete transition from the traditional voluntary funding to almost complete funding by the state. The voluntary hospitals of all religious persuasions, however, continued to receive both financial and practical support from volunteers and various groups. The working group were also asked to set up a structure with a particular ethos ('the position of the Adelaide as a focus for Protestant participation in the Health services and its particular denominational ethos must be continued at Tallaght'). They felt that a Charter would cope with this requirement most readily and concentrated on adapting the Adelaide Charter.

It was agreed *inter alia* that

(1) the history of the Meath and NCH would be included in the introduction;
(2) that the powers needed updating;
(3) that the objects should include:

>(a) to ensure that all medical and surgical procedures which are legal in the state would be available in the hospital as a matter between a patient and his or her doctor;
>(b) to provide for the treatment of illnesses requiring medical or surgical relief either gratuitously or otherwise;
>(c) to provide as far as possible for the health, happiness and welfare of children and others accepted as patients;
>(d) to manage the new hospital in the interests of patients;
>(e) to provide instruction in medicine and surgery;
>(f) to accept students for training in medicine, surgery and other relevant disciplines;
>(g) recognising the fundamental principle on which the Adelaide was established, to maintain the new hospital as a focus for Protestant participation in the health services, preserving its denominational ethos; while maintaining this focus and preserving the denominational ethos, freedom of conscience and the free profession and practice of religion by all within the institution are equally affirmed and guaranteed;
>(h) to develop the tradition of support groups for the hospital's activities;
>(i) to continue close co-operation with the Eastern Health Board in providing complementary services;
>(j) to solicit and receive subscriptions and gifts . . . and generally to do all things necessary or expedient for the proper and effective carrying out of any of the aforesaid objects.

The existing hospital boards were to remain constituted as before and to focus on particular aspects of medicine in support of the new hospital. In particular, the NCH Board was to place special emphasis on medical work for children, and the Meath Board on medical research. The special area of concentration for the Adelaide was to be determined later.

Regarding medical education, the new hospital was to have a faculty of medical science within which there would be a single college of nursing and a school of postgraduate medical studies. The college was to comprise the Meath School of Nursing and the Adelaide School of Nursing. Entrance to the college was to be through the schools which would be autonomous for this purpose and for certain aspects of nurse education. The working group recommended that the Meath and NCH set up foundations similar to the Adelaide Society to administer their assets after the move to Tallaght. There would be a paediatric committee for the new hospital on which the NCH would be strongly represented. Future changes in the Charter would have to be separately approved by the Adelaide Society and the Meath and NCH Foundations.

An important innovation was a proposal to appoint a president of the hospital to whom appeals could be made if the Charter or its spirit appeared to be violated. The President was to be appointed by the Adelaide Society. The Board Chairman would rotate, with the Adelaide having the first three-year term. The first heads of the two nursing colleges would be from the Meath and Adelaide respectively and the Matron of the hospital would be chosen in open competition by the Board. Subsequent heads of the nursing school were to be appointed by the Adelaide Society and Meath Foundation respectively.

The proposed Board membership was as follows: Adelaide 4, Meath 4, NCH 3, TCD 2. This formula was acceptable to the Meath and NCH but not to the Adelaide which wanted a majority. An alternative was put forward whereby TCD would reduce to 1 member and the Adelaide increase to 5 members provided that a CEO was appointed, a common budget established, beds were pooled, a single nursing school was established and the merger was progressed as quickly as possible. The suggested name of the new hospital was the Tallaght Adelaide.[2]

The Meath reaction came in a letter dated 31 May 1991 from the acting Chairman of the Board of Management, Professor Brian Keogh. In this he reiterated the Meath Hospital's commitment to the concept of joint management before Tallaght Hospital was built, stating that the preferred option was to amalgamate and form a partnership. He drew attention to the fact that the Meath employed more staff and treated more patients than the other two hospitals combined. It also provided wider services and had a larger financial allocation than the other two hospitals together. In the context of the Meath's pre-eminent and long standing contribution he pointed out the considerable concessions already made by the Meath to further the single management concept and asked that its position receive the same consideration as had been given to the Adelaide, during discussions at the working group and before. He went on to quote the Minister for Health Rory O'Hanlon's remarks during a Senate debate on the Adelaide Hospital, on foot of a motion by Senator David Norris. The Minister had stated that he 'recognised the importance of the Adelaide tradition and he wanted to see the Adelaide tradition continued at Tallaght and his belief (was) that this could be done and an acceptable Board of Management could be established which would accommodate the traditions and rights of all three hospitals'.

The Meath Board suggested the following modifications: (1) the hospital name and Chairman should be decided by the new Board; (2) the President might be termed a Visitor as in a university setting and (3) the powers of the President/Visitor should be clarified.

The 4:4:3:2 Board membership was acceptable subject to some clarifications. Professor Keogh stressed that amalgamation must be, and be seen to be, a partnership, a 'meeting of the ways' and stated that 'nobody could argue that the Meath Hospital had not already met the Adelaide Hospital more than half way in these discussions and proposals'.

Meanwhile, the Tallaght Hospital Board continued with the development and planning permission was secured in 1990. The Department of Health suggested that the hospital be built in one phase but with a reduction to 600 beds. The Dublin Hospitals Advisory Group, chaired by David Kennedy, were already considering emergency services in the Dublin hospitals. They were asked by the Minister for Health, Mary O'Rourke, to include a review of the Tallaght project in these considerations. This was disappointing as it was felt that eight years hard work by the Tallaght Hospital Board and the staff of the three hospitals was being set aside. A smaller hospital was suggested for Tallaght which had a final cost estimate of £118 million. The DHAG agreed to review and make recommendations on the function, scope and scale of the new hospital.

There followed an in-depth appraisal of the Tallaght project. Options ranged from scrapping it altogether, and refurbishing the existing hospitals, to proceeding with the full initial brief. The existing hospitals, when inspected, were clearly incapable of being refurbished to a satisfactory standard for modern healthcare. The older parts of the Meath were in a particularly poor state. The west wing of the hospital had been built in Dean Swift's vineyard over a tributary of the river Poddle which gave rise to flooding occasionally. It was reputedly haunted by Stella's ghost. During the appraisal, however, it became clear that other Dublin hospitals would not have been unhappy if Tallaght Hospital did not proceed and a rigorous defence of Tallaght and its constituent hospitals was required.

The Kennedy Committee recommended that the development proceed with a markedly reduced bed complement of 427 beds compared to the 830 envisaged in the original brief. There was a parallel downsizing of support services but the acute bed complement of St Loman's Psychiatric Hospital was included. Regrettably some proposed new services appropriate to a new teaching hospital, e.g. a department of clinical photography, were excluded and there was a proportionate reduction in the size of some departments, particularly outpatients. This resulted in the hospital opening with fewer outpatient facilities than in the base hospitals and the requirement of additional building when the hospital opened.

Throughout this time the Meath Board and staff members continued to be concerned about the terms of the proposed Charter. The staff felt under pressure from working in an overcrowded old hospital and many had the additional burden of planning their departments and work arrangements at Tallaght. Furthermore, many felt that too many concessions had been made to the Adelaide and others feared for their jobs and promotional prospects in the new hospital. On 3 September 1992, the Chairman of the Adelaide, Professor David McConnell, announced that the Meath was thwarting the efforts of the Adelaide to protect its rights. Next day, the Chairman of the Meath Hospital Board, Peter Houlihan, rejected the claims and reiterated the provisions already agreed in the Kingston Report, in particular the adoption of the Adelaide Charter, the recognition and acceptance of the 'fundamental principle', agreeing to equal representation despite being the largest and acute hospital, the appointment of a president of the hospital to protect the Adelaide ethos, the Adelaide to have chairmanship for the first three-year term, and the protection of the Adelaide nursing school. In the light of these and other concessions, the Meath Board were 'surprised and deeply disappointed' by the remarks made by the Adelaide Chairman. Mr Houlihan re-stated the commitment of the Meath to creating a successful partnership with all the parties involved in the Tallaght project.

There was much media attention and public relations activity at this time. Furthermore, the Adelaide situation became an issue in the ongoing search for a peaceful solution to the conflict in Northern Ireland. It had been pointed out by Adelaide representatives that special provisions had been made for the Mater Hospital, Belfast, by the authorities in Northern Ireland and they wanted a similar approach in the Republic. The Adelaide issue arose at talks between the British and Irish governments and also at European level. Despite the increasing misgivings of the Meath staff, but taking into account the sensitivities of the unresolved situation in the North, and in an effort to finally get Tallaght Hospital built, the Meath proposed on 11 June 1992 that 'the Church of Ireland Archbishop of Dublin or an equally independent and representative figure should be appointed President of the new Tallaght hospital'. It called on all interested groups to show the necessary flexibility to get this urgently needed major public facility underway as soon as possible.

On 8 February 1993 Nicholas Jermyn, Secretary-Manager of the Meath, replied to an article by D. Kiberd in the *Irish Press* entitled 'The Adelaide objects—A test of our pluralism'. In this article Kiberd had quoted from a sermon by the Rev. Kenneth Kearon, Dean of Residence in Trinity College Dublin[3] in which he stated, *inter alia*, 'the Adelaide does not enshrine Protestant ethics. It stands against enshrining any denominational tradition in its practices'. Jermyn went on: 'We fully subscribe to the Adelaide approach. It stands against enshrining any denominational tradition in its practices; that is our approach also. We respect all traditions therefore we are confident that we can create a successful working partnership with the Adelaide.'

At the request of the Minister, Brendan Howlin, on 1 April 1993 representatives of the Meath Board met with the MANCH joint management facilitators David Kingston and David Kennedy to explore the ethos issue, and to establish ground rules for further discussions and the handling of media issues. This had become necessary in the light of the public relations campaign being conducted by the Adelaide and the possibility of their withdrawal from the project as had been suggested by the Minister for Health, John O'Connell. The Meath representatives were sufficiently reassured of the sincere intentions of the facilitators to see fair play to all parties that they re-entered discussions with the other hospitals. This led to negotiations hosted by David Kennedy at Irish Life headquarters culminating in Heads of Agreement dated 19 May 1993.

In addition to the items already agreed in 1991 the Church of Ireland Archbishop of Dublin, Dr Donald Caird, had agreed to act as President of the hospital. The Adelaide and the Meath would have 6 representatives each, and the NCH 3. The Minister for Health would appoint 8 additional representatives, 6 of whom would be on the nomination of the President of the hospital, 1 from the local authority and 1 from a third level medical training school. The increased size of the proposed Board—similar in size to the Meath Board which had also been set up in difficult circumstances in 1950 [see p 46]—offered the flexibility to meet all representational requirements.

The President's nominations were to 'reflect both the position of the hospital as a focus for Protestant participation in the health services and also the need to have regard to all communities served by the hospital'. The name of the hospital would be 'The Adelaide and Meath Hospital'. The name of the paediatric unit should include the name of NCH. It was also agreed that the Adelaide would have the right to admit up to 40 suitable applicants each year to the nursing school and that a modern nurse uniform be designed for all student /trainee nurses. This would recall the traditional characteristics of the Adelaide uniform. The working party members were to strongly recommend acceptance to their boards.

Further amendments were sought by the Meath following representations from the unions who were concerned for their jobs, promotional prospects and nursing issues in the new hospital. Meanwhile in February 1993, the new Minister for Health, Brendan Howlin, had announced that the building of a 467-bed hospital would begin in Tallaght as soon as possible. This would include 60 children's beds and a 10-bed psychiatric unit. He asked that proposals for the functional content of the revised hospital be submitted as soon as possible and generally he injected much needed urgency into the project.

Hospital staff and the small staff of the Tallaght Hospital Board worked tirelessly to ensure that the revisions in the functional content were truly reflected in the drawings of the departments affected. An additional 46 psychiatry beds were approved by the Department of Health facilitating the closure of the unsuitable St Loman's Hospital.

The contract was signed with Laing Paul Joint Ventures in October 1993 and work began on site in October 1993. After many years of negotiation with Trinity College Dublin a teaching agreement was finally signed with the hospital in October 1995. This cleared the way for the building of additional academic facilities adjoining the educational complex already on site. Construction of this building was delayed but finally started in February 1999 and was available for use in September 2000.

There was continuing disquiet among Meath staff who felt that their concerns were being ignored. At the January 1995 Board meeting Chairman Gerry Brady reported no progress on the Charter since the previous meeting. The subgroup of the Board had completed their consideration of the draft Charter and a further meeting under Professor

Kennedy's chairmanship was planned. There was also reference at this meeting to the 'horrific' conditions in the Meath A&E due to a shortage of beds with patients waiting for up to 24 hours. It was predicted that the problem would be worse at Tallaght which would have fewer acute beds and no step down facilities. The Medical Board had pointed out that there were 107 private beds in the existing hospitals and that the issue of private beds at Tallaght was not being addressed. At the February 1995 Board meeting the Charter subgroup presented a document entitled 'Adelaide Charter Draft June 1994 Proposed amendments agreed by Subgroup of Meath Hospital Board'. This was the product of regular meetings over the previous 15 months facilitated by Professor Kennedy with representatives of the other two hospitals. In its deliberations the subgroup were grateful for legal advice from John O'Connor—the hospital solicitor. The areas of difficulty were:

(a) the preamble to the Charter;
(b) the concept of merit in the Tallaght Hospital situation and how the Charter could guarantee that all staff appointments would be based on merit;
(c) the rights of existing staff at the Meath and how these could be carried forward, without prejudice, to Tallaght;
(d) the nursing difficulties which would arise with three schools within one college;
(e) representation of medical consultants on the Tallaght Hospital Board by election from the Medical Board as at the Meath.

During a long but constructive discussion it emerged that the preamble might be acceptable as an appendix and that the trades unions had requested a meeting with the chairmen of the boards of the three hospitals to put their concerns regarding their members. The Chairman underlined the urgency of resolving these matters in the light of progress with the new building. It was pointed out that the amendments to the July 1994 Heads of Agreement had been proposed in order to avoid future problems in the new hospital and that once these were part of a Charter they would be difficult to change. It was suggested that after two or three terms of the new Board the Charter should be reviewed. A member of the subgroup was of the view that negotiations were still ongoing and that the Board should endorse the work of the subgroup saying unanimously that they were not happy with the draft Charter and that they were sending their representatives back to Professor Kennedy to see what progress could be made on the suggested amendments. The

Chairman concluded the meeting by reminding members that:

(a) the Board rejected the draft Charter based on the recommendation of the subgroup;
(b) the contentious matters would be taken back to Professor Kennedy to effect the changes required;
(c) bye-laws had to be provided before the Meath could conclude its deliberations on the amended Charter.

While the Board was rejecting the draft Charter in its then form it was also proposing some changes. It was not 'closing the door, it was making proposals'. The draft Heads of Agreement as amended by the subgroup and a summary of comments in a letter dated 10 February 1995 from John O'Connor were sent to Professor Kennedy. In his reply to Meath Hospital Board Chairman, Gerry Brady, in March 1995, Professor Kennedy painted the broader picture, pointing out that the final decision on the contents of the Charter

> . . . will not be taken by the three hospitals or myself but by the Government and the Oireachtas . . . the process in which we are currently engaged is useful in trying to present an agreed position to Government by the three hospitals on the detailed contents of the Charter. However, this will not be decisive in determining what will go into the Charter. In this context I should point out that the Minister for Health will certainly wish to address a number of substantive issues in the Charter which have not been considered at all in the discussions to date between the hospitals.
>
> I think it is also important to understand that the Heads of Agreement are formally part of the Government decision to proceed with the hospital. It is therefore a waste of time to try to change the substance of the Heads of Agreement. The only circumstances in which I could envisage any modifications being acceptable to the Government would be if they were agreed by all three hospitals and not in conflict with the substance already agreed.

He went on to comment without enthusiasm on the amendments proposed by the Meath. He dismissed the proposal that the history of the hospitals should be located in a schedule at the end of the document and suggested that in the event of disagreement the matter should be left to the parliamentary draftsmen. Kennedy felt that deletions referring to paediatric medicine and surgery and nursing and to the paediatric medical advisory committee would not be acceptable to the NCH representatives. He felt that there might be a solution to the representation of the Medical Board members but warned that the Meath suggestion of a pro rata Meath 60 : Adelaide 40 : NCH 21 recruits to the nursing school was clearly a change in the Heads of Agreement and as such would be rejected by the Adelaide. Finally, he proposed a meeting of the three Chairmen to try to reach agreement or 'at least a minimal level of disagreement' which he would report to the Department of Health.

Following the meeting between Professor Kennedy and the three chairmen, further problems arose. It was reported in the *Tallaght Project Newsletter*, Issue No. 2, May 1995, that

> ... Professor Kennedy and the three hospital chairmen have agreed a wording for the full text of the Charter following a consideration of the amendments proposed by the Meath Hospital. This agreement has been reported to the Minister. The Boards of the Adelaide and NCH have confirmed their approval of the new draft Charter. The process for its consideration is in place in the Meath Hospital.

In reality the Meath Board had not considered the outcome of the meeting between Professor Kennedy and the chairmen. A letter was sent to Gerry Brady on 22 May by four Board members reminding the Chairman that he had no mandate from either the subgroup or the full Board to agree to any form of words. They underlined a number of issues of continuing concern to the hospital staff 'which had not been addressed or resolved to the extent that we can support the adoption of the Charter as it stands'. They concluded: 'We do not consider that the views of the Meath Hospital have been adequately reflected in the draft Charter.'

Subsequent to a Board meeting Gerry Brady, in his reply to Kennedy's letter of 2 May 1995, stated that he was not empowered to agree any document until it had been passed by the Charter subgroup and the Board of Management of the hospital but that he was willing to recommend a particular course of action to the Board which might or might not be consistent with the text of the new draft Charter.

This did little to allay the concerns of the Meath staff. The hospital Board sought submissions from the unions; the unions held meetings of their members who had robust views of the Charter and Heads of Agreement and these were conveyed to the Board. For instance, IMPACT expressed the view that there were implications in terms of contracts of employment, transfer of contracts etc., all within an ethos which is termed Protestant, and stated that all matters were subject to labour laws and industrial relations procedures and not subject to interpretation or ethos. They concluded:

> This document is flawed both in its sentiments and in its basis of constitutionality

and legality; that the sentiments expressed therein are in no way appropriate to a 21st century, publicly funded institution and that a new document reflecting the fundamental principles of a pluralist and democratic state should replace it.

SIPTU concluded that:

> The document was flawed in so many respects that it should be torn up and a new document, setting general guidelines, be put in place—in effect a statement of principles. This document should look forward not backwards and should reflect the aspirations of a modern democracy for a hospital, which after all, is to operate in the context of a new century and well beyond.

The Irish Nurses' Organisation replied on behalf of nurses expressing their serious concern at the implications of putting in place the proposed Charter. There were also expressions of mutual support between the unions.

The Meath Board Chairman, Gerry Brady, pointed out that many of the provisions of the draft Charter were not in dispute. The areas of continuing disagreement related mainly to recruitment and conditions of employment, including promotional prospects, appeal mechanisms etc. However, he wrote to the Minister on 17 July 1995 stating that the Board were unable to accept the draft Charter in its present form. The Board reiterated their total and absolute commitment to the Tallaght Hospital project and endorsement of the principles which constituted the Heads of Agreement including the principle of maintaining the hospital as a focus for Protestant participation in the health services and preserving its particular denominational status. The Board included its reservations and recommendations. The letter also sought to refute ill-informed, unbalanced and at times hostile comment in sections of the press.

The ceremonial laying of the foundation stone by Dr Michael Woods took place in late 1994 followed by the topping out ceremony in 1995. The base hospitals finally agreed the governance structure of the new Adelaide and Meath Hospital, Dublin Incorporating the National Children's Hospital (AMNCH) in late 1995. This was helped by the provision of an industrial relations protocol parallel to the Charter to mollify the concerns of the unions and staff on their terms and conditions of employment. Although the enabling legislation was complex and took time the AMNCH Board finally became a statutory body with responsibility for the three transferring hospitals on 1 August 1996 and for the new hospital from 'Transfer Day'. Dr David Mc Cutcheon, who had experience of hospital amalgamation in Canada, was appointed as CEO to AMNCH. The first three departments were handed over by the contractors in 1996.

However, functional deficiencies in the hospital, as built, became apparent and had to be rectified. These included provision of a separate paediatric outpatient department and a multi-storey car park and the rearrangement of the operating theatres. The staff of the radiology department strongly advocated the provision of a picture archiving and communications system (PACS) for the digital dissemination of x-ray images throughout the hospital. The AMNCH board borrowed the money to cover the difference between the cost of PACS and that of the lowest tender for a conventional film-based system and the hospital became the first film-less hospital in Ireland. The initial proposed opening day in January 1998 came and went. After a further six months' frantic activity preparing for the move, while maintaining existing services in the old hospitals, the hospital finally opened on Midsummer's Day 1998 with the transfer of patients and staff from the old hospitals. The move went smoothly and most of the staff adapted readily to their splendid new environment. Some, however, missed the intimacy and camaraderie of the old hospitals—and the proximity to Grafton Street!

In the early days there were financial and consequent governance problems. These were gradually overcome and although the hospital has not yet (2005) reached its full potential much has been achieved. The differences surrounding the Charter and Heads of Agreement have been largely overcome as the transferring hospitals have had to focus their efforts on co-operating to run the fine hospital at Tallaght. Bringing on to one site the activities of four hospitals with varying cultures, against the backdrop of a financially strapped health service, was in itself a complicated task. It is well to remember that the Tallaght Hospital development took place before the advent of the Celtic Tiger boom. The ethos question provided another obstacle which had to be negotiated against the background of much political and social change in the island of Ireland. It is a testament to the good sense and tenacity of the many active participants in the development process that a fine hospital is now providing a comprehensive range of medical services at the new Adelaide and Meath Hospital, Dublin Incorporating the National Children's Hospital at Tallaght. The Meath, with its broad representation of public representatives, volunteers and staff, contributed generously and constructively to the development of the new hospital and in its residual role the Meath Foundation will continue to promote and support the AMNCH in the future.

References

[1] Letter from Liam Flanagan, Secretary of Department of Health, 18 December 1988.

[2] Kingston Working Group Report 6 May 1991.

[3] Also quoted by Senator David Norris in an article in the *Journal of the Irish Colleges of Physicians and Surgeons* Vol. 20, No 2, April 1991.

9. Mercer's Hospital

J. B. Lyons

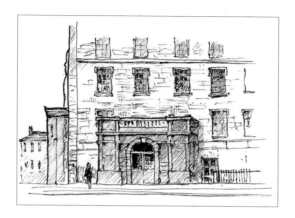

'There are nineteen hospitals in Dublin and all unmergeable into one.'

Oliver St John Gogarty *As I Was Going Down Sackville Street*

'We are . . . compelled to hold the view that the day of the small hospital is passing or past.' These prescient words were spoken by Robert James Rowlette (1873–1944). The occasion of their utterance was a celebration in 1934 of the bi-centenary of Mercer's Hospital. They are less efficient than larger hospitals, he explained with inescapable logic:

> That is the view taken by the Governors of Mercer's Hospital [he continued] with the full support of the members of the Medical Staff, and within recent months they have decided to explore, in association with the governing bodies of two other hospitals of similar scope, Sir Patrick Dun's Hospital, and the Royal City of Dublin Hospital, the possibility of an amalgamation of these three institutions into a hospital of some 450 or 500 beds.[1]

The 'At Home', in the course of which Rowlette, an honorary physician to Mercer's, was one of the speakers may not have been the ideal or most tactful forum for discussion of the hospital's amalgamation or closure, and those present who actually cherished the place for its neatness and small size, may well have believed the physician had a bee in his bonnet concerning bed numbers. He had devoted his presidential address to the Royal Academy of Medicine in Ireland's Section of State Medicine, in 1920, to 'The Problem of the Dublin Voluntary Hospitals'.[2] Two of them he regarded as having 'an adequate number of beds to render the medical service adequate', but there were eight clinical hospitals in Dublin 'with an average of perhaps 120 beds in each'. Why, he had asked, shouldn't all or some of these several institutions come together in one or two larger buildings? This would achieve greater economy and efficiency.

> The primary object of the voluntary hospitals [Rowlette declared] is, no doubt, to furnish medical treatment and care to the sick poor who cannot provide these necessities for themselves. Other functions, at one time secondary, have now become equally essential. Of these the chief are the education of the medical student and the advancement of medical knowledge.

He had no fault to find with the care devoted to the ailing ('Our medicine is sound and safe') but posed a more difficult question: What have our voluntary hospitals done in recent years to advance knowledge? He wasn't 'going back to the generations of Cheyne and Graves, of Stokes and Corrigan, but dealing with the decades in our immediate memory'. What recent advances had been made in Dublin in medicine or surgery? He couldn't think of any! A glaring defect was the lack of expert laboratory assistance in Irish hospitals.

Amalgamation (or 'federation' as it came to be called), was not to be achieved without an unconscionably protracted incubation period. 'RJR', as Rowlette was commonly called by his familiars, continued to be the principal spokesman for Mercer's, and a major force in ensuring survival of a project which was not without its opponents. He was not a member of the Board of Governors but his opinion was valued, and he was often invited to attend their meetings and advise on this point or that.

According to Gogarty (ENT surgeon to the Meath) the unmalleable nature of the capital's hospital system resulted from the fact that so many grants and endowments were denominational. There was, he said, a greater vested interest in disease than in Guinness's Brewery.

R. J. Rowlette

If we are to recognise Rowlette's pre-eminence in the process of amalgamation it is appropriate to supply an outline of his career. He was born in Carnacash, County Sligo in 1873. He studied philosophy and medicine at TCD (BA, 1895, MB, 1898), proceeding MD (1899) and elected FRCPI (1913). For a time he was lecturer in pathology at Queen's College, Galway, later settling in Dublin and becoming physician to Jervis Street and Mercer's hospitals, editor of the *Journal of the Medical Association of Éire* and Irish editor of *The Medical Press and Circular*. As a centenary tribute he wrote and published *The Medical Press and Circular, 1839–1939*.

An accomplished orator (awarded a gold medal in 'the Hist'), Rowlette was drawn to medical politics, representing TCD in the Senate. In due course he became President of the Royal College of Physicians of Ireland but was fated to die in office on 13 October 1944.

'What were his qualities?' The question was posed, and answered, by his obituarist, William Doolin, Editor of the *Irish Journal of Medical Science*:

> They were many, and all essential elements in his equipment. 'His mental abilities were large, and they became the more robust as the more weight was imposed on them.' So wrote Morley to his mother, describing Lincoln. Word for word, the description applies no less aptly to Rowlette. In good sense and knowledge of the ordinary man he had no rival. His own mental discipline was stern, which made him invaluable in council, where few knew better than he the value and the use of evidence; a master of debate, his even-tempered balance and his clear sense of logic helped him ever to 'keep the doors of his mind open'; his judgment was lit by the light of humility, his justice tempered by a deep humanity. And he was utterly free from those deadly foes to all who would give counsel—pride and prejudice. Here, all felt who sat with him through hours of often tedious debate,
>
> > *. . . was one whose even balanced soul*
> > *Business could not make dull, nor passion wild;*
> > *Who saw life steadily, and saw it whole.*
>
> It was in his few spare hours of relaxation—talks in his study of an evening, or, less frequently of late, sitting in the afternoon sun in the Square, that one came to know him more intimately. There one found a wholly delightful companion, a ready and informing talker, a kindly listener, with an inexhaustible fund of recollections of men and events garnered from his many contacts with all sorts and conditions of men through the years. For music and the theatre he had little time and less inclination; books had been always his chief source of distraction, his favourite authors, Trollope and Tolstoy. A star performer on the track in his youth, his chief relaxation had been to foster and encourage the development of Irish athletics through the years of his maturity; here, he was made free of the sodality of youth, and here, in the graphic phrase of one who knew him only as a guide to Irish youth, he 'was the brains and soul of Irish athletics for five and twenty years'. How wide was his authority in this sphere was evidenced by his selection to act as Hon. Physician to Olympic teams from Britain and Ireland at the successive Games held at Antwerp, Rotterdam, and Paris.[3]

Rowlette was not, of course, the first in Dublin to strive for hospital reform, though it is likely that his endeavours were largely unknown to the doctors of a later generation who were to face a self-imposed task with fresh enthusiasm in 1957. It seems in fact that the Charitable Infirmary (Dublin's first voluntary hospital) had hardly come into existence in Cook Street before the founders were seeking for radical ways to improve it. Only four beds were provided there at its opening in 1718, but it accommodated 50 patients in larger premises in 1728.

Mercer's Hospital was named for a charitable spinster, Mary Mercer (d. 1735), who had donated a stone house (originally intended for the general care of poor girls) but opened as a hospital on 11 August 1734, with beds for ten patients; 'an Additional Building [to] contain 30 more Sick Poor' was provided in 1740. A newspaper advertisement designed to attract subscribers in November 1745 stated: 'Patients lodged & taken care of in the Hospital last Year, 264. Now under Cure in the Hospital, 56'. In 1811 the RCSI decided not to recognise any hospital which had fewer than 20 beds.

Mercer's attained its centenary labouring under a debt 'upwards of £300', which led to an examination of 'the Accounts and affairs of the Hospital generally and the present system of Expenditure.'[4] For years it had an average of 100 to 120 pupils annually and 'was the first Hospital in this City in which clinical lectures were delivered.'[5] It boasted the best locality in the city for a hospital 'being in an impoverished and thickly inhabited district near the great thoroughfares . . . and within five minutes walk of the five principal Schools of Dublin.'[6] A small sum would permit the addition of a moderate number of lock and fever wards but an appeal towards this modest end was unsuccessful.

An enquiry in October 1848 from the Central Board of Health, as to how many cholera patients might be accommodated, led the Governors prudently to reply that they did not think themselves justified in admitting patients with cholera 'as they are of opinion that their doing so would deter those Patients for whose relief the Hospital has been established from seeking relief therein'. When asked by the Lord Mayor on 24 February 1855 what accommodation the hospital could provide for the sick and wounded from the Crimean War, the Governors offered 'to accommodate 40 of the wounded Soldiers and Sailors from the Crimea on the Government providing the necessary expenses'.[7] The first Ladies Visiting Committee (Mrs Shaw, Mrs Osborne, Mrs La Touche and Mrs Longfield) was established in April 1858 and they issued recommendations for the supervision and purchase of linen and blankets. Their report in this area caused the Matron to be reprimanded.

Lord Spencer's plan

A tangible example of constructive reform, which preceded Rowlette's, was encountered at a meeting of the Dublin branch of the British Medical Association in 1888, when Edward D. Mapother supported Lord Spencer's plan to amalgamate the Richmond Hospital and Dr Steevens' Hospital on a site near Christchurch Cathedral, 'and the simultaneous fusion of several of the other smaller hospitals, with the view of saving working expenses and aggregating a larger number of cases suitable for scientific observation'.

He opened his address as follows:

> The number of hospitals, general and special, will bar all progress unless consolidation or, at least association is brought about . . . A line drawn N.W. to S.E. [he pointed out] from the Midland Bridge, N.C.R., to Leeson Street Bridge, fairly bisects the city. The hospitals which might thus group with Trinity College would be the Mater, Rotunda, Jervis-street, Sir Patrick Dun's, Baggot-street, St Joseph's, the Adelaide, and Mercer's; and with the College of Surgeons, the Richmond, Coombe, Meath, Cork-street, and St Vincent's, each group containing about 550 beds occupied, but let the selection be by fitness, affection, or in any other way.[8]

The Central Hospital

The dull uniformity of the topics which came up for discussion at the Board of Governors monthly meeting in Mercer's was enlivened on 2 December 1924 by details relating to a resolution of the Board of Representative Governors of the Associated Dublin Clinical Hospitals. Submitted by its Honorary Secretary, Dr Horace Law, an ENT surgeon, it stated as follows:

> Resolved, that in view of the possibility of obtaining a sufficient Grant for the erection and endowment of a Central Hospital in Dublin, the Boards of Governors of the several Dublin Clinical Hospitals are invited to consider, whether, if such grant is forthcoming, they would wish to join in discussing a scheme of amalgamation.

The Registrar was instructed to communicate with Dr Law, intimating Mercer's eagerness to participate in any such discussion.

The draw for Ireland's first hospital sweepstake (the 'Iodine Sweep') took place in Jervis Street Hospital in 1925. The Public Charitable Hospitals Act (1930) legalised sweepstakes; six hospitals profited from the first official Irish sweepstake on the Manchester November Handicap, 1930, sharing almost £132,000. The Governors in Mercer's declined to participate, but before long some of them were having second thoughts. At a special meeting in April 1931, with the Protestant Archbishop of Dublin in the chair, Captain Gordon Ferrier proposed that the hospital, so straitened for funds, 'do take part in the Sweepstakes'. The meeting was adjourned to enable the Board to have the opinion of the medical staff. The latter strongly favoured participation, but at the reconvened meeting Captain Ferrier was persuaded to withdraw his motion. The principle was wrong, a majority urged, and must be opposed. Sweepstakes were having a demoralising influence.

The voice of reaction (as we now see it) was weakening. The matter was reconsidered and on 5 September 1933, supported by a letter from RJR (acting Honorary Secretary of the Medical Board) the Governors decided that the hospital should 'go into the Sweep'. By failing to do so, Mercer's was losing £2,236 10s 2d per annum. Voting was 8 for, 6 against. Emboldened, perhaps, by the promise of funds, it was agreed to spend £350 on the ECG department and to purchase a portable ECG machine for £250.

In the early 1930s Mercer's appointed new representatives to discuss amalgamation. Arising out of a letter from Dr T. Gillman Moorhead, the Chairman of the Board of Governors (Reg. H. Keatinge) explained on 5 December 1933 that members of the Hospitals Commission, having heard Professor Leonard Abrahamson's recent address, asked that a scheme for the amalgamation of certain hospitals might be submitted to them. It was then proposed that Mr Keatinge, the Chairman, Mr W. B. Brooks, Mr G. L. O'Connor and Dr R. J. Rowlette 'be appointed representatives to enter into conversations with the Boards of other hospitals to discuss the desirability or otherwise of amalgamation.'

The Hospitals Commission in 1934 sanctioned the expenditure by the hospitals concerned of £1,000 to investigate legal and other questions. A special meeting of the Board of Governors attended by members of the Medical Board was held on 17 July 1934 and it was unanimously agreed 'That the Governors of the Hospital are in favour of an Amalgamation with one or more Dublin hospitals provided that such amalgamation can be adequately financed and that the ultimate detailed scheme of amalgamation meets with the approval of the Governors.'[9]

With the support and encouragement of the Department of Local Government and Public Health planning continued through the 1930s.

A letter addressed to Professor T. G. Moorhead, MD, from the Secretary of the Hospitals Commission, dated 26 January 1934, was read at the Governors' monthly Board meeting on 6 February. It indicated that the Commission was now ready to proceed with the investigation of the legal position of the hospital relative to the proposed amalgamation. The matter of appointing a solicitor to undertake the investigation was discussed, and the house committee was empowered to engage one, having taken suitable advice. There was, too, at this juncture the matter of the bi-centenary to consider.

The Draft Bill

Not until 5 July 1938 was the draft Bill, prepared by the amalgamation committee, placed before the Governors, at their Board meeting. His Grace the Archbishop of Dublin, was in the chair and the following members of the Medical Board were in attendance: Sir John Lumsden, Dr R. J. Rowlette, Mr J. Seton Pringle, Dr Gibbon Fitzgibbon. A discussion took place on the draft Bill, prepared by appointed representatives of Mercer's, Sir Patrick Dun's and the Royal City of Dublin Hospital, which provided for the amalgamation of the three hospitals. Mr R. Keatinge (Honorary Secretary of the Amalgamation Committee) read the report, from which it appeared that the Minister for Public Health strongly favoured a scheme of amalgamation.

Mr W. B. Brooks proposed (1) that after amalgamation Mercer's Hospital should be used as an auxiliary hospital, staffed by its medical staff, and rooms provided for private patients, and (2) that Mercer's should retain its funds, that if this suggestion were not carried out, the funds [should] be handed over for use as pensions for the nurses, or possibly to augment salaries and (3) that the Minister be asked to provide £2 million as endowment for the amalgamated hospitals. The proposals were seconded, for purposes of discussion, by Canon E. G. Sullivan, MA, but after considerable debate they were not carried.

Doubtless the Second World War contributed to the unwarranted delay, but in 1944 a letter from Dr T. G. Moorhead intimated at last that the government was now in a position to proceed with the Bill. Once more Mercer's was pledged to amalgamate. On 27 May 1947 the Governors elected their representatives to the Amalgamation Committee: P. J. Cahill, James Forsyth, and T. M. Lyle; doing likewise the Medical Board appointed Mr T. Bouchier-Hayes and Dr Joe Lewis. But the best laid plans of mice and men . . . RJR had died, and for unstated reasons, the amalgamation planned by his colleagues in Mercer's and elsewhere failed to materialise.

The seven hospitals

A glittering idea, and a new beginning were the opportunities and rewards that now awaited whatever courageous souls were sufficiently brave to exploit them. According to one account: 'In 1957 four doctors from some of the hospitals now federated met informally and agreed that a move should be made to bring together the small Voluntary Hospitals of Dublin.'[10] They were W. George Fegan, Peter B. Gatenby, Stanley McCollum, and John Sugars. Seven hospitals were invited to participate: the Adelaide, Dun's, the Meath, Mercer's, the National Children's Hospital, Baggot Street and Dr Steevens', all of which agreed to do so. A joint committee of lay and medical representatives was formed under the chairmanship of Mr Robert Woods, ENT surgeon to Dun's.

At the Governors' Board meeting on 10 June 1958 it was confirmed that 'the Hospitals Merger Scheme' had been discussed with all members of the honorary medical staff and met with their approval: 'it is agreed that it now be put on record that this Board approves in principle the entry of this Hospital into a Hospitals Merger Scheme and in pursuance of this, it is prepared to enter into negotiations for the purpose of formulating an acceptable scheme.' Captain Colville was appointed to represent the governors; Dr P. A. McNally and Mr J. E. Coolican were to represent the honorary medical staff.[11] The joint committee met several times in 1958 and 1959.

At a special meeting of the Board of Governors held on 4 February 1959, the following resolution was proposed by Mr James Forsyth, seconded by Mr C. W. Fulcher and passed unanimously: 'that the Board of this Hospital will join with other hospital Boards in inviting the Minister for Health to summon a conference to discuss the preparation of legislation for setting up a New Combined Hospital.'

The governors received a letter on 6 October 1959 from the Minister for Health, enclosing a draft scheme of legislation for a Bill to provide for the federation of certain hospitals. Progress, inevitably, continued to be slow. No attempt is made here to record all stages of the long-drawn-out affair, but it may be recalled that the vitally important Hospital Federation and Amalgamation Act became law on 8 July 1961.

Students

In the first half of the 20th century, Dublin medical students paid fees to one teaching hospital but had access to all. Tradition linked certain hospitals to one or other of the schools, quite unofficially. This pleasant but lax system was replaced in the 1950s by an arrangement whereby the affiliation of the schools was officially regulated. St Laurence's (the Richmond) Hospital, the Charitable Infirmary in Jervis Street, and Mercer's were the general hospitals which became associated officially with the RCSI. Before long, however, Mercer's (by then a member of the Federated Dublin Voluntary Hospitals) opted to accept students from Dublin University.

This came about when Professor Gatenby's offer to take students from Mercer's coincided with a mood of disaffection towards the College of Surgeons which had sent Mercer's an unrelieved group of its weaker students. (At 'Surgeons' the students were encouraged to express a preference, and those with the highest marks were given first claim on the hospital of their choice. It so happened that in a particular year none of the better students had selected Mercer's; the academic records of all those directed there were abysmal.) It was regretfully decided that the time had come for a change of academic allegiance. In January 1969 the governors recommended that a teaching connection be established with the Trinity School of Physic.

In so doing, it should be pointed out, it was renewing a link fashioned long ago, for Mercer's was the first hospital associated with the School of Physic. Later, as we shall see, it was to revert to a permanent relationship with the RCSI, when the college seized the opportunity to purchase Mercer's for use as a library.

Mercer's had given its consent readily in 1958 to what was often miscalled the 'Hospitals Merger Scheme'. Captain J. C. Colville, RN, Dr P. A. McNally and Mr J. E. Coolican represented the hospital on the negotiating committees; joined by Brigadier Stanley Clarke, CBE, DSO, and Mr R. E. Jacob, they were Mercer's first representatives on the Central Council of the FDVH.

It was by now well understood that Mercer's, the smallest in the group, could not hope to continue its function as a hospital; the best that could be hoped for was its sale to a sympathetic purchaser with a liberal function in mind and that meanwhile its day-to-day running would be hampered as little as possible. It was vulnerable in certain respects: clinical teaching was dominated in the Federation by Trinity College but students came to Mercer's from the RCSI; pathology, a developing subject, was similarly situated but many specimens had to be processed (and paid for) in 'Surgeons'.

Urbane, compassionate, knowledgeable, 'Paddy' McNally's accomplishments were based on professional competence and he was gratified when appointed associate Professor of Medicine in the RCSI and later in TCD. His geniality and sincerity appealed to students, and he was one of the few Dublin teachers to have been president of 'the Bi' in two schools. His presidential address: 'Medical care: can we afford it?' was published in *The Irish Times*. He was the founder and first president of the Irish Epilepsy Association.[12]

Problems with pathology

The teaching connection with the RCSI necessitated the referral of tissue specimens, biopsies and the like to the department of pathology in the College of Surgeons. A charge was levied, though the same service was carried out at no further cost under financial arrangements already established with the Federation's laboratories. This 'irregularity' proved irksome to the Central Council and moves to make Mercer's fall into line (which it was powerless to do) caused tension in the hospital. Eventually the situation provoked an outburst from Professor McNally who, on 27 November 1967, proposed a motion defending the status quo: 'That the present satisfactory and efficient pathological services in Mercer's Hospital which are of benefit to patients and staff alike be left undisturbed.'

> It appears to us [Mc Nally continued] that all seven hospitals are to be Federated but Mercer's is to be more Federated than the others. We find it difficult to understand the expenditure of £250,000 by the Adelaide if it intends to move and we question if this expenditure fully complied with requirements of the Act. . . . The recent expenditure by Sir Patrick Dun's of £5,000 without even getting prior approval from the Council has surprised us as the eventual post facto approval did not. However, when a point arises vital to the professional status and financial welfare of the staff of Mercer's and costing a negligible sum for an efficient pathological service of benefit to the patients and staff, this arouses the necessity of a couple of committees talking and meeting over several years and not reaching any satisfactory conclusion. We do not believe that if the professional welfare of the medical staffs of the Adelaide, Sir Patrick Dun's, Meath, Royal City of Dublin, Dr Steevens' or the National Children's Hospital were involved, it would arouse such opposition, controversy and discussion.[13]

McNally's aggressive argument prevailed. The site of the new hospital also gave rise to endless debate. The Central Council had decided in 1964 that five hospitals be merged into one on the Dun's site (which later proved impossible); Steevens' was to be an orthopaedic centre; the Meath a centre for genitourinary and gynaecological surgery. Finally, however, St James's (formerly St Kevin's) emerged as the favoured focus for development. The St James's Board met for the first time on 2 July 1971. 'So, after many years of countless meetings and discussions, the Federated Hospitals . . . at last [had] a definite prospect of new hospital construction.'[14]

The main business of the monthly Board meeting at Mercer's on 25 November 1971 was to consider a proposed recommendation to the Central Council on the question of amalgamation of Dun's, Royal City of Dublin and Mercer's, resulting from a meeting held between representatives of the three hospitals on the previous evening.

After prolonged discussion, the following resolution was proposed by Mr Hall, seconded by Mr Carter, and passed unanimously:

> The Boards of Sir Patrick Dun's Hospital, Mercer's Hospital and the Royal City of Dublin Hospital agree to the Principle of Amalgamation of their respective Boards with a view to a unified move to a new hospital. They recommended that consideration be given to the best method of advancing the removal of these to a new hospital at St James's and that a joint working party be set up to investigate this resolution.

A copy of the resolution was forwarded to the Central Council, with the recommendation that the working party should consist in the first place of one lay and one medical member from each hospital.

Closure and dispersal

Irritation, even anger, was experienced in Mercer's in the late 1970s when rumours of impending closure started to circulate, the justification offered being a falling bed occupancy, and Comhairle na nÓspidéal's insistence that the city had too many acute beds. The building of the new hospital had not even yet begun; its completion was not expected before 1987. Consequently the staff was inclined to adopt a 'head-in-the sand' attitude; the rumours initially were found to have little substance, and many doctors shared the delusion that they were fully protected by the terms of the Act, that was conceived in the spirit of a gentleman's agreement, and would even now be honoured. But when interviews with a Transfer Committee were arranged it became clear that there was serious business afoot.

The Matron, Ms P. M. Taafe, took up the post of Matron at Baggot Street; most of the nurses went to St James's or to Dun's. Three consultants retired under the terms of the common contract, another took up a career outside medicine. Five moved to Dun's (where I may say we were graciously received and dealt with fairly); two to Steevens'; one to Baggot Street; and Dr Peter Daly, who had represented his colleagues so painstakingly on the Transfer Committee, took a post as oncologist at St James's.

A meeting of the Section of the History of Medicine of the Royal Academy of Medicine in Ireland was held in the hospital on 18 May 1983. The actual closure was phased over a few weeks in May 1983, teaching and outpatient sessions continuing well into the month. Ambulatory patients were sent home, others were transferred elsewhere.

Mercer's last patient was a member of its surgical staff. Mr Richard Brownell Brenan lay dying from cancer on 28 May while the nurses who tended him stole about quietly, aware how eerily their footsteps sounded in the empty building. Dick Brenan succumbed that evening— *Requiescat in pace!*

Sale

On 7 July 1983 the Governors agreed to place the premises of Mercer's on the market for sale. Messrs Osborne King & Megran, the agents handling the transaction, received enquiries from both property developers and institutional clients. The Irish Medical Association suggested Mercer's should be a geriatric home . . . Rumours circulated. Early in January 1984, an *Evening Herald* columnist reported that the final price (£1.25 million) paid by the RCSI 'was hammered out over Christmas dinner in the Berkeley Court Hotel'.

The actual price was lower than the columnist's inflated figure, the event less festive than his imaginary occasion. He had, however, picked the right purchaser. The College of Surgeons, so closely linked to Mercer's down the years, was now to become united with it indissolubly, and henceforth the former hospital was to be known as the Mercer's Library. Space was utilised, too, for a well-appointed department of general practice, directed by Professor William Shannon, and for a residential function for students and visitors.

The new library was opened to readers on 9 April 1991. The Mercer Building was officially opened by Her Excellency the President of Ireland, Mary Robinson, on Thursday, 12 September 1991.

References

[1] R. J. Rowlette 'The Future of Mercer's Hospital' *Irish Journal of Medical Science* 1935 pp 22–3.

[2] *Idem* 'The Problem of the Dublin Voluntary Hospitals' *Dublin Journal of Medical Science* March 1920 pp 9–24.

[3] W. Doolin 'In Memoriam Robert James Rowlette' *Irish Journal of Medical Science* 1944 pp 583–4.

[4] J. B. Lyons *The Quality of Mercer's The Story of Mercer's Hospital 1734–1991* Dublin: Glendale Publishing 1991 pp 67.

[5] *Ibid.* p 71.

[6] *Ibid.* p 71.

[7] *Ibid.* p 70.

[8] E. D. Mapother 'Our Hospitals and the Interests of Patients and Pupils' *Dublin Journal of Medical Science* 1888 LXXXV pp 110–122.

[9] Mercer's Hospital Minutes Board of Governors 17 July 1934; in RCSI Mercer Library Archives.

[10] P. B. B. Gatenby *History of the Federated Dublin Voluntary Hospitals (1961–1971)* Federated Dublin Voluntary Hospitals and St James's Hospital, 10th Anniversary Celebration, Dublin 1971 [Commemorative publication] pp 14–17.

[11] Patrick A. McNally, MD, Ph.D, FRCPI, the eldest of the family of Walter and Molly McNally was born in Wardner, Idaho, USA, in 1909 but was reared in Dublin. Educated at Clongowes and Trinity, he had the *savoir faire* that can be imparted to a son by a successful father. (Walter MacNally was an acclaimed 'Irish baritone' becoming a wealthy cinema owner when moving pictures replaced vaudeville). McNally was Vice-President of the RCPI. Trained in general surgery, chest surgery and vascular surgery, 'Jack' Coolican was the son of J. H. Coolican, honorary surgeon to Mercer's and Peamount.

[12] I succeeded Patrick McNally as President, and was followed by John Kirker.

[13] See J. B. Lyons *The Quality of Mercer's* p 166.

[14] Gatenby, P. B. B. *op. cit.* p 17

10. *The National Children's Hospital*

Hilary M. C. V. Hoey and Meadhbh M. O'Leary

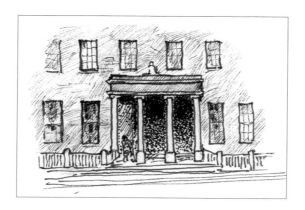

The National Children's Hospital first started in a house in Pitt Street, Dublin, in 1821. It was the first children's hospital in Great Britain and Ireland[1] and was founded by three distinguished Dublin doctors, Sir Henry Marsh, a Trinity graduate, and Sir Charles Johnston and Sir Philip Crampton, both of whom were surgeons at the Meath. The hospital was then known as The Institution for Sick Children, Pitt Street. On 31 December 1834, Sir Lambert Ormsby merged the Pitt Street Institution with the National Orthopaedic and Children's Hospital in Adelaide Road under the name of the National Children's Hospital, following which both institutions worked under one management with combined staff. In 1887 the National Children's Hospital moved from Pitt Street and Adelaide Road to Harcourt Street.

The objectives laid down for the hospital in 1821 were:

(1) to provide free medical and surgical aid to sick children;
(2) to give students the opportunity to acquire knowledge of infantile diseases, which clinical instruction alone can impart;
(3) to educate mothers and nurses regarding the proper management of children in both health and disease.

The founders clearly recognised that child health requires dedicated trained staff and separate facilities for children, and their ambitions could scarcely be improved upon today 185 years later.

Many famous physicians and surgeons were associated with the hospital including William Stokes, Richard Evanson, Henry Maunsell, Fleetwood Churchill, Abraham Colles and Charles West. Dr Charles West later founded the Hospital for Sick Children, Great Ormond Street, London, in 1852.

A number of seminal paediatric books and publications have been produced from the National Children's Hospital. Dr Richard Evanson and Henry Maunsell wrote one of the first paediatric textbooks in English, *The Practical Treatise on the Management of Diseases of Children*. This book went through many editions in Great Britain and Ireland and also in America and Germany. Dr Fleetwood Churchill, as a result of a request from America, published *Diseases of Children* in 1850. This also ran to many editions, both here and in America, and was translated into several European languages. These two books alone brought world renown to our hospital.

The first book on paediatric ear, nose and throat surgery was written by T. G. Wilson. The first books on neonatal paediatrics were written by Robert Collis who also played a major role in setting up the cardiac unit at Johns Hopkins. Robert Collis was a household name in this country. He was known not only as a paediatrician but also as an author, playwright and international rugby player. He took a special interest in the case of Christy Brown who was born with severe spastic cerebral palsy and became a very talented and famous writer. Robert Collis was instrumental in setting up the Marino Cerebral Palsy Clinic in Bray. Together with Patrick McClancy, consultant paediatrician at the National Children's Hospital and the Rotunda, and surgeon Nigel Kinnear, he travelled to the Bergen-Belsen transit camp after its liberation by the British forces in 1945 where he set up a hospital in Belsen for orphans of the holocaust. In 1957 he went to Nigeria where he created three university departments of paediatrics in Ibadan, Lagos and Zaria. His autobiographies, *The Silver Fleece* and *To be a Pilgrim,* epitomise this era.

More recently, many books and papers have been published by the staff; these include: *Epilepsies in Childhood* by Professor Niall O'Donohoe, now in its third edition; *The Irish National Growth Standards for Children from Birth to 18 Years* by Professor Hilary Hoey; *Medical Management Guidelines for Children and Adolescents with Down's Syndrome in Ireland* by Joan Murphy, Hilary Hoey, Edna Roche and Magued Philip. Professor Prem Puri has written many major definitive books and literature on paediatric surgery. Professor Michael Fitzgerald has written extensively; his books include the six volume *Irish Families under Stress.*

Robert Steen was appointed to the Chair in Paediatrics in Trinity College Dublin in 1960, and the Department of Paediatrics has since been based in the National Children's Hospital. He was the first Professor of Paediatrics in the University of Dublin and the first and only paediatrician to date to become President of the Royal College of Physicians of Ireland. He subsequently became President of the British Paediatric Association.

Dr Marie Lea-Wilson graduated from Trinity in 1928. She became a house officer in the National Children's Hospital and in 1933 was appointed a consultant. She remained on the staff until she died at 82 years in 1971. She purchased the painting 'The Taking of Christ', attributed to the Dutch painter Gerrit van Honthorst, in Edinburgh for £8 10s and presented it to the Jesuits in Leeson Street. The Jesuits later invited the National Gallery in Dublin to assess it and when it was found to be a Caravaggio they placed it on loan to the gallery.

Eric Doyle was appointed Lecturer in Paediatrics in 1960; in 1971 he was appointed Professor of Paediatrics in Trinity College, based in the National Children's Hospital. He was also a consultant paediatrician in the Rotunda. He had a special interest in neonatology and established the first paediatric intensive care unit in Dublin in the National Children's Hospital. He also had special interests in coeliac disease and congenital heart disease. He was elected President of the Irish Paediatric Association and was also President of the Dublin University Biological Association.

In 1971 Dr Raymond Rees was appointed a consultant paediatrician. He had a major interest in paediatric nephrology and coeliac disease. He was President of the Irish Paediatric Association and in 1976 founded the Junior Irish Paediatric Association, an all-Ireland society which met for the first time in the National Children's Hospital in November 1976. Its members are registrars and house officers of the children's hospitals, the neonatal departments of the maternity hospitals and the provincial paediatric units. Its officers are drawn from non-consultant hospital doctors with the exception of a consultant chairman. Two meetings are held annually, a general paediatric meeting in November in association with the Irish Paediatric Association, and a neonatal meeting in April. Short papers are delivered and there is a guest lecture from an invited speaker. A medal is presented for the best paper and subsidiary prizes are awarded including bursaries to junior doctors who are going abroad to attend an overseas meeting or to study some new technique in diagnosis or treatment.

In 1965 Professor Ian Temperley and Raymond Rees established the first paediatric haematology service in Ireland that included the treatment of leukaemia; and in 1971 Professor Temperley founded the National Centre for Children with Haemophilia. In 1976, together with Dr Gordon Mullins, he performed the first bone marrow transplant in Ireland in the National Children's Hospital.

Dr Mervyn Taylor was appointed consultant and senior lecturer in 1972. He did much work on the prevention of cross infection in hospital and pioneered research on the benefits of welcoming parents to stay with their children demonstrating that this resulted in a shorter stay. He conducted important research in a wide range of subjects including respiratory disorders, asthma, allergy, toxocariasis, meningococcal disease and normal blood values for children.

The second hospital for children in Dublin, the Children's University Hospital, Temple Street, was founded in Buckingham Street in 1872 by a charitable group of people led by Mrs Ellen Woodcock. In 1876 it was taken over by the Sisters of Charity and moved to Temple Street.[2]

St Ultan's Hospital was founded in 1919 by Dr Kathleen Lynn, Dr Alice Barry and Madeleine Ffrench-Mullen. Negotiations to merge the National Children's Hospital with St Ultan's took place in the early 1930s; however, this merger was opposed by Archbishop Byrne as there was a perceived need for a Catholic hospital for children on the south side of the city. Subsequently, Archbishop John Charles McQuaid in 1938 purchased 16 acres in Crumlin and Our Lady's Hospital for Sick Children opened in 1956.

In 1952 the National Children's Hospital was registered under the Companies Acts, as an association limited by guarantee. In 1961, it became federated with six general hospitals, most of which were traditionally associated with the Trinity medical school, to form the Federated Dublin Voluntary Hospitals group governed by Central Council. In 1960s the boards of St Kevin's (later St James's), St Ultan's and the National Children's Hospital, with Federation approval, proposed that a new children's hospital be built on the St Kevin's site to replace the children's beds in the Federated Group including the children's unit (36 beds) and neonatal unit in St Kevin's. This was rejected due to the cost and the proximity to Our Lady's Hospital for Sick Children in Crumlin.

In 1969, the Minister for Health, Mr Flanagan, appointed a study group chaired by Professor Conor Ward to advise on children's hospital services with particular reference to Dublin. Recommendations from this group included that the hospital beds of the National Children's Hospital (91 beds/cots), St Ultan's (93 beds/cots), Our Lady's Hospital for Sick Children, (324 beds/cots), the beds in St Kevin's (40 beds/cots plus neonatal unit) and St Columcille's paediatric units be integrated in the South Dublin Regional Centre on the site of Our Lady's Hospital for Sick Children. Following this report negotiations took place to merge the National Children's Hospital with Our Lady's on the Crumlin site. There were regular enthusiastic meetings of joint medical and hospital board committees; however, these negotiations failed in 1975 due to irreconcilable differences relating to membership of the board of the new merged hospital.

In 1977 it was proposed that the National Children's Hospital move to St James's; however, following the decision to merge the Adelaide and the Meath on a new site in Tallaght, the move was changed to Tallaght. This was in keeping with the Comhairle na nÓspidéal report on the development of hospital paediatric services, published in 1979, which recommended that a paediatric unit or hospital should ideally be part of a general hospital and on the same site.[3] The locating of a children's hospital on a general campus allows for shared use of expensive laboratory and radiological technology, enhances academic interchange, facilitates student teaching, and eases the transfer of children during or after adolescence to the appropriate adult services.[4]

St Ultan's Hospital merged with the National Children's Hospital and moved to Harcourt Street in the 1980s. Drs Rose Barry, Pauline O'Connell and Barbara Stokes moved their sessions to Harcourt Street; they brought with them their very broad paediatric expertise particularly relating to ambulatory paediatrics, and the management of disability, developing the services for children with disability set up by Drs Robert Collis, Mary O'Donnell and Dympna O'Hagan.

In 1987 the general paediatric unit in St James's closed and its work was transferred to the National Children's Hospital.

In 1998 the National Children's Hospital moved to the new Tallaght hospital, named The Adelaide and Meath Hospital, Dublin Incorporating The National Children's Hospital, where there are dedicated facilities and staff for paediatric care. It is part of a major university hospital with a brief to provide high quality health care to the very large Tallaght catchment area, where 40 per cent of the population are children. As recommended by the British Paediatric Association in 1994 and by other international organisations, it is a comprehensive children's department within the hospital. The children's services are managed by the management team, the National Children's Hospital committee, and by the board of the hospital. There is a major commitment to child health as enshrined in the new Charter of the hospital which clearly states that it ordains 'To promote and develop paediatric medicine and surgery in the State by developing the work heretofore carried out by the National Children's Hospital and to associate all paediatric services with the name of the National Children's Hospital'.[5]

The Charter is committed to maintaining the excellent standards of the paediatric nursing school, which was founded in 1884, and was the first in Ireland. The Charter ordains 'to maintain and develop sick children's nursing within the College of Nursing and to associate such sick children's nursing with the name of the National Children's Hospital'.[6] The National Children's Hospital Committee as defined by the Charter, 'subject to the superintendence of the Hospital Board', is 'responsible for all paediatric services, and services relating thereto provided by the Hospital'.[7]

In Tallaght there is a local community of approximately 125,000 children under the age of 14 years, the fastest growing and one of the largest child populations in Europe. This is also a very deprived local community. The hospital aims to provide comprehensive quality care for acute and chronic medical and surgical problems. At present, despite the small number of staff, the National Children's Hospital treats over 75,000 children per year. It has large tertiary services including endocrinology, diabetes, respiratory medicine and surgery. Numerous children are referred from all over Ireland and also from abroad.

Paediatric medicine, surgery (general, gynaecology, ophthalmology, orthopaedics, otorhinolaryngology, urology), anaesthesia and psychiatry are provided to the highest standards at the hospital by consultants of international standing, together with highly qualified enthusiastic staff in paediatric nursing and multidisciplinary care including medical social work, nutrition, occupational therapy, physiotherapy, play therapy, psychology, speech and language therapy. There is a designated paediatric accident and emergency department with dedicated staff and facilities for children which was established by Dr Mary McKay. There are first class laboratory (chemical pathology, histopathology, microbiology) and diagnostic services on site including a dedicated paediatric radiology department led by Dr Eric Colhoun. The children's services are supported by excellent medical records, information services and clerical administrative staff.

The Council for Children's Hospital Care, chaired by Professor Helen Burke, was established in 1999 by the Minister for Health and Children. The main objectives of the council are to advise on child health issues and to promote collaboration in the delivery of paediatric services with particular reference to hospital care for children. Its membership comprises the chairmen of Our Lady's Hospital Crumlin, the National Children's Hospital at Tallaght and the Children's University Hospital, Temple Street, together with the chief executive officers, directors of nursing, the chairpersons and secretaries of the Medical Boards from these three hospitals and a representative from the Eastern Regional Health Authority. The council has made many positive changes relating to collaboration within child health care.

The National Children's Hospital, together with the Meath and Adelaide Hospitals, has a very long and distinguished history in medical education. This was illustrated in a recent editorial in the *American Journal of Diseases in Childhood* entitled 'The "new" curriculum: is it new?' where the author described how the new methods of medical education such as problem solving sessions, small group discussion, and independent learning, which are being advocated as new methods of teaching in medical education centres in universities such as McMaster, Dundee and Maastricht, were in fact previously described and implemented 200 years ago in Dublin by Robert Graves, William Stokes, Robert Adams and Abraham Colles in the Meath, the Adelaide and the National Children's Hospital.[8]

The National Children's Hospital is to the forefront of medical education. The Trinity department of paediatrics is based there and all Trinity students obtain the majority of their paediatric training on site. There are also excellent postgraduate paediatric training programmes including an MSc programme in paediatrics developed with the help of Dr Edna Roche; the department was awarded the contract for the national training programme for public health doctors and nurses for child health surveillance in 2003. The first clinical skills laboratory in Ireland was developed for the TCD Faculty of Health Sciences by the department of paediatrics in the National Children's Hospital in Harcourt Street and transferred to a purpose built facility in Tallaght.

Over the years the hospital has won a significant reputation for research, both nationally and internationally. Extensive collaborative research is conducted by many members of the staff, including work on endocrine disorders, growth, development, nutrition, diabetes, respirology, nephrology, urology, psychiatry, and other areas. Substantial research grants have been awarded for a wide range of research topics including Down's syndrome, growth and diabetes. The world recognised procedure to correct vesico-ureteric reflux, the STING (Submucosal Teflon Injection and Guaranteed Irish), was developed by Professor Prem Puri together with Professor Barry O'Donnell of Our Lady's Hospital

Crumlin. (Puri and O'Donnell, together with Stanley McCollum, Ray Fitzgerald and Eddie Guiney had of course over the years provided a comprehensive paediatric surgical service to the hospital.) Treatment for this condition previously required major abdominal surgery with a two-week stay in hospital, but with the STING procedure this can now be performed as a simple day-case. The hospital board and the TCD Faculty of Health Sciences have recently supported the proposals for an institute of child health and adolescent health and that of a resource centre for children and adolescents with Down's syndrome. Paediatric research is a fundamental element of research in adult medicine including cardiovascular disease and cancer prevention.

The National Children's Hospital is now located in an architecturally superb university hospital. The staff of the four very distinguished hospitals (the Adelaide, Meath, NCH and St Loman's) are establishing a centre of excellence in collaboration with other Irish and international hospitals and universities in clinical medicine, medical education and research. Services for adolescents provide a challenge and present new opportunities for both the paediatric and adult services. The combination of paediatric and adult services allows the smooth transfer of children with chronic disorders. The hospital in Tallaght, with a wide range of multidisciplinary academic departments on site, presents a unique opportunity to develop and provide a seamless service from birth to old age, integrating primary care, public health and hospital services.

Appendix: Office-holders National Children's Hospital

Chairmen of the Board of Governors

1962 Mr W. M. Anderson
1964 Mrs D. B. B. Kingsmill Moore
1966 Mr Luke Dillon-Mahon
1968 Mr Fred O'Donovan
1974 Mr W. D. Fraser
1977 Dr Maurice Hegarty
1981 Professor Eric Doyle
1984 Mr T. A. McManus
1988 Mr M. A. Cole
1991 Mr T. A. McManus
1993 Mr Salters Sterling

1999 Mr Denis Reardon
2006 Mrs Melissa Webb

Chairmen of the Hospital Committee

1998 Mr Salters Sterling
1999 Mrs Melissa Webb
2002 Mr Gerry Brady; Vice-Chairman Ms Estelle Feldman

Chairmen of the Paediatric Medical Advisory Committee

Professor Stanley McCollum
Professor Eric Doyle
Professor Eddie Guiney
Professor Ian Temperley
Dr Raymond Rees
Mr Walter Doyle Kelly
Mr David FitzPatrick
Dr Eric Colhoun
Dr Mervyn Taylor
Dr Peter Greally

House Governor/Secretary-Managers

1965 Col. Learmont
1965 Mr Donal O'Brien
1967 Col. D. Affleck Graves
1978 Mr Des Rogan
1986 Mr Derek Dockery
1994–8 Mrs Catherine McDaid

Matrons

1930 Miss Delia Hastings
1969 Miss Anne Quigley
1980 Mrs Betty Brady
1988 Miss Ann Taylor
1992 Mrs Catherine McDaid
1994 Mrs Maura Connolly, Matron and Manager

Professors and Heads of Department of Paediatrics, TCD

1960 Professor Robert Steen
1970 Professor Eric Doyle
1980 Professor N. V. O'Donohoe
1991 Professor Hilary M. C. V. Hoey

Henry Marsh Chair of Child and Adolescent Psychiatry, TCD

1997 Professor Michael Fitzgerald

References

[1] E. E. Doyle 'Coming of Age', *J. Irish Med Assoc.* 1979; 72: 6-13.

[2] *The Children's Hospital Temple Street, The Post-Centenary Years 1972–2002*, Dublin: Blackwater Press 2002.

[3] *Development of Hospital Paediatric Services* Dublin : Comhairle na nÓspidéal 1979.

[4] D. G. Gill 'The development of Dublin's children's hospitals'. *J. Irish Coll. Physicians* Summer 1991; 20: 252–253.

[5] AMNCH Charter Clause 5 (p).

[6] *Ibid.* Clause 5 (q).

[7] *Ibid.* Clause 16 (6a) .

[8] Corrigan, J. 'The "new" curriculum: Is it new?' *American Journal of Diseases in Childhood* 1992; 146: 909.

II. *The Royal City of Dublin Hospital, Baggot Street*

Gerry Gearty

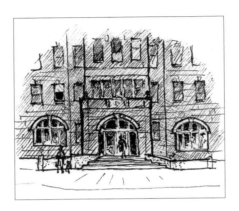

The immediate effect of the Federation Act 1961 was the takeover of all consultant appointments. Baggot Street, of course, was represented on appointment boards etc. This did not bother people too much and senior medical and surgical registrars working their way through the system in the old traditional style were gradually accommodated within the new system without too much difficulty.

My appearance as the first federated appointment to Baggot Street was trouble free—indeed the senior physicians, particularly Victor Synge, were very actively interested in new developments and Robert Wilson was quite happy to go along with the general ideas. The development of cardiology there owes a lot to their encouragement and co-operation.

The surgeons, on the other hand, felt that the whole scheme was outrageous and always laid into Professors Jessop and Gatenby on their regular peacekeeping missions to Baggot Street. Though loud in their comments and criticisms it is fair to say that in their actions they were actually supportive of the new developments even to the extent of making beds available for specialist development. They realised, I am sure, that major plans would not mature within their working lifetime—as indeed turned out.

With regard to the eventual transfer to St James's this proposal came rather late in the day as some previous ones had come and gone—Sir Patrick Dun's, Clonskeagh, and Cherry Orchard, for example. In 1968 the FitzGerald Report recommended the transfer of the Federated Hospitals, dividing them between a site at Elm Park beside St Vincent's and the site of St Kevin's in James's Street. In 1969 Central Council commissioned a feasibility study by Llewellyn Davies Weekes. This firm had been responsible for producing a planning study for the Milton Keynes new town so came with a considerable reputation. It seems that their conclusion was that the best sites for the Federation would be at Cherry Orchard and St Kevin's, as it then was.

The Cherry Orchard option came to nothing but in 1971 the Order for the establishment of St James's on the St Kevin's site was signed. The concept of moving to St James's did not engender either particular enthusiasm or objection. Indeed Keith Shaw had been doing some sessional work there from an early stage and I had visited on occasion. Cardiac surgical activity, of course, had increased since the establishment of the cardio-thoracic unit which had opened in 1959. Keith Shaw, Rory Childers and Terence Chapman were instrumental in this, aided by David Hogan whose appointment in 1960 as anaesthetist provided essential expertise in that field. I was appointed in 1963 to replace Childers who had left to take up a post in Chicago.[1]

Open cardiac surgery was also being developed in the Mater by Keith Shaw's colleague Professor Eoin O'Malley. In 1971 the Federated Hospitals reached an agreement with the Mater authorities to develop a joint unit for open heart surgery at the Mater, to which both Shaw and Hogan were appointed. Patients were still investigated in Baggot Street, had their operations in the Mater and returned to Baggot Street for post-operative care and rehabilitation. Coakley notes that the hospital activity level remained high and indeed in 1986 over 6,300 patients were admitted, an increase of almost 20 per cent over five years and that a new cardiac rehabilitation class was introduced in 1982.[2]

However, even then, in 1982, the future of the hospital was in doubt. In his annual report for that year the Chairman, R. C. Lewis-Crosby, commented that the hospital 'in common with other institutions in the health care area was suffering from a scarcity of funds . . . there is much talk about possible reductions in services'. He commended the staff of the hospital for their commitment and concern and went on to discuss the hospital's future:

It is now well established and generally accepted that the services presently provided by this hospital, Sir Patrick Dun's and Mercer's will move to a new hospital at St James's. The first firm move in that direction came with the announcement early this year that Mercer's Hospital has decided to close. Present plans suggest that, while some services from here may transfer on completion of stage 1C of the new hospital, i.e. 1986, our hospital will continue to provide an acute medical service up to ten years hence and perhaps beyond.

The continuation of acute services was not, however, to last that long and despite a submission to the Department of Health in 1987, *Royal City of Dublin Hospital—A New Future,* suggesting that the hospital would continue to provide non-acute services benefiting the community, closure was imminent. Despite the fact that the facilities in St James's were not yet adequate to receive the transferring workload the hospital activity was reduced gradually and on 4 December 1987 the last patients were transferred to St James's.

The Board of Baggot Street continues to operate and meets regularly, concerned now with the intelligent dispersal of the significant funds which were raised by the sale of the old nurses' home and, more recently, leasing the hospital building to the Eastern Health Board. Major health centres are planned for Pearse Street and Ringsend in co-operation with the Health Board and local general practitioners. Also research funds are distributed regularly, mainly to our colleagues in St James's, particularly those with a previous association with Baggot Street.

The hospital continues to function somewhat along the lines outlined in the 1987 plan and remains the property of the Board. It is interesting to reflect on the fact that of all the seven hospitals which formed the Federation, only the Royal City of Dublin and the Meath survive, providing patient care, albeit in a somewhat altered state.

References

[1] *Editor's note:* Coakley comments : 'Gearty and Shaw worked closely to build up one of the finest cardiac units in these islands . . . new techniques such as echocardiography were introduced over the next decade and saphenous vein grafting was a major innovation for suitable cases of coronary artery disease'. Davis Coakley *Baggot Street—A Short History of the Royal City of Dublin Hospital* Dublin: 1995 p 87.

[2] *Op. cit.*

[3] Royal City of Dublin Hospital *Annual Report* 150th Anniversary 1982 p 3.

[4] *Op. cit.* p 4.

12. Sir Patrick Dun's Hospital

Donald G. Weir*

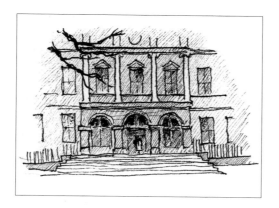

Sir Patrick Dun's was from its inception the flagship hospital of the Trinity medical school. The financial resources used for its construction were derived from a bequest from Sir Patrick Dun (1642–1713), whose main intent had been to provide for the remuneration of the clinical professors of the university and the Royal College of Physicians of Ireland (RCPI). However, due to the acrimonious nature of the relations between the two bodies as to where their relevant professors should deliver their lectures, it was eventually agreed to use part of the Dun estate to build a new hospital specifically for the teaching of medical students. It would appear that such instruction began with the opening of Sir Patrick Dun's in 1808, but it was not until 1820 that it became a routine event. Although clinical teaching was subsequently conducted in other Dublin hospitals the board of the college specifically resolved that 'no University Professor of the School of Physic shall be allowed to hold an appointment to any clinical hospital other than Sir Patrick Dun's Hospital'. This was followed by a similar decree from the RCPI concerning the King's Professors who were also paid for by the Dun bequest. This principle, however worthy, was difficult to maintain in practice although, as outlined in the *History of the Medical School in Trinity*

* The author is very grateful for the help and constructive criticism given by John Goodbody and John Kirker in the writing of this chapter.

College Dublin by T. P. C. Kirkpatrick (1912), many professors did transfer from other hospitals to Sir Patrick Dun's.

The hospital is also the place where Countess Markievicz died, and where it is reputed de Valera surrendered to a posse of British infantry in 1922, amongst whose number was Charles McDonogh who later became the radiologist to the hospital. More recently, in 1972, Dun's served as the frontline hospital to look after the victims of the bomb blast outrage in Nassau Street, although it was only afterwards that Dublin hospitals were specifically designated for such emergency duty.

Until its closure in 1986 Sir Patrick Dun's remained the main centre of the university for undergraduate medical training, and a wide variety of very eminent and diverse personalities served within its portals as professors of the university, details of whom can be found in Professor Peter B. B. Gatenby's *The School of Physic Trinity College Dublin* (1994). This chapter will deal specifically with the last 25 years of Sir Patrick Dun's existence as an acute frontline hospital.

'St Patrick's', as the patients insisted on calling Sir Patrick Dun's, was a very happy hospital; the porters, nurses and doctors had good working relationships and even the patients seemed satisfied. Indeed from its inception in 1808 till its closure in 1986, actions for medical negligence or malpractice against the hospital or any of its staff scarcely feature in the records. The pursuit of such actions today may be due to the changing mores of patients and the law over the last 20 years, but the fact that there used to be so few reflects the more leisurely pace of medicine in those days and the availability of beds for sick patients as and when required. The relative equanimity of Sir Patrick Dun's was also due to the benevolent governance of the hospital by its Medical Board under the guidance throughout these years of John Goodbody, its honorary Secretary from time out of mind, the board of governors, run in later years by its CEO Eamon Stubbings, and the nursing staff, led by the matron, Kathleen Brennan, a lady of quite exceptional sagacity and commonsense. Under her guidance the hospital collected arguably the finest nursing sisters in Ireland at that time; indeed some, like Ann Dixon, Marie Stapleton and Olive Doyle, subsequently transferred to St James's where they continued to look after the patients of Dublin with great distinction. It was a time when the practice of medicine was both a pleasure and an honour.

One of the traditions that was peculiar to Dun's passed into history 25 years ago. This was the greeting received by each member of the visiting consultant staff on arrival at the hospital each morning. The porter would deliver a long and loud roll on a large hospital gong and a number of beats that depicted the seniority of the entering consultant. The most senior surgeon or physician who was distinguished by the relation to the roll, got one beat, the next most senior two beats and so on down the line. The gong was kept in the entrance hall of the hospital especially for this purpose. This informed the nursing staff of the imminent arrival on their respective wards of the relevant consultant. However, the porters (at the behest of the Medical Board,) discontinued the practice in 1972, to the dismay of the nursing staff who professed to finding it very helpful!

Another quaint practice at Dun's was that for many years the resident medical staff of the hospital used to carve their names on the coffee table in the consultants' meeting room. Many of them subsequently

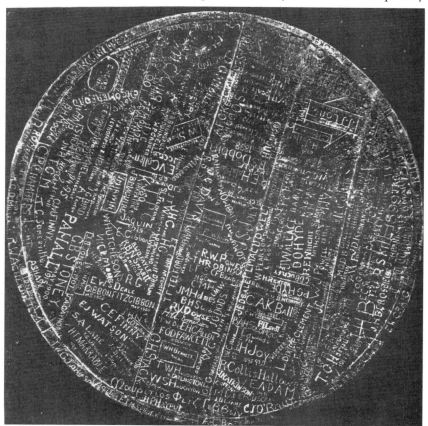

The famous table-top in the consultants' meeting room, scarred with the names and initials of hundreds of residents.

went on to become prominent figures in their own right in Irish medicine. This practice was so popular that extra leaves had to be added to
the top of the table! Following the closure of the hospital for acute medicine in 1986 this table was moved to the Royal College of Physicians as a
memento of the hospital.

The 1960s and 1970s were a time of concentration of the resources in
Trinity medical school. These years saw the creation of the Federated
Dublin Voluntary Hospitals (FDVH), a loose collection of those Dublin hospitals associated with Trinity. This event was spearheaded by a
group of dedicated consultants, hospital board members and TCD professors, including in particular Peter Gatenby and Jerry Jessop. The details of these events are covered elsewhere in this book. The objectives of
the FDVH were twofold: (1) to allow the evolution of the developing
specialties in medicine and surgery within the FDVH, which created a
complementary system within the group, and (2) to demonstrate the
necessity for their amalgamation on one, or at most two, new hospital
sites.

Sir Patrick Dun's was given the role of developing vascular surgery
under the direction of George Fegan (a member of staff from 1950 and
Professor of Surgery in TCD from 1967 to 1975) whose special expertise
lay in his revolutionary techniques for the management of varicose veins,
a subject on which he became a world authority and about which he
lectured extensively. In the evolution of this work he was ably assisted
by Paddy Byrne PhD, the chief technologist to the department from
1970, who has been responsible for shepherding a vast array of surgical
graduates through their postgraduate degrees in Dun's and subsequently
St James's. The other mega star of the unit was Mary Henry who later
became a consultant in both Tallaght and the Rotunda. She has been
elected to the Senate as the TCD representative on a number of occasions; this has allowed her to have a significant influence on a wide
range of political issues, especially those with a medical slant. The unit
was complemented by Jimmy Milliken who became the vascular surgeon and not only took over the varicose vein unit when George Fegan
retired but also, with Gregor Shanik, developed the field of arterial surgery and especially the treatment of abdominal aneurysms. Nigel Kinnear,
Regius Professor of Surgery, TCD (1967–73), a former Dun's student,
had pioneered this operation in Ireland at the Adelaide.

Fegan was also responsible for the restoration of the derelict basement areas of Dun's. This allowed the development at one end of an
undergraduate teaching facility for Trinity medical students and a can-

teen which greatly enhanced the family atmosphere of the hospital. The other end became the new gastrointestinal endoscopy unit and the hospital's administrative centre.

The other developments in the surgical area were otorhinolaryngology, a specialty of the hospital since the days of Sir Robert Woods; he was succeeded by his son Bobby who was appointed in the 1940s. Bobby Woods became renowned for his development of the technique of stapedectomy of the middle ear. This specialty continued to evolve under the guidance of Walter Doyle-Kelly, Frank O'Loughran and Thomas Wilson (after the closure of Mercer's) and subsequently Hugh Burns. Louis Werner and John McDougald ran a large ophthalmology outpatient clinic which was much valued by patients and students alike.

In the medical area the senior physician was J. A. (Jackie) Wallace, who was for many years the Trinity medical school lecturer in toxicology and jurisprudence, a position he filled with great fervour, imagination and humour. One example was his lecture on phosphorus poisoning which amongst other effects produces diarrhoea. He claimed this was the only way you could truly get 'a flash in the pan'! He was also for many years the medical practitioner to the students in Trinity College, and was frequently to be seen doing the rounds of his patients on his bicycle.

R. H. (Robbie) Micks had been the senior physician for many years leading up to this period. He was a supremely dedicated and conscientious physician and teacher, and an early advocate of optimum care for diabetes. As professor of Materia Medica and Pharmacy (1945–66) his textbook lasted over many editions and was valued far beyond his own medical school, being translated into a number of languages..

John (Joe) Kirker was a neurologist who was not only an expert physician but also largely responsible for the introduction of electroencephalography into Ireland, of which he remained the leading exponent for many years. He later became president of the Royal College of Physicians. He was renowned for his witty asides. On one occasion when his team was presenting a case of a left sided Graham Steel syndrome, a student asked him what would happen if the patient got it on both sides, to which Joe replied, 'I rather feel that that would be a capital offence'!

Raymond Rees, although also a consultant paediatrician at the National Children's Hospital, ran a paediatric ward at the top of the stairs on the first landing. This facility addded greatly to the range of services offered by the hospital.

The other development was in gastroenterology, which followed the evolution of flexible endoscopy. In 1962 I introduced flexible endoscopy to Ireland in the Meath; and when I transferred to Dun's in 1967 I set up the first Irish endoscopy unit with a day ward attachment.

This unit operated in association with surgeons Tom O'Neill and David Lane, and became the major gastroenterology centre of the FDVH. Tom O'Neill was a most energetic and highly organised surgeon who established a well deserved reputation for his management of chronic peptic ulceration using his particular variation of the partial gastrectomy operation. David Lane had also moved to Sir Patrick Dun's from the Meath in the early 1970s, and his arrival brought not only a formidable surgical expertise which greatly enhanced the standing of the unit, but also a calmness and maturity which was much appreciated. When time permitted he would find an isolated part of the hospital where he practised his oboe, an instrument he played with great artistic ability. Indeed, as he played, it gave everyone the comforting feeling that everything was under control in the hospital.

Graham Neale, who was primarily associated with St James's as the professor of clinical medicine (1976–80), also had an attachment to the gastroenterology unit. He had an international reputation as a physician, nutritionist and gastroenterologist. During the brief time that he was in Ireland he did much to resolve medico-political problems within the FDVH, and to ease the transfer of these hospitals to the new St James's.

Napoleon (Nap) Keeling was briefly attached to the Dun's gastroenterology unit in the early 1980s, although his main attachment was to St James's. While at St James's he developed the technique of operative intervention ERCP for the first time in Ireland.

The anaesthetic unit was run by Frank de Burgh Whyte (until his untimely death in 1976), in conjunction with John Goodbody, Brendan Lawless and Lesley Fox. This group was the first to develop a purpose built recovery room in the surgical area. They also had one of the first intensive care units, and ran the only preoperative assessment clinic in Dublin. They were probably the first department to set up a formal joint department with St James's.

The pathology division was initially centred on the Trinity campus, and its members were allocated to individual federated hospitals. Dermot Hourihane was assigned as histopathologist to Dun's, along with Niall Gallagher (cytologist). Hourihane, who later became professor and head of department in Trinity, was instrumental in developing the depart-

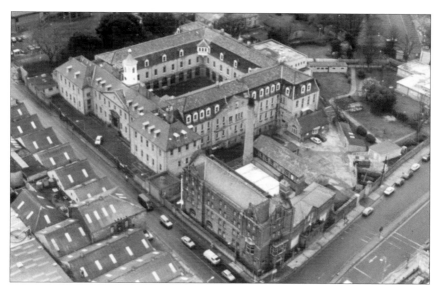

Dr Steevens' Hospital as it was in 1988, with the Nurses' Home and chimney stack still in place (Bobby Studios)

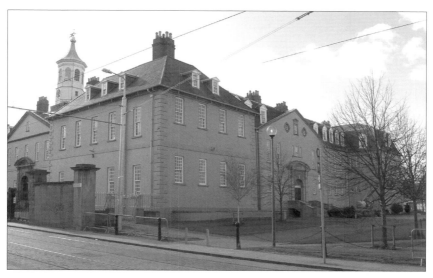

Dr Steevens' in 2005, showing the new west-facing entrance (Michael Pegum)

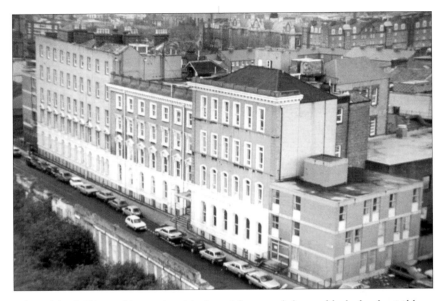

The Adelaide Hospital in 1998, with the residence and theatre block clearly visible at rear (Bobby Studios)

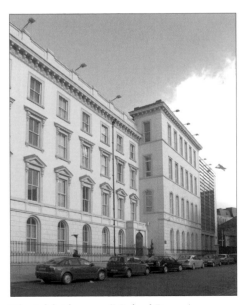

The Adelaide 2005 (Michael Pegum)

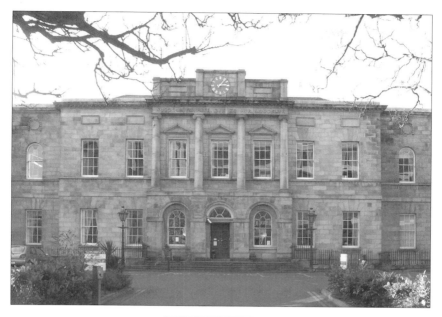

Above *Sir Patrick Dun's Hospital 2005 (Michael Pegum)*

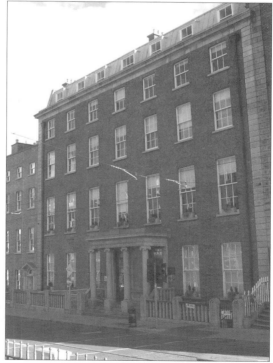

Right *National Children's Hospital 2005 (Michael Pegum)*

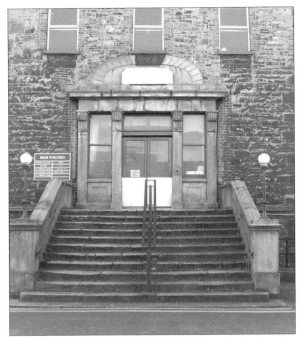

The Meath Hospital 2005 (Michael Pegum)

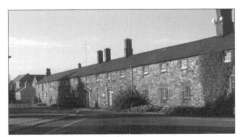

The Foundling Hospital (Davis Coakley)

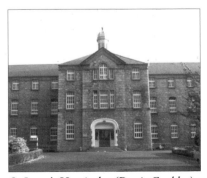

St James's Hospital 7 (Davis Coakley)

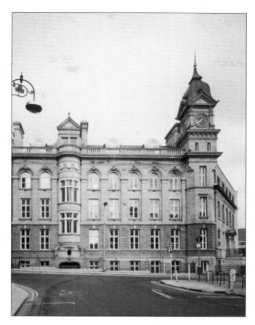

Mercer's Hospital circa 1980 (Davis Coakley)

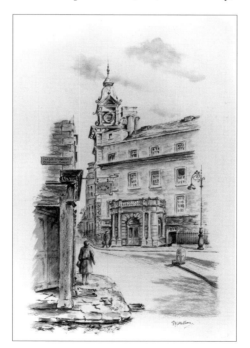

Mercers' (S. K. Mellon—courtesy J. B. Lyons)

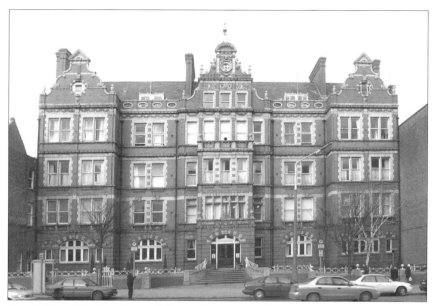

Royal City of Dublin Hospital, Baggot Street 2005 (Michael Pegum)

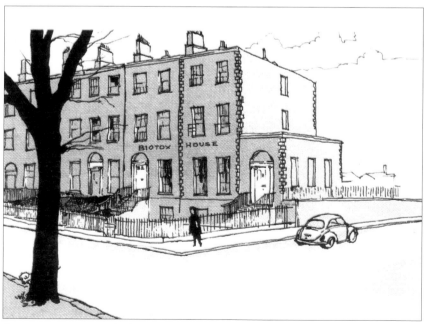

*Biotox House 82 Ranelagh Road—the first offices of FDVH were located here
(Thomas Wilson)*

Some of the original protagonists of federation

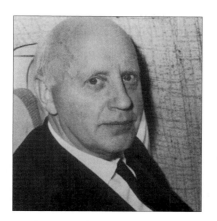

Prof. W. J. E. (Jerry) Jessop (Bobby Studios)

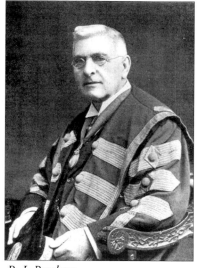

R. J. Rowlette (Mercer's—courtesy J. B Lyons)

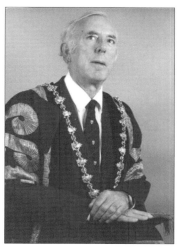

Stanley McCollum (courtesy McCollum family)

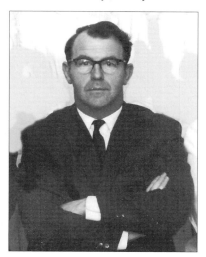

George Fegan (Michael Pegum)

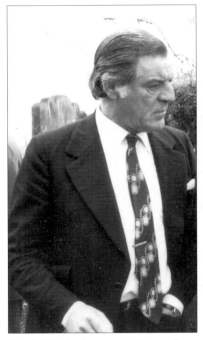

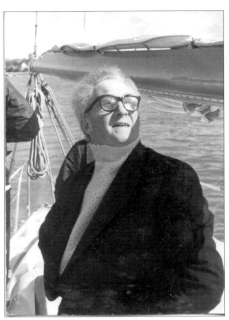

Sandy McVey (courtesy J. Bonnar)

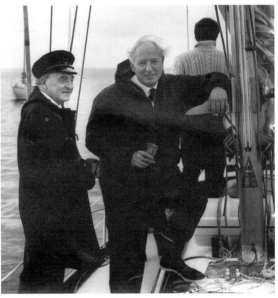

Above and left *Two nautical obstetricians: Ninian Falkiner and (facing) Rory O'Hanlon (courtesy J. Bonnar)*

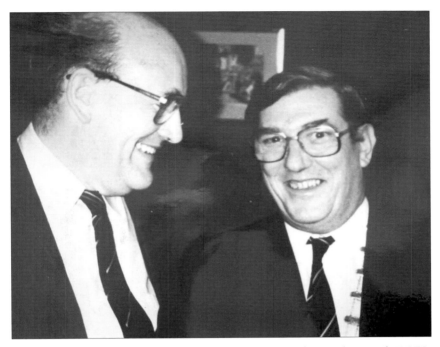

THE FEDS IN PICTURES

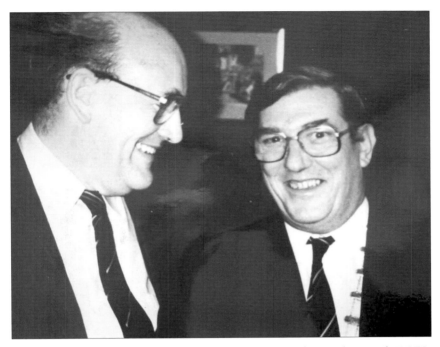

Prof. Bill Watts, Provost TCD and some time Chairman of Central Council FDVH, with Prof. Tom Hennessy, President RCSI 1993/94 (Bobby Studios)

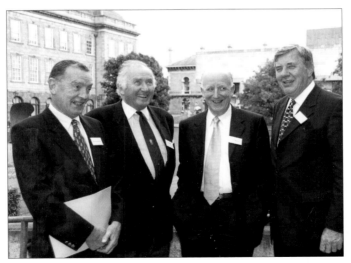

A posse of professors and deans—Dermot Hourihane, Donald Weir, John Bonnar and Ian Temperley (courtesy J. Bonnar)

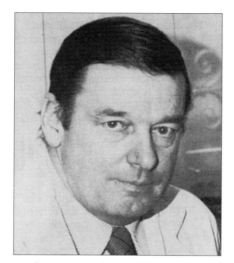

Prof. Peter Gatenby

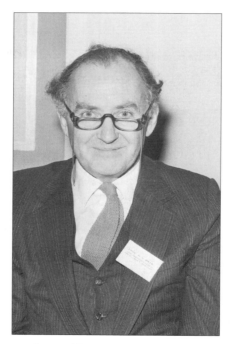

Prof. Donald Weir (Bobby Studios)

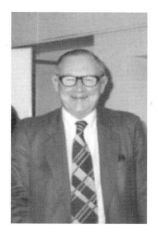

A radiological trio (Bobby Studios) Above *Shan Henderson,*
Below left *David McInerney* Below right *Gerry Hurley*

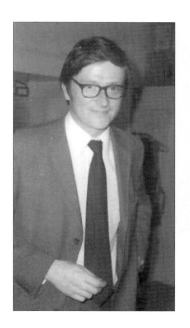

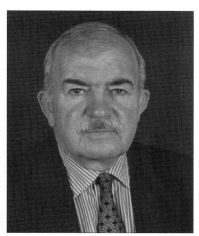

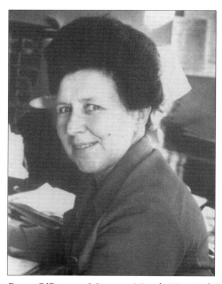

Betty O'Dwyer, Matron, Meath Hospital (courtesy Michael Butler)

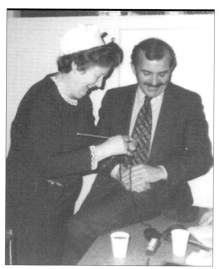

Below *Miss M. Mansfield, Matron, Adelaide Hospital, and Gerry Hurley at a fund-raising knit-in (courtesy Gerry Hurley)*

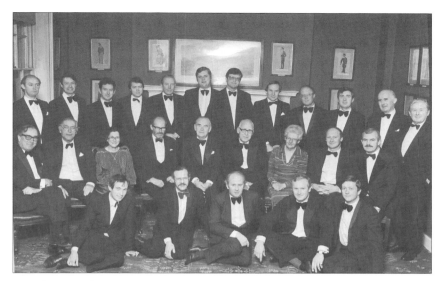

Meath Hospital Medical Board Dinner in the early 1980s
Back row: *John Barragry, Michael Pegum, Michael Cullen, Karl O'Sullivan, Derek Robinson, John Fitzpatrick, George Mellotte, Bill Beesley, Frank O'Loughran, Brian Keogh, Joe Galvin, Gerry Owens*
Second row: *Victor Lane, Sholto Douglas, Una O'Callaghan, Brian Mayne, Dermot O'Flynn, Brandon Stephens, B. Brennan, Michael Butler, Gerry Hurley*
Front row: *Colm O'Morain, Arthur Tanner, Sam Hamilton, Frank Keane, David McInerney (Michael Walshe)*

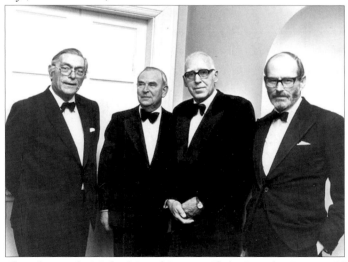

Also taken at the Medical Board Dinner: Sholto Douglas, Dermot O'Flynn, Brandon Stephens, Brian Mayne (Michael Walshe)

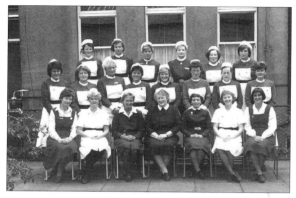

Adelaide Hospital senior nursing staff and tutors circa 1982
Back row *Iris Gordon, Ruth Hipwell, Jenny Herbert, Eileen MacDonnell, Mildred Maxwell, Marion Wilson*
Centre row: *Denise Barkman, Olive Glen, Kathleen Wilkins, Linda Johnston, Audrey Fennell, Sylvia Armitage, Maura McGettigan, Shirley Wilkinson*
Front row *Joan FitzPatrick, Ann Gillespie, Valerie Adams, Eileen Mansfield (Matron), Yvonne Seville, Maura Donohoe, Barbara Lennon (Arthur Ogilvie)*

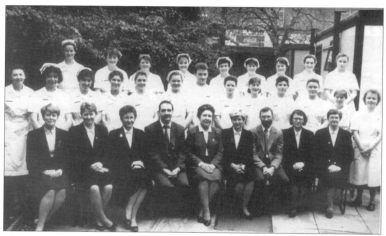

Meath Nursing School, 1989 Intake—Graduation 1992
Front row: *Mary Briscoe (Tutor), Angela O'Donoghue (Tutor), Margaret McCarthy (Tutor), Michael Coughlan (Tutor), Elizabeth O'Dwyer (Matron), Mary Cotter (Tutor), Liam Plunkett (Tutor), Mary Lennon (Tutor), Angela Hoey (Prinicpal Tutor)*
Middle row: *Eileen Devane, Anne Heavy, Catherine O'Connor, Rosaleen Davey, Eileen Doyle, Maeve O'Reilly, Frank Hynes, Catherine Rooney, Marie Owens, Siobhan Ryan, Orla Bohan, Anne Marie Hughes, Joanna O'Donnell*
Back row: *Susan Dillane, Marguerite Brady, Alison Grace, Sheila Barton, Yvonne Burke, Eileen Lynch, Martina O'Dowd, Geraldine Cox, Bernadette Murphy (Michael Walshe)*

[XIV]

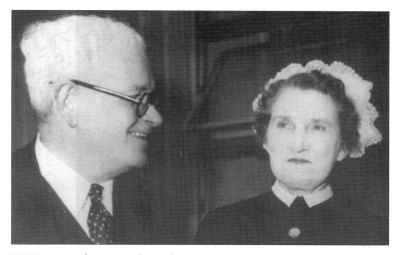

T. J. D. Lane sharing a joke with Matron Ann Magee in 1965

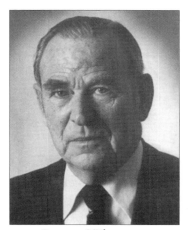

Dermot O'Flynn

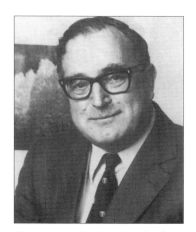

Victor Lane (courtesy Michael Butler)

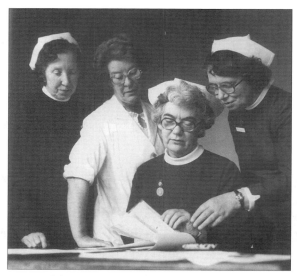

Sisters of the Meath GU Department in 1980: Maura Dunne, Eileen Sheridan, Marie Cooney, Maureen Fallon (Bobby Studios)

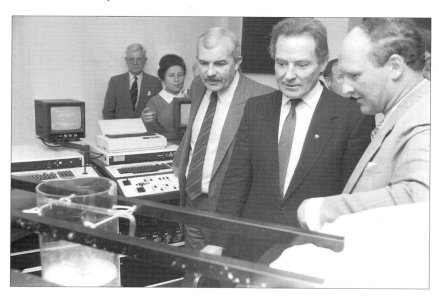

Inauguration of lithotripter, Meath Hospital: Niall Tierney, Dept. of Health, Betty O'Dwyer, Gerry Hurley, Rory O'Hanlon (Minister) Michael Butler

Opening of the Renal Dialysis Unit, April 1987 Meath Hospital

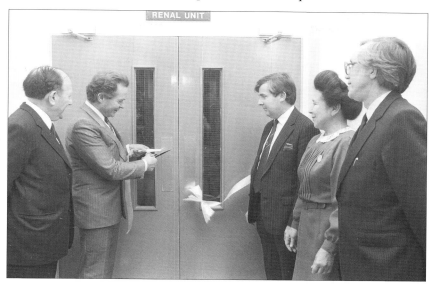

*Harold Ellis, Minister for Health Rory O'Hanlon, Brian Keogh, Betty O'Dwyer,
Eddie Thornhill*

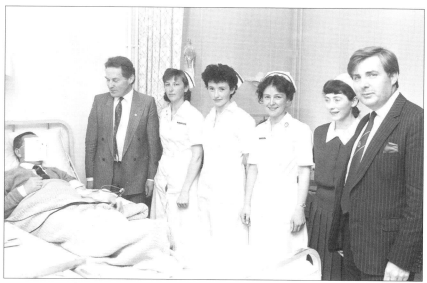

*At a patient's bedside: Minister Rory O'Hanlon, Brid Brennan, Mary Dineen,
Collette O'Farrell, Anne Murphy, Brian Keogh (Bobby Studios)*

At an FDVH Conference

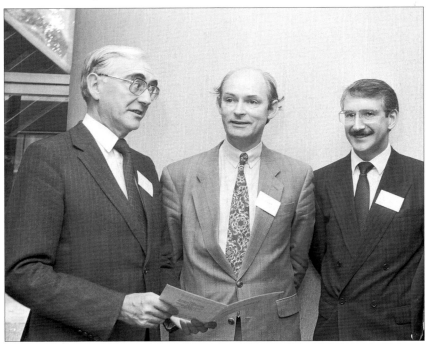

Desmond Dempsey, John Barragry, Ronnie Grainger (Bobby Studios)

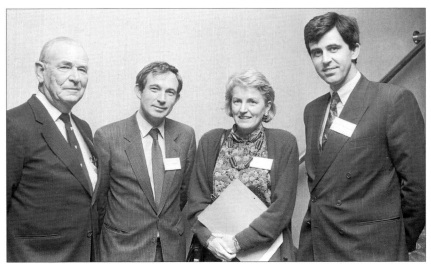

*Dermot O'Flynn, Colm O'Morain, Hilary Hoey, Ted McDermott
(Bobby Studios)*

Baggot Street Groups

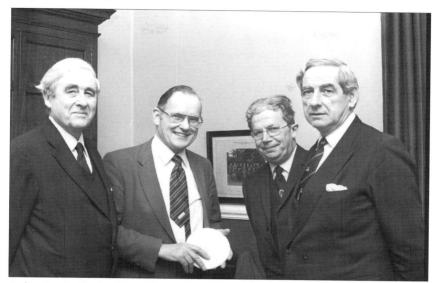

Robin Lewis-Crosby, Gerry Gearty, David Hogan, Frank O'Reilly, Pro-Chancellor TCD (Bobby Studios)

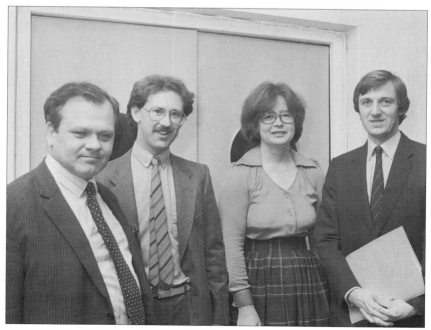

R. Quill, Tony O'Flaherty, Doreen Dowd, Dermot Moore (Bobby Studios)

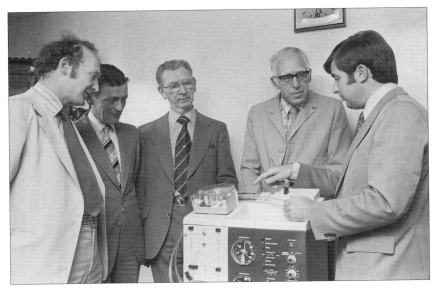

Dialysis demonstration—Michael Butler, Departmental official, J. Colfer (Meath Secretary-manager), Brandon Stephens, Brian Keogh (courtesy Michael Butler)

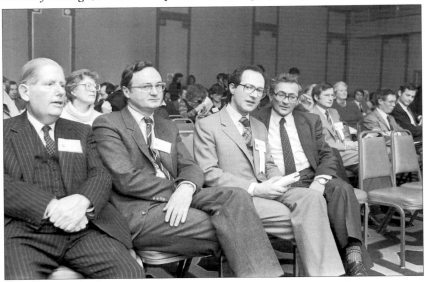

Front row: *Walter Verling, Conor Keane, Derek Freedman, Tom Quinn (Johns Hopkins University) (Bobby Studios)*

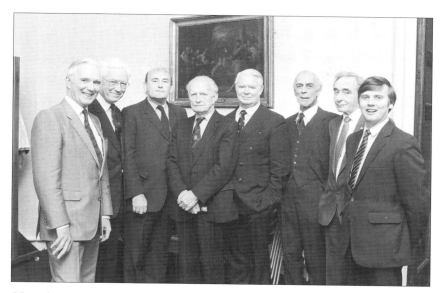

Mercer's group—Joe Matthews, Jack Coolican, Bill Watts, Prof. Thomas Gilmartin, Paddy Matthews, Michael Solomons, Joe Timoney, Peter Daly

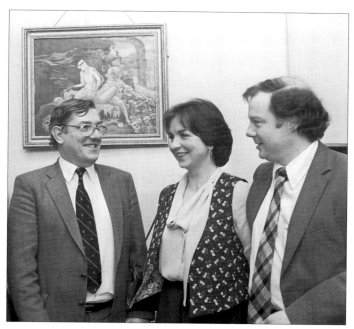

Baggot Street group—Tom Hennessey, Katherine McAleer & Carl O'Malley (Bobby Studios)

Two Adelaide groups

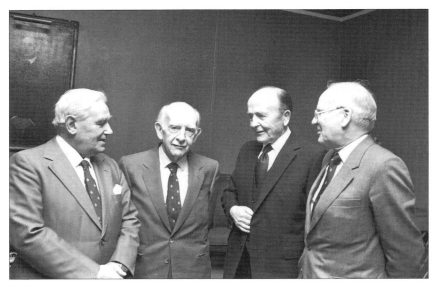

Eric Fenelon, David Mitchell, Basil Booth, Chairman, Adelaide Board, Robin Nelson (Bobby Studios)

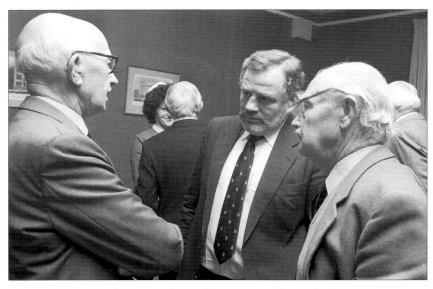

Vernon Harty, David FitzPatrick, Nigel Kinnear (Bobby Studios)

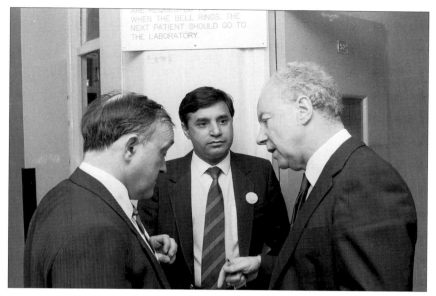

Paediatric surgeons at the National Children's Hospital: Eddie Guiney, Prem Puri and Barry O'Donnell (Bobby Studios)

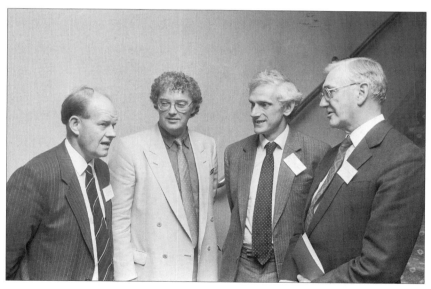

Mervyn Taylor, Derek Dockery, Gerald Tomkin, Desmond Dempsey (Bobby Studios)

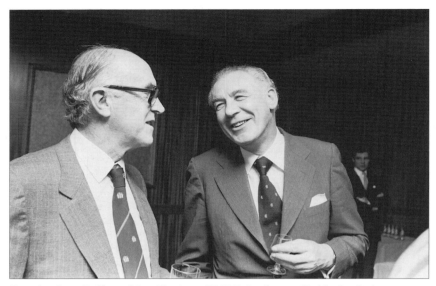

Brendan Prendiville and Ian Howie at FDVH Conference (Bobby Studios)

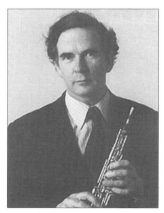

David Lane—oboeist (Bobby Studioes)

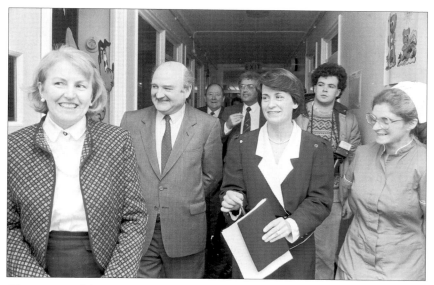

The opening of the NCH Mother and Child (Steen) Wing: Hilary Hoey, Barry Desmond, Minister for Health, Betty Brady, Matron, Eileen Manifold

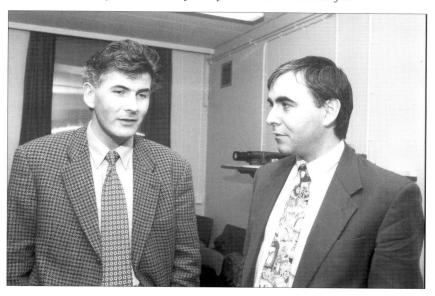

Peter Greally and Prof. Des O'Neill (Bobby Studios)

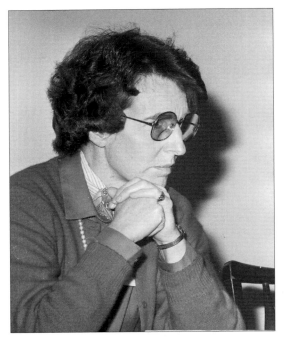

Miss Peta Taafe, Matron of Mercer's Hospital and then Baggot Street

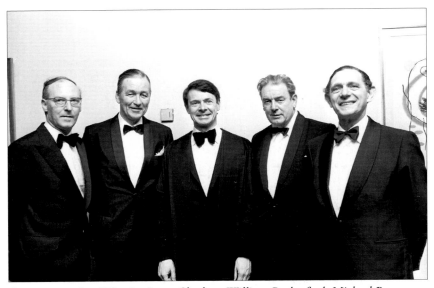

Opening meeting 'Bi' 1980: James Sheehan, William Rutherford, Michael Pegum, Peter Gatenby, Alan Apley

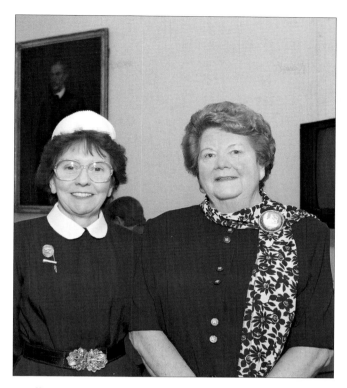

Yvonne Seville, Matron, Adelaide, and J. J. Baker, Nursing Committee Adelaide (Arthur Ogilvie)

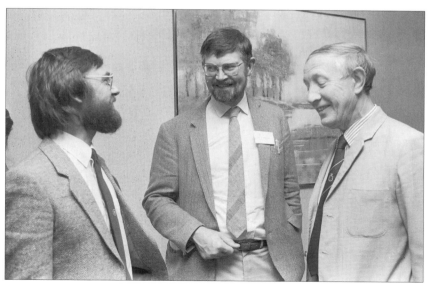

Derek Taylor, George Donald, Eddie Martin (Arthur Ogilvie)

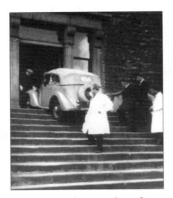

Parking at the Meath in former times

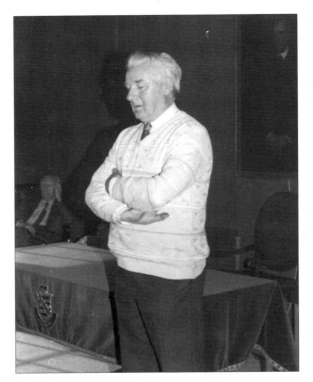

Joe Cowell, Adelaide Head Porter, reminisces (courtesy Adelaide Society)

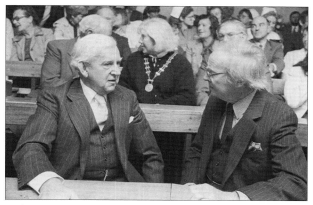

Stalwart NCH Chairmen—Prof. Eric Doyle and Maurice Hegarty

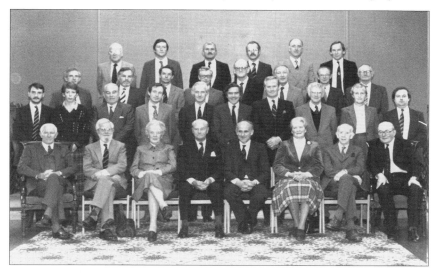

Adelaide consultant staff about 1980.
Back row: *Robin Nelson, David McInerney, Gerry Hurley, Arthur Tanner, John Bonnar, Bill Beesley*
Third row: *Gerald Tomkin, David FitzPatrick, Marcus Webb, John Goodbody, Keith Shaw, Eddie Martin, Ian Graham, Shan Henderson*
Second row: *Declan Magee, Barbara Eagar, Eric Fenelon, Colm O'Morain, Frank Allen, Huw Rolf, Frank Keane, John McDougald, Mary Martin, Paul Bowman*
Front row: *Dick Baker, John Sugars, Sheila Kenny, Nigel Kinnear, Paddy Moss, Adelaide Chairman, Helen Watson, David Mitchell, Joe Eustace*
(Arthur Ogilvie)(courtesy Adelaide Society)

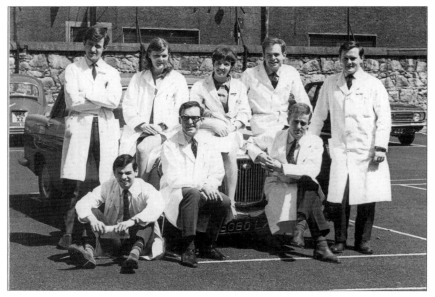

Adelaide intern staff 1968—the scanty numbers were typical. Back row: *Liam Diskin, Oonagh Brownlee, Heather Anderson, David Dorman, Hugh O'Neill* Front row: *George Borrett, Brendan Donaghy (Arthur Ogilvie) (courtesy Adelaide Society)*

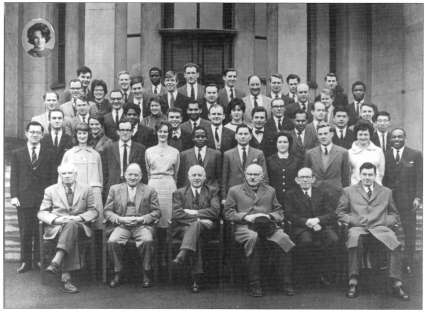

Final Year 1964 These classes had many more non-Irish students than today and many fewer women. Front row: *Prof. Jack Henry, Prof. John (J. B.) Fleming, Prof. J. Jessop, Prof. Victor Synge, Prof. Davy Torrens, Dean, Prof. Peter Gatenby*

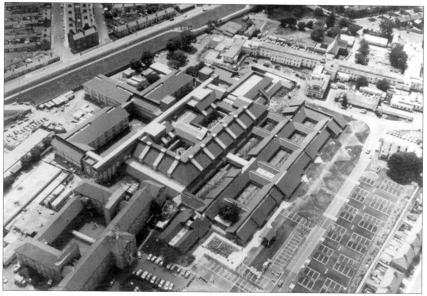

St James's in the late 1980s showing the old and the new, showing the extensive new developments and (lefthand corner) the old Hospital 3 building dating from the 19th century, still in use but soon to be demolished. (courtesy Paul O'Hare)

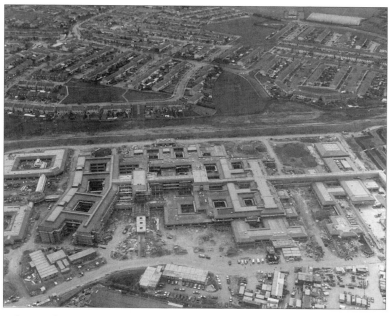

The new hospital at Tallaght in the process of construction

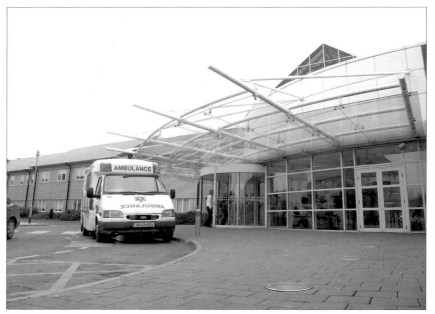

The new entrance to St James's was constructed on the site of the old Hospital 3 building and opened in 2004 (courtesy Paul O'Hare)

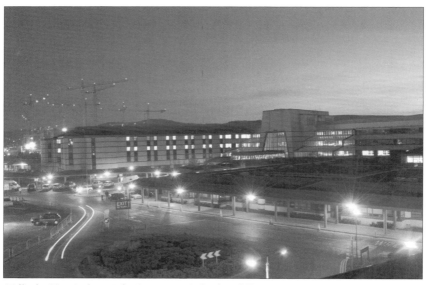

Tallaght Hospital at night (courtesy Michael Walsh)

ment of immunology which at the time was unique in the Republic. He also acted as a catalyst for the movement of Dun's, along with the other designated hospitals, to St James's by arranging for the pathology department to be moved from Trinity into the Central Pathology Laboratory building on the St James's campus in 1976.

The radiology department was run by Shan Henderson following the traditions set up by Charles McDonogh, one of the pioneers of Dublin radiology. With the arrival of Noel O'Connell 'x-ray meetings' became a prominent feature of the proceedings of the hospital, a tradition carried on by Pat Freyne in later years.

Another feature of the *modus operandi* of the hospital that was ahead of its time was the mutually collaborative use of general practitioners in the services offered to Dun's patients. In particular, GPs for many years were the backbone of the varicose vein clinics; Vincent Pippet became an expert endoscopist; Neville Boland ran an allergy clinic for many years; Norman Jackson was one of the first pure specialist dermatologists,(he was also a competitor in the Monte Carlo Rally,) while others helped in the STD clinics run by H. G. (Bunny) Ellerker and latterly by Derek Freedman and Alex Whelan (who became a world authority on immunology).

The 1970s and 1980s were a time of severe national financial austerity which led to the closure of Mercer's in 1983. The consultants were given the choice of either transferring directly to St James's or of joining Dun's for the remaining years of its existence. The younger consultants tended to opt for St James's whilst those closer to retirement came to Dun's where they were made very welcome. These included surgeons Thomas Wilson and Jack Coolican, who was also assigned to the Adelaide, and physicians J. B. (Jack) Lyons and Joe Timoney. Jack Lyons was appointed professor of medical history in the Royal College of Surgeons and his writings both before and since his time in Dun's have done much to record the evolution of medicine in Ireland.

During the 1970s the hospital acquired a reputation for postgraduate training and many graduates of both UCD and TCD, who subsequently became eminent consultants in Ireland and elsewhere, served as research fellows and non-consultant hospital doctors at Dun's.

Because the hospital had originally been built as a teaching hospital for the professors in Trinity medical school using the estate of Sir Patrick Dun, it was possible to persuade the Charitable Commissioners that since the medical school was moving to the St James's campus it would be appropriate that resources released from the sale of Dun's should be transferred to St James's. Initially, the funds derived from the sale of the nurses' home on Lower Mount Street were used to fund the construction of the Dun's research laboratories, which were sited on the roof of the Central Pathology Laboratory at St James's. These laboratories were officially opened in 1982 by Provost W. A. Watts. The associated scientific exhibition and seminar were attended by many eminent professors of clinical medicine from the United Kingdom and by representatives of the Wellcome Trust. These were the first such laboratories to be constructed on a hospital site in Ireland and as such were of enormous importance to the evolution of clinical research in this country. It is hard to remember the relative dearth of any such activity then as compared with the flourishing state of clinical academic medicine in Ireland today. The medical/legal/political battles to acquire the Dun's research laboratories were long and tedious; they were spearheaded by John Scott, professor of experimental nutrition, TCD, Dermot Hourihane, at that time dean of the medical faculty, TCD, and myself.

Subsequently, in 1987, the main buildings of Sir Patrick Dun's were sold. After considerable discussion it was decided by the governors to allocate one third of the proceeds of the sale to the Royal College of Physicians to promote postgraduate medical training, and two thirds to a new Trinity College building at St James's which would house facilities for the teaching of undergraduate medical and nursing students. Once again there were many tedious legal battles fought for these rights. There were further difficult negotiations to acquire an appropriate area on the St James's campus from the Eastern Health Board to allow the construction of the new medical school building. This story is recorded in more detail elsewhere in this book. Suffice it to say that the bulk of the revenues required for this building came from the sale of Sir Patrick Dun's, the Chester Beatty Fund in TCD, and funds specifically earmarked by the Department of Health for the construction of the nursing school.

The Dun's building had been purchased by Austin Darragh. He was a past student of the hospital and had developed a thriving private drug testing facility with contracts with leading international pharmaceutical companies. He transferred this business to the Dun's building, which he lavishly restored and redecorated. It was subsequently sold on to the Eastern Health Board for administrative offices and as such it remains today.

*A selection of the graduate alumni of Sir Patrick Dun's known to the
author*

Surgical
Bill Beesley, consultant surgeon, Tallaght Hospital
Gary Brow, consultant surgeon, Loughlinstown Hospital
Michael Fox, consultant surgeon, St Michael's Hospital
Tom Hennessy, Regius Professor of Surgery TCD (1976–98) at St James's;
  international reputation in the management of oesophageal cancer
George Patrikios, consultant surgeon, Zimbabwe and South Africa
Michael Pegum, orthopaedic surgeon, Tallaght Hospital
Robert Quill, senior lecturer and consultant surgeon, St James's
Julian Sommerville, urologist, UK
Ian Wilson, general surgeon, Kilkenny

Medical
Bernadette Carr, prominent member of the VHI administration
Gary Courtney, consultant gastroenterologist, Kilkenny Hospital
Peter Daly, Professor of Oncology TCD, at St James's, an authority on
  the molecular genetics and management of breast cancer
Con Feighery, Professor of Immunology, TCD, at St James's, and
  international expert on coeliac disease
Michael Goggins, Professor and Director of the Molecular Genetics Unit,
  Johns Hopkins Hospital, USA
Dermot Kelleher, Regius Professor of Medicine, TCD, founder of the
  Institute of Molecular Medicine at St James's
Ciaran Kelly, Professor of Gastroenterology, Harvard University Hospital,
  USA, expert on infections of the gastrointestinal tract
Deirdre Kelly, Professor and Director of the Gastrointestinal Paediatric
  Department, Birmingham University Hospital, UK, expert on
  paediatric gastroenterology, and author of the standard textbook on
  paediatric hepatology and liver transplantation
Nick Kennedy, Senior Lecturer in Human Nutrition, TCD
Michael Lucey, Professor of Medicine, Wisconsin Medical University
  Hospital, USA, and President of the American National Liver Transplant
  Society
Shaun McCann, Professor of Haematology TCD, Director of the National
  Bone Marrow for Leukaemia Unit in the Durkan Institute at St James's,
  and author of a popular undergraduate textbook on haematology
David Nunes, Consultant Gastroenterologist, Boston City Hospital, USA,
  expert on viral infections of the liver

Peter O'Connor, consultant emergency medicine physician, Mater Hospital

Christine O'Malley, Vice-President Irish Medical Organisation

Kevin Ward, consultant physician, Waterford Hospital, and director of a clinical undergraduate teaching unit of an offshore American medical school

Marjorie Young, consultant dermatologist, Tallaght Hospital, and lecturer in medical jurisprudence, TCD.

PART THREE:

THE DEVELOPMENT
OF SPECIALTY UNITS

In this section developments in many of
the specialties are recounted. Unfortunately it has not been possible to include
all specialties; among the omissions are
A&E services, ophthalmology and respiratory medicine—to mention a few.
There is also no account of psychiatric
services or the transfer of St Loman's to
Tallaght. The editor apologises for these
omissions and craves the indulgence of
the reader and members of these groups
which all play a vital role in the comprehensive services provided by St James's
and AMNCH.

13. Age-related health care

Des O'Neill

The concept of specialist care services for older people is relatively new in the Irish healthcare system but it has been embraced over the last three decades by central government.[1] *The Years Ahead*, the blueprint for the development of services for older people, was published in 1988 and adopted as government policy in 1993.[2] This specified that there should be a dedicated department of geriatric medicine in each general hospital. A dedicated service in the current successor to the FDVH is relatively recent; indeed, the Meath and the Adelaide were the last teaching hospitals in Dublin to appoint a geriatrician to their staff.

Up to that time, the hospitals were fortunate to have consultation services from the geriatricians in St James's. In the first instance these were provided by Dr J. Flanagan and subsequently by Professor Davis Coakley and Dr J. B. Walsh. The first post created was designed to incorporate sessions with St James's as an interim measure until the opening of the new hospital in Tallaght. It also incorporated sessions with the Eastern Health Board, which indicates the strong commitment to promoting a practice which prioritises the setting up and development of community services. The co-operation with both institutions has continued: weekend cover is shared with St James's and consultant input into the nursing home situated in the old Meath represents an ongoing commitment to shared care with the current successor to the Eastern Health Board.

The rationale of specialist geriatric medicine may seem unclear to lay, and indeed some medical, readers: don't all doctors look after older people? However, older people not only present with diseases that are largely specific to them (such as stroke and dementia) but these illnesses may present in atypical ways in later life: for example, a stroke can occur without weakness of an arm or leg and a heart attack can occur without chest pain. Two other issues are also important: illness may present as, or be accompanied by, loss of function such as immobility, confusion or incontinence. This implies a two-fold imperative: to discover the cause of such functional loss and to provide a care pathway that includes a strong rehabilitative component. Multiple studies have shown that the geriatric medicine model can

provide a better form of service to frail older people.³ Institutional resistance can occur, especially as a result of ageism, that form of discrimination
that refuses to acknowledge the special needs of older people. However,
such resistance was also common to the development of paediatric medicine a century ago and a strength of purpose and a critical mindset will be
crucial to the wider development of specialist medicine in Ireland.

First unit for the elderly, Meath

The first unit was based in the ground floor of west wing 1 in the Meath
and opened in August 1993. The department was fortunate to build on the
excellent medical and nursing traditions of the Meath. However, from the
point of view of the facilities it was fortunate that this was to last only five
years, as the physical setting was totally inappropriate for the care of older
people. One of the first priorities when setting up the new unit in the
Meath was the development of the multi-disciplinary team—this in the
setting of a general hospital which had only one therapist in each of the
disciplines of speech and language therapy and occupational therapy. The
staff now includes clerical/administrative support, one therapist in each of
the disciplines of physiotherapy, occupational therapy, speech and language
therapy, clinical nutrition, and a social worker. The majority of staff is
trained in specialist nursing care for older people. Currently, the unit in
Tallaght, directed by clinical nurse manager Sean O'Brien, is a training site
for the TCD Diploma in Gerontological Nursing.

The service quickly developed and was soon able to show a practice that
reflected a rehabilitative and community focus. Over the course of one
year, this 17-bedded unit referred more people to community rehabilitation services than the 350 beds of the general hospital. While the in-patient
focus was in the Meath, consultative practice was offered to the Adelaide
and developed into a weekly service. A major development was the linking
of the service with Naas and the provision of three sessions from 1995 with
Patricia McCormack. This was of particular note as it enabled the development of the first acute stroke service in Ireland, albeit catering for approximately 50 per cent of those with stroke. The background to this development was the recognition in the early 1990s that people who have had a
stroke will benefit significantly from having their care given by a specialist
with expertise in stroke and associated multi-disciplinary team. With the
co-operation of the departments of gastroenterology and cardiology and
Professor G. Tomkin, the service quickly proved its worth, reducing the
inpatient mortality from 15 per cent to 9 per cent in a matter of years.⁴

The team was also involved in the design and commissioning of the purpose-built unit in the new hospital in Tallaght and was happy to move to it in June 1998. This necessitated a temporary siting of the diabetic service which was resolved when the diabetic day care unit was opened in May 2002.

What's in a name?

Although the specialists involved are still called geriatricians, the team was aware that many older people are unhappy with the label 'geriatric' largely as a result of ageist abuse of the term. Therefore, as a result of a poll which explored the preferences of a group of older people who were service users, a preference was distinguished for the title of Age-related Health Care. This has been the name of the department since this time. With the move into the new hospital, it was felt that the name of the unit, representing the last major development in the Meath, should reflect this and with the blessing of the Stokes family, it was named the William Stokes Unit. As the practice and research in the unit has a strong neurosciences orientation, we wished to reflect this as well and we are happy that a link has developed with the Mitchell family who were so central to the recording of the history of the Adelaide. The Mitchell family presented a specially commissioned piece of garden furniture for the garden courtyard, and it is hoped that the garden will be named the Mitchell Garden.

Further developments

The psychiatry of later life service based at Tallaght began in November 1998 under the direction of Greg Swanwick with a psychiatric liaison service to those over 65 years of age admitted to the hospital. The team has been expanded to include two non-consultant hospital doctors, two community mental health nurses, a social worker, and an occupational therapist. Unfortunately, the six-bed inpatient unit has yet to be commissioned; however, a day-hospital in Sheaf House next to the hospital opened at the end of 2003. In addition to the liaison service, a community based service with domiciliary assessments and day-hospital support is now available to older people with new onset mental health problems who live within the catchment area. The focus for research has been post-stroke depression in collaboration with age-related health care. This work has been supported by a grant from the Meath Foundation and has led to presentations at international meetings and the award to Leona Judge of the poster medal at the All-Ireland Institute of Psychiatry meeting in 2003.

Research and policy—national

The unit has been fortunate to make a significant contribution to national, European and international gerontology in a relatively short period of time. Research has been a key priority of the department since its inception and every profession within the multi-disciplinary team has contributed to research projects that have been presented at national and international levels. During the life of the National Scientific Meeting of the Royal College of Physicians, the William Stokes Unit had the highest number of research presentations from any department of geriatric medicine in Ireland. It has also had a high profile at the Irish Gerontological Society since 1994; I am serving as Secretary to the Society at the time of writing. The unit successfully hosted the Irish Gerontological Society Annual Scientific Meeting in 2003, and the department secretary, Marian Hughes, was instrumental in ensuring that this was very well organised, with simultaneous publication of the abstracts in the *Irish Journal of Medical Science* for the first time in the history of the Society.

I was also the Medical Director of the Alzheimer Society of Ireland from 1993 to 2004 and chaired the Council on Stroke of the Irish Heart Foundation. This has resulted in the production of the first national report on the development of stroke services in Ireland which has been instrumental in promoting developments in this area.[5] The unit has also received an €800,000 grant from the Irish Health Research Board (in conjunction with the Royal College of Surgeons in Ireland and Queen's University, Belfast) for research on healthy ageing, and in particular on how older people adapt to stroke. Another area of expertise has been the difficult area of elder abuse; I chaired the Irish government's working group on elder abuse and the report was adopted as government policy immediately after its publication.[6] It resulted in the immediate release of €800,000 of revenue by the government. I also chair the national implementation group to ensure that this government policy is implemented. The unit has also had the first website for gerontology and geriatric medicine in Ireland, active since 1996. The neurosciences profile has resulted in neurosciences and ageing being recognised by the hospital as one of the four main pillars of research activity. Monthly research seminars are held and the unit is linked with Trinity College Institute of Neurosciences (www.tcd.ie/Neuroscience).

Research and policy—European

As a founder member and representative of both the Geriatric Medicine Section of the European Union of Medical Specialists and the European

Union Geriatric Medical Society I formulated a joint response to the United Nations 2nd Declaration on Ageing.[7] A key element of responding to the opportunities and challenges of an ageing society is the training of an adequate number of professionals with sensitisation and expertise in gerontology. A further involvement has been with a European initiative to build capacity in gerontology at a postgraduate level. This has been funded by the Public Health section of the European Commission (DG V), in the first instance as a developmental project and secondly as a European Masters degree. The William Stokes Unit hosted a module of this degree in the summer of 2004, the first William Stokes Summer School in Ageing and Health. This brought leaders in Irish gerontology together with other European experts. The proceedings will be published as an update in Irish gerontology.

Research and policy—international

One of the key research interests of the department has been transportation and ageing, and in particular the medical aspects of fitness to drive. A number of international panels and working groups, including the OECD, the US Transportation Research Board and the World Health Organisation are concerned wih this issue, and I participate in their activities, sitting on the OECD editorial panel for their report on ageing and transport,[8] on a panel of the OECD and the Massachusetts Institute of Technology looking at technology, ageing and transport (http://web.mit.edu/ctl/www/research/utc/re_utc-symposium.htm) and on the Committee for Safe Mobility for Older People of the US Transportation Research Board which is involved in the preparation of a US government report on transportation in an ageing society[9] as well as the 2004 WHO report on traffic safety.[10]

The future

While the unit has gained a national and international profile, our core clinical practice relates to the provision of assessment, rehabilitation and health promotional services for the hospital's catchment area. The challenge for the future lies not only in the increasing sophistication and depth of needs of older people but also in the rapid expansion in the ageing population that we serve. Currently there are 17,000 people over 65 in the catchment area; there are another 17,000 in the 55–65 age group, representing a major augmentation in demand. Plans have been made with the Eastern Regional Health Authority to expand the services but this process is slow. A post promised by the Department of Health in 1999 only finally materialised in 2004! This post will be linked with Peamount, in the expectation of developing extended-care facilities, respite care and low-grade rehabilitation. We believe that our emphasis on teamwork, education and research will help us to adapt and respond creatively to the increasing pressures that the hospital will face in the future.

References

[1] O'Neill, D., O'Keeffe, S. 'Health care for older people in Ireland'. *J Am Geriatr Soc* 2003 Sep; 51(9):1280–6.

[2] Working Group on Services for Older People *The Years Ahead* Dublin: Government Publications, 1988.

[3] O'Neill, D., Hastie, I., Williams, B. 'Developing specialist healthcare for older people: a challenge for the European Union'. *J Nutrition, Health and Ageing* 2004, 8, 109–115.

[4] Collins, D. R., McConaghy, D., McMahon, A., Howard, D., O'Neill, D., McCormack, P. 'An Acute Stroke Service: Potential to Improve Patient Outcome Without Increasing Length of Stay'. *Ir Med J* 2000, 93, 247.

[5] *Towards Excellence in Stroke Care* Council on Stroke, IHF, 2001.

[6] Working Group on Elder Abuse, 1999–2002 *Protecting Our Future* Dublin: Government Publications 2002.

[7] O'Neill and O'Keeffe *op. cit.*

[8] OECD Working Group, ERS4, on Ageing and Transport *Ageing and Transport: Mobility Needs and Safety Issues* OECD, 2002.

[9] O'Neill, D., Dobbs, B. 'Medical aspects of fitness to drive'. In Transportation Research Board. *Transportation and an Ageing Society: A Decade of Experience.* Washington (in press).

[10] Hakamies-Blomqvist, L., O'Neill, D. 'Older people and road traffic injury'. In Peden, M., Scurfield, R., Sleet, D., Mohan, D., Hyder, A. H., Jarawan, E., Mathers, C. (eds.), *World Report on Road Traffic Injury Prevention* Geneva: WHO, 2004, p 47.

14. Anaesthesia

Joseph Galvin

Many of the Federated Dublin Voluntary Hospitals were built in the 18th century and were considered to be obsolete by modern standards in 1968. The seven hospitals that formed the Federation in 1961 were all on the south side of the Liffey and consisted of:

	Beds
Dr Steevens'	203
Meath	282
Adelaide	154
Mercer's	124
National Children's Hospital	91
Baggot Street	193
Sir Patrick Dun's	168
Total	*1,215*

The Federated Dublin Voluntary Hospitals Group was formed by agreement among the seven hospitals, passed by an Act of Parliament in July 1961. The object of forming the group was to build a new hospital on the west side of Dublin to which all seven hospitals were expected to move. There were many objections to closing so many hospitals in the centre of Dublin and moving them to the western suburb. City councillors and politicians and public bodies joined in the protest.

The next proposed location for the new hospital was the Sir Patrick Dun's site, between Grand Canal Street and Lower Mount Street—it was considered ideal and near Trinity College. Mr George Fegan, surgeon at Sir Patrick Dun's, was a leading force in the acquisition by the Federation of many properties surrounding the site, with the agreement of the Department of Health.

Plans were drawn up for a 750-bed hospital on the site. Planning permission was sought, expectations were high. It seemed an ideal location in those days, the mid 1960s, so near the centre of the city and on the site of one of the former hospitals. Dismay descended on the group when the news reached us that Dublin Corporation refused planning permission on the grounds that they intended to run a new road through the site! To this day, no road has been built.

The search continued for another site, and the next to be considered was on Mespil Road off Leeson Street where Tullamaine, a residential house and junior school belonging to Wesley College, was considered ideal. Efforts were made to acquire the site but it was discovered that Mr P. V. Doyle had bought it for a new hotel—the Burlington.

Efforts continued and this time the Clonskeagh Fever Hospital came under scrutiny. When negotiations began to acquire the site, the Department of Health said it was not a good idea since it was so near the planned new St Vincent's on Merrion Road.

The Department of Health, under Minister for Health Sean Flanagan, set up a consultative council, chaired by Professor Patrick FitzGerald, with the following terms of reference:

> To examine the position in regard to general hospital in-patient and out-patient services in the state, and to report and outline on the future organisation, extent and location of these services, taking into account the changing pattern of demand, the impact of developing specialisation, and the introduction of new techniques, so as to secure, with due regard to the national resources, that the public was provided in the most effective way, with the best possible services.

The first meeting of the council was held on 20 November 1967; its report, *Outline of the Future Hospital System,* was published in June 1968. The following are some of the council's findings:

(1) Public patients comprised about 90 per cent of the public hospitals, and most of the consultant medical staff of the voluntary hospital were unsalaried and were appointed on the traditional basis of having a specified number of beds allocated to them.

(2) Certain recommendations were made on the size of hospitals: a hospital based on a population of 120,000 people should have at least 300 beds.

(3) Major hospitals should be regional hospitals with 800 beds and should be referral centres, with more specialisation.

(4) The minimum consultant staffing of a general hospital should be:

    3 physicians
    3 surgeons
    3 anaesthetists
    2 obstetrician-gynaecologists
    2 radiologists
    2 pathologists

(5) Dublin should have two regional hospitals and two general hospitals.

(6) It was also recommended that 'All existing hospital consultants be approved and invited to enter into contracts with the Regional board on terms which would take into consideration their present contracts, or terms of appointment, either formal or implied, without detriment to the position of any existing consultants.'

As time went on, meetings were held, and councillors and TDs protested against the local hospitals being closed.

In Dublin, instead of two regional hospitals and two general hospitals, agreement was reached on six hospitals, three on the north side—Beaumont, the Mater and Blanchardstown—and three on the south side—St Vincent's, St James's and Tallaght. The closing of certain county hospitals is still causing great problems.

Plans were made for the development of St Kevin's and a London firm of architects was instructed to draw up plans. Today St James's, as it is now called, is the largest and one of the best equipped hospital in the country. It has about 12 operating theatres, post-operative recovery rooms, intensive care units, and a cardiac intensive care unit.

Many of the wards are called after certain surgeons e.g. Keith Shaw, or after hospitals like Dun's, Mercer's etc.

The Adelaide, Meath and National Children's Hospital was planned for Tallaght in the 1980s and all members of the staff of the three hospitals and hospital boards put forward ideas. Special meetings were held at the National Children's Hospital on Saturday mornings so that all the units had their needs met. But despite the careful planning some of the theatres were too small, especially the orthopaedic theatre, and alterations had to be made.

From the anaesthetist's point of view the induction rooms, recovery areas and intensive care units attached to the theatres are excellent.

The hospital building has a beautiful modern design with a wide entrance hail with fountains and flower beds, lifts to every floor, and excellent information centres in the main hall, a very modern radiological department and a large accident and emergency centre. It serves a large catchment area—Kildare, Carlow, Wicklow and west Dublin.

These two centres, St James's and the Adelaide, Meath and National Children's Hospital at Tallaght, are a great asset to Trinity for teaching and a wonderful asset to our city of Dublin.

The move of staff to the new hospitals was carefully planned. From 1961 all new consultant appointments were made by the Federated Dublin Voluntary Hospitals so that most of the consultants could not object to being moved and were on equal terms. Within the hospitals, staff were encouraged to form surgical, medical and anaesthetic units.

The development of the accident and emergency hospitals in Dublin in 1967 encouraged co-operation within the Group. The accident service developed in Dublin following calls for a better service at night from 6 p.m. to 9 a.m. and at weekends from 6 p.m. on Friday to 9 a.m. on Monday. Dr Steevens' and the Meath were the two Federated Hospitals selected.

The Mater, Jervis Street and St Vincent's also shared duty. It started with two nights on and two nights off call and every second weekend. Extra junior staff in the form of registrars were provided by the Department of Health to ensure that each hospital was covered while on duty with anaesthetic and surgical and medical staff.

The service worked well until the bombing started in Dublin between 1968 and 1974. The bombing at the quay outside Liberty Hall took place about 6.30 one evening. We at the Meath were not on call but got about 30 cases, mainly glass injuries to the face and hands. Only two cases had to go to theatre that night but several cases were admitted.

The worst bombing was in 1974. It occurred at 5.30 pm. There were three separate incidents—Parnell Street, North Earl Street and South Leinster Street, near the Moyne Institute in Trinity College.

The Meath and Jervis Street were on call, but the ambulances could not get to the Meath due to congestion in the city. The Parnell Street bomb victims went to the Mater mainly, but some patients were treated at the Rotunda, one male patient being admitted there. Jervis Street was inundated with cases. Brandon Stephens from the Meath travelled to Jervis Street to give a hand and he later described the scene: 'It was like a battlefield, bodies everywhere.'

The victims of the South Leinster Street bombing were taken to Sir Patrick Dun's which was not on call. The hospital staff, like all the Dublin hospitals that night, reported for duty to give a hand.

The staff of the Meath, all the consultants and junior staff off duty reported for duty and stayed most of the night. Matron Betty O'Dwyer opened the canteen and served refreshments. It was a dreadful night. Following the confusion and congestion of traffic on the night of the car bombs in Dublin the Department of Health opened more hospitals for emergency services. Now the six hospitals in Dublin provide 24 hour, 7 days per week accident and emergency services.

Development of anaesthethics

From the anaesthetist's point of view it is interesting to note that the first consultant-anaesthetist in Dublin was appointed to Dr Steevens' Hospital in 1899—Percy Kirkpatrick. He was 30 years of age, and did not retire until he was in his 80s.

The first recorded anaesthetic was given in the Richmond by Dr McDonald, a surgeon, on 12 October 1846, within months of the first ether anaesthetic given by Morton in Boston in 1846, at the Massachusetts Hospital. Eleven days earlier Lister had given an ether anaesthetic in Edinburgh.

The Federation's department of anaesthetics gradually developed from 1968 onwards and helped to unite all the consultants in anaesthesia with regular monthly meetings held at Sir Patrick Dun's. Having one department of anaesthetics within the group facilitated the move of anaesthetists and junior staff to St James's and Tallaght.

Memories go back to 1951 when the Meath had a beautiful tree-lined avenue, with tennis courts on the left of the avenue as you entered; Bert Keating, the head porter, lived in a cottage on the right as you entered. Bert was always in the front hall of the hospital, dressed in dark blue livery, and red waistcoat with brass buttons. He would sound the gong when a consultant came in the morning, or any time of the day. The gong could be heard all over the hospital, everyone was then on tenter-hooks! When Bert Keating died he was never replaced. He knew everything about the place and anywhere any consultant could be contacted any time of the day.

The main boardroom, situated on the left of the main hall, was the meeting room for all consultants every morning. Coffee was served from 10.30 a.m. onwards, lunch was served from 1 p.m. Cecil Robinson was Secretary of the Medical Board and could always be contacted every morning in the boardroom. He kept a detailed note on every undergraduate student, and would send out notes to students who had not paid their fee for the year for attending the hospital tuition. Dr Robinson maintained discipline in the hospital and investigated every complaint that was made against a student or a nurse or a doctor. He organised the annual dinner at the Kildare Street Club every year. Dr Robinson died in 1974 and for years his son, Derek Robinson, organised the dinner, which was later moved to the University Club on St Stephen's Green.

Another memory of the early 1950s is that only the consultants had cars, and they had a parking place opposite the main steps to the hospital. There were only about ten cars parked there. Further up outside the west wing you could see 50 to 80 bicycles piled up against the wall, depending whose clinic was on that morning.

It was not unusual in the 1950s to have more than one surgeon per theatre. In the main section of the Meath Hospital there was a major theatre and a minor theatre. The major theatre was on the first floor above the hall—it was very large. As a student one would go occasionally to watch a surgeon operate—nearly always the one who had given the clinic that morning. He would say at the end of the clinic, 'If you would like to see me operate, come to theatre, and put on a gown and mask.'

The theatre often had three operations going on at the same time. I remember one morning Mr T. J. D. Lane operating in one corner, Mr Montgomery in the centre, and Mr Stokes operating in another corner. It was a large theatre, that could accommodate them. There were three anaesthetists, Silver Deane-Oliver, Bertie Wilson and Maureen Murphy. The patients were put asleep in a small anaesthetic room before entering the theatre.

The washing area for the surgeon and his assistant was in the theatre, at a large window with a good view of the grounds below. Outside the theatre, there was a wash-up room for instruments, next door to that room was a little tea-room for nursing staff. Upstairs there was the 'bird's nest' for the surgical staff etc.

The theatre in those days had its own autoclave which sterilised all the instruments and anaesthetic equipment; needles and syringes were washed and boiled. Later this autoclave was replaced by a central sterilising unit in the hospital and disposable syringes and needles were introduced about 1968.

The minor theatre on the ground floor was used on Mondays and Thursdays for ENT and on Wednesdays and Fridays for gynaecology. This theatre was independent of the major theatre. It was run by Sister Lyons who was also sister to the male and female ward on the same landing—generally known as 'the accident landing'.

The main hall and entrance to the hospital was large and square, with beautiful Italian tiles, with the hospital crest in the centre, and statues of Graves and Stokes. On the right side of the hall as you entered, there was a large fire grate; its warming fire was very welcoming as you entered the building. This was later replaced by a gas fire, as were the fire grates in other parts of the building.

It was not unusual in the earlier part of the 19th century to have operating rooms attached to surgical wards, both here and in Britain. Today, they are all arranged in theatre suites, with anaesthetic rooms, recovery areas, and intensive care units.

The west wing was known as 'the fever wing' but in the 1950s it mainly had TB and medical cases which were looked after by Brendan O'Brien and Brian Mayne.

Gradually the site was built on. When the genitourinary wing was built and opened in 1955, the whole picture changed. It was a very modern unit with twin theatres, and a smaller theatre for minor operations, and a recovery area—all due to the ideas and planning of T. J. D. Lane. The unit became world-renowned, and like the Rotunda attracted doctors from many parts of the world. Beside the new unit was a new nurses' home with lecture theatres, reception room and recreation room for the nurses. It was completed in 1955 and opened with a big party. Prefabs started to appear and the medical professorial unit at the back of the west wing for Trinity College where Professor Gatenby held weekly teaching meetings on a Tuesday morning. This was a great asset to the hospital and he developed many specialised medical units within the hospital.

A shortage of space led to more prefabs for the physiotherapy unit and gradually the site was overdeveloped. One of the last buildings to be developed was the administration red building on the right of the avenue, a gift from two Board members.

In the late 1960s, the hospital was able to get extra space at the old TB clinic at the far end of the grounds behind the west wing, and it was used for extra clinics.

Another great development in the 1980s was that of the gastrointestinal unit under the direction of Colm O'Morain.

Unit after unit appeared over the years. Pathology was so big it was shared by the Federated Group. The radiology department grew and grew. In the 1950s the surgeons mostly read their own x-rays but that changed when Sholto Douglas was appointed, followed by Gerry Hurley in the late 1970s, and later Noel O'Connell, from Baggot Street and Dun's, transferred to the Meath.

To accommodate the orthopaedic unit from Steevens' in the 1980s, extra theatres had to be built at the Meath. Some of the staff from Steevens' joined the Meath, namely John McElwain and David FitzPatrick, orthopaedic surgeons, and John Gately, radiologist.

Intensive care units gradually developed in the 1960s at the Adelaide, Meath, Steevens' and Baggot Street. Ward nurses in rotation spent time in the units. Later, special nurses were allocated and trained in intensive care nursing. A cardiac unit was also developed in the west wing. This was one of the areas in which co-operation between the Adelaide and the Meath was to become closer.

One of the best units in the Federated Group was designed for the Meath by Peter Morck, funded by the Chester Beatty Fund in the early 1980s. It was near the theatre area—a large, bright unit, fully equipped and well maintained.

Nearly all the hospitals in the Group had intensive care units. The Adelaide ICU was run by Sheila Kenny, the unit in Baggot Street (the chest unit for Keith Shaw) was run by David Hogan, in Steevens' by Eddie Delaney, and in Dun's by John Goodbody. Sheila Kenny was a pioneer in many areas as well as intensive care. One of these was one of the first mechanical ventilators which she developed with Mike Lewis, one of her registrars; it was often used for long periods for postoperative ventilation. She also developed hypotension techniques and was one of those instrumental in the establishment of the Faculty of Anaesthetists in the Royal College of Surgeons in Ireland.

The establishment of the British National Health Service in 1948 by Aneurin Bevan did much to improve health and medical treatment and the development of special units and intensive care in new hospitals. Doctors who had served in the 1939–45 war came home to Britain and started research units at Oxford, London, Cardiff, Manchester, Liverpool, Glasgow, Edinburgh and Belfast.

Many of the Dublin anaesthetists formed the Dublin Anaesthetists Travelling Club. Visits were made to units in Britain and Europe— Paris, Stockholm, Madrid, Copenhagen, and also to the US—Stanford University, Seattle and Massachusetts General Hospital, Boston.

The visit to Madrid coincided with the great contaminated oil disaster in the late 1970s when patients were poisoned with commercial oil used for cooking. They developed paralysis of the muscles with severe wasting. About 100 were on ventilators throughout Madrid, and many more never recovered. It reminded many of us of the polio disaster that hit Ireland in the 1950s when large numbers of patients developed respiratory paralysis. They were mainly treated in Cherry Orchard on ventilators—the Radcliffe ventilator. Some patients never came off the ventilator; one survived for nine years. Great credit was due to care given by Desmond Gaffney from the Peamount thoracic unit and the Richmond Hospital. Dr Gaffney later transferred to the Regional Hospital in Cork as consultant anaesthetist.

To get money for new equipment was almost impossible in the 1960s and 1970s, but thanks to the various committees, especially the Ladies' Committee at the Meath, running various functions with the help of the nursing staff and Matron, money was raised.

There are many consultant names I have not mentioned. They were the hard-working surgeons and physicians. To do justice to the various surgeons, physicians, anaesthetists, nephrologists and radiologists would require a much larger paper.

One physician I must mention is Cyril Murphy, physician in the 1950s at the Meath. He was very keen on medical students observing everything. He used to give a clinic on examination of the urine—all the different colours and tastes. In those days, each ward had its own laboratory outside the ward, consisting of an examination bench, where urine, blood and specimens were examined.

Dr Murphy would hold up some urine in a beaker, he would dip his index finger into the beaker, then taste it on his tongue, saying, 'It is sweet, it must have sugar in it.' He would then get the students to do likewise.

Students would all dip their fingers in the urine, place it on their tongues, and spit it out saying it was horrible; to which Dr Murphy would reply: 'If you were watching and observing me you would have noticed I put my index finger in the urine, but my middle finger on my tongue.'

Dr Murphy's wife was a consultant anaesthetist at the hospital and when Cyril died she resigned and went to India where she developed a large teaching hospital.

During the early 1950s all medical schools and hospitals were inspected by American assessors. When one consultant physician was asked where was the post mortem room he replied: 'I don't know—none of my patients ever go there!'

There are a lot of old memories of the Dublin hospitals. Fortunately many of the older members who had spent 25 or so years retired before 'the move' came.

15. Cardiac services

Gerry Gearty

Cardiology has a long and honourable tradition in the Federated Hospitals. Indeed William Stokes (of the Meath, 1804–87) is rightly considered the father of Irish cardiology. His textbook *Diseases of the Heart and Aorta* (1854) was a quite remarkable contribution to the literature of the day. Nevertheless the common cardiac problems were within the comfortable competence of the general physician till around the mid 1950s.

The Irish Cardiac Society was established by P. T. O'Farrell, (St Vincent's) in 1949. Founder members from the Federated Group included B. Mayne (Meath), R. E. Steen (National Children's Hospital), V. M. Synge (Baggot Street), J. A. Wallace (Sir Patrick Dun's), J. Lewis (Mercer's) and later, R. S. W. Baker (Adelaide) and B. Pringle (Dr Steevens'). Brian Mayne was first secretary of the society and his meticulous scripts adorn and endure in the minutes of this body.

The 1940s were exciting times. The chest surgeons had discovered the heart and these adventurous pioneers were repairing congenital defects and attacking stenotic valves. Murmur markers were not enough. Specialist investigations were required to provide the road maps to define precise anatomy, pathology and haemodynamics. The specialist cardiologist emerged to meet this demand.

Robert Wilson, in his reminiscences published on the occasion of the 150th anniversary of Baggot Street (1832–1972), recorded the birth of cardiology there.

Terence Chapman (assistant physician, 1954) was full of new ideas. Through his imagination, initiative and energy the cardiopulmonary departments were started. 'We need a pulmonary surgeon. Shaw is very good, the Board should invite him to join us.' Keith Shaw, who had recently completed his specialist training in London was appointed as chest surgeon in 1958.

Robert Wilson, Terence Chapman and Keith Shaw visited Brussels to attend the World Congress of Cardiology in 1958. They chose an NEP six channel photographic recorder to monitor and record the ECG and pressure patterns during cardiac catheterisation. At Baggot Street a large basement room became available with the opening of the new outpatients' complex and accident department on Haddington Road. This area became the cardiopulmonary unit. Keith Shaw found an abandoned x-ray screening table at Blanchardstown, borrowed a Shonander split film angiogram unit, added an oximeter and other odds and ends, and we were ready for action.

Carmel Lynch was the sister-in-charge, Columba Wrenn chief radiographer and Patricia Clifton first secretary. Charles O'Neill conducted the electronic orchestra.

Rory Childers, subsequently professor at Chicago, was our first cardiac specialist. The unit was officially opened by Walter Sommerville, a TCD graduate and then a leading London cardiologist, on 11 May 1959.

With the passage of the Hospital Federation and Amalgamation Bill (1961), Central Council assumed control of all consultant staff in the Federated Group. A cardiologist assigned to Baggot Street was the first appointment under this new regime.

The surgical dimension

Keith Shaw had tasted the excitement of heart work in London and was keen to develop this field. The records of the Irish Cardiac Society indicate that T. C. G. O'Connell (St Vincent's), E. O'Malley (Mater), and Maurice Hickey were reporting their experiences in repairing congenital heart lesions in June 1950 and March 1955.

Robert Steen already had a special clinic for congenital heart disease at the National Children's Hospital, with a growing surgical waiting list. Soon PDA ligation, resection of aortic coarctation, pulmonary valvotomy and closure atrial septal defect featured regularly on operative lists, as did the dramatic Blalock Taussig shunt turning blue babies (Fallots tetralogy) pink by diverting left subclavian artery blood flow into the left main pulmonary artery. Many of these procedures were carried out using induced hypothermia techniques developed by Sheila Kenny. Acute rheumatic fever was still common so that its unpleasant cardiac consequences, particularly mitral stenosis, demanded attention. This latter problem was treated by closed mitral valvotomy with index finger snared in left atrial appendage and a Tubbs dilator introduced via the apex of the left ventricle guided into the narrowed mitral orifice to split the fused cusps. This tricky procedure produced excellent results in expert hands. I remember one such case in a pregnant women with pulmonary oedema where the procedure was carried out, skin to skin in 40 minutes: Keith Shaw, of course.

It was now becoming clear that open heart surgery would be required for many complex congenital defects and valve replacement. Thus a system of cardiopulmonary bypass was required. The many technical challenges posed by this advance were already being addressed by Shaw and his research team from the animal lab. David Hogan supervised the anaesthetic aspect, Cliff Dawson, our chief laboratory technician, developed perfusion techniques and Charles O'Neill was in charge of electronic development.

Translating experimental routines into clinical practice requires time and space. Our twin theatres were fully booked but Saturday morning was free! Open heart surgery then soon became a weekly feature. Intensive care facilities were non existent so that the theatre area became the ICU for the weekend. A strict rule was that we had to be out before 8 a.m. on Monday! Our first series, 28 patients, including six complete repairs of Fallots tetralogy, were reported at the Irish Cardiac Society on 5 March, 1969.

With limited room for expansion and increasing demand accentuated by the perfection of valve replacement and the emergence of vein graft surgery, surgical services were now under considerable pressure. This, of course, was a national problem. Keith Shaw and Eoin O'Malley proposed a national open heart unit, an idea fully supported by the Department of Health leading to the setting up of such a unit in the Mater in November 1971. The first report from this joint unit was presented to the Irish Cardiac Society on 10 April, 1974. This listed 277 open heart procedures mitral aortic and tricuspid valve replacements and 66 complex congenital defects.

The emergence of intensive coronary care

During my registrar years (1953–63) heart attack was managed on the acute medical service (oxygen, morphia and prolonged immobility). Global hospital mortality ranged from 30 to 35 per cent with substantial death rates prior to hospital admission. Recorded mechanisms of death were obscure: 'heart failure', 'this heart was too good to die'. ECG monitoring eventually demonstrated the critical role of ventricular fibrillation (VF). Animal work had described effective open chest electrical defibrillation and this was extended to human cases. External DC shock was successfully applied to humans but it was not until effective CPR, closed chest cardiac massage and ventilation was developed that a practical system of VF management evolved.

This led to the rapid development of effective intensive coronary care. In 1965 Meltzer published his manual for nurses highlighting the essential central role of the specialist nurse in the coronary care unit.

The concept of modern coronary care was introduced to Dublin at a mass meeting at St Vincent's Hospital on St Stephen's Green, organised by the Irish Heart Foundation on 20 October, 1967 and addressed by Desmond Julian. This stimulated great activity. Everybody naturally wanted a coronary care unit. Buying a defibrillator, now essential in all acute hospitals, and ECG monitors was straightforward enough. However, ensuring adequate trained staff at all times proved difficult.

The Federated Group was facilitated by special courses for nurses at Baggot Street, a scheme subsequently adapted and developed by the Heart Foundation. Soon efficient units were functioning at Baggot Street and the Meath (Brian Mayne and W. Fennell) and the other Federated Hospitals had somewhat smaller multi purpose units dealing also with medical intensive care and post-operative care.

Mobile intensive care

Our colleagues at the Royal Victoria Hospital Belfast, Pantridge and Geddes, extended the coronary care unit concept to address early mortality prior to hospital admission. Their rapidly available, appropriately equipped, medically staffed ambulance units made an important impact on survival figures, confirming the central critical role of ventricular fibrillation and extending widely our knowledge of events during the critical early hours of heart attack. This idea held widespread appeal but general application of the plan proved difficult, particularly with regard to medical staffing.

In co-operation with the Heart Foundation and Noel Gleeson of the Stillorgan Ambulance Service, we developed a system of rapid response staffed by specially trained ambulance personnel backed by a rota system of CCU beds in the south city. This innovative approach proved valuable and was reported in the *British Medical Journal* in 1971.

Coronary artery surgery

Surgical attempts to improve obstructive coronary artery disease advanced spectacularly with Favaloros vein graft techniques. Now accurate definition of coronary anatomy became essential. Sones had introduced coronary angiography via brachial arteriotomy. However, Judkins' femoral artery approach with pre-formed catheters was soon preferred. Following a month in London, courtesy of the WHO, at the Royal Hammersmith and King's College Hospital, coronary angiography was introduced at Baggot Street in 1972 and vein graft surgery commenced at the national unit.

PTCA—percutaneous transluminal coronary angioplasty

Andreas Grunzig reported his successful development of coronary angioplasty, balloon dilation of obstructive coronary lesions. This exciting advance expanded rapidly aided by his week-long tutorial and live demonstrations, initially at Zurich and soon at his new department in Emory University, Atlanta.

Following a most rewarding month I spent in Atlanta, (April 1982) percutaneous transluminal coronary angioplasty was introduced at Baggot Street later that year. The work built up rapidly extending soon into unstable coronary situations and was the basis of many reports and publications such as a paper in the *British Heart Journal* IN 1986—'PICA in unstable angina comparisons with stable angina'.

The highlights of the decades which dominated our workload were undoubtedly intensive coronary care, mobile care, coronary angiography and PICA. Other exciting developments along the way included cardiac pacing, a most rewarding relatively minor procedure, Rashkind atrial septostomy for infants with transposition of the great vessels, who arrived in their incubators from the Rotunda Hospital, and DC cardioversion for atrial fibrillation and flutter.

The emergence of echocardiography was a major advance and greatly helped by Noel Cahill's Chicago acquired expertise. Our flirtation with aortic valvuloplasty was short lived.

Much of the burden was carried by our junior staff, whom I recall with gratitude and affection—Pat Moloney, Noel Cahill, John Irwin, Peter Quigley, David Gilligan and Paul Geuret. I hope they remember our annual soirée at the Beaufield Mews.

Consultant associations increased over the years with the appointment of Brian Maurer, Ian Graham and Michael Walsh.

Saturday mornings were devoted to teaching following the example of Brian Mayne at the Meath and encouraged by the success of Edward Martin's 9 a.m. neurology sessions at the Adelaide. There was the extra incentive of morning coffee courtesy of Nelly Stewart at 10.30 a.m. followed by case and data evaluation till noon and then informal data review for about an hour.

Transfer of services to St James's Hospital

Baggot Street closed as an acute hospital facility in December 1988. We joined our Baggot Street, Sir Patrick Dun's and Mercer's colleagues in the new St James's. A traumatic experience, perhaps, but nevertheless remarkably smooth and gentle since we had been working harmoniously as colleagues for many years. It has been a great joy to experience the first-rate expansion of laboratory and coronary care unit facilities there in recent years, particularly the development of open heart surgery—appropriately a lasting memorial to the wonderful work of Keith Shaw.

Research presentations/publications

Here is a selection of the more interesting papers.

(1970) 'Nutritional and epidemiologic factors related to heart disease'. (The Ireland Boston Diet Heart Study) *World Review Nutr Diet* 12: 1-42.

(1971) 'Pre-hospital Coronary Care Service'. Gearty G. F., Hickey N., Bourke S. J., Mulcahy R. *BMJ* 3: 33.

(1981) 'Urgent surgical intervention in unstable angina'. Quigley P., Gearty G. E., Shaw K. M. *Journal Irish Medical Association* 74: 360.

(1982) 'Q fever endocarditis'. Tobin M. J., Cahill N., Gearty G. et al. *American Journal of Medicine* 72: 396-400.

(1982) 'Partial ideal bypass in familiar hypercholesterolaemia'. Kelly D., Lane D., Gearty et al. *Irish Journal of Medical Science* 343-7.

(1986) 'PICA in unstable angina'. Quigley P., Erwin J., Gearty G. E. *British Heart Journal* 55: 227.

(1988) 'Balloon aortic valvuloplasty'. Moore D., McDonald K., Gearty G. *Irish Journal of Medical Science* 272.

16. Cardiology

Ian Graham

Developments in cardiology during the 20th century were mirrored by developments in the Federated Dublin Voluntary Hospitals. While heart failure, rheumatic valvular disease and the main congenital heart diseases were well described by the 1920s, it was only from then on that the magnitude of the problem of coronary heart disease began to be appreciated. Up to the 1950s, treatments were essentially palliative. By the 1970s, the concept of acute coronary care had been developed, as well as the idea of early mobilisation of subjects recovering from myocardial infarction. From spending six weeks in bed, it became apparent that a policy of early mobilisation and discharge within about a week was not only realistic but beneficial. The development of coronary arteriography and coronary artery bypass surgery from the 1970s onwards transformed the management of coronary artery disease; the aetiology and management of cardiac rhythm disturbances were elucidated, and pacemaker treatment became an everyday occurrence by the 1970s.

From the Second World War onwards, it became apparent that the atherosclerosis underlying coronary disease was not necessarily an inevitable occurrence. Meticulous epidemiology indicated that most atherosclerosis is environmental in origin, although with much of the individual variation being genetically determined. It is now clear that atherosclerosis can be prevented, or at least deferred, in most people.

Until the 1970s, most cardiology services were delivered by physicians with a special interest in the field. Major contributors included Professor V. Synge and G. Gearty in Baggot Street, Dr R. Kirker in Sir Patrick Dun's, Professor Peter Gatenby in Dr Steevens', Robert Steen in the National Children's Hospital and Professor David Mitchell in the Adelaide Hospital.

The Meath was historically a great contributor to both cardiology and medicine. This was initiated by the appointment of Robert Graves in 1821 and William Stokes in 1826. Both were gifted teachers. Trousseau described Graves as 'a perfect clinical teacher'. As noted by Peter Gatenby in his history of the Meath, Stokes published his *An Introduction to the Use of the Stethoscope* while a student in 1825. His *Diseases of the Chest* was published in 1837 and his description of the slow pulse and syncope, now known as

Stokes-Adams Syndrome, in 1846. His famous book on disease of the heart and the aorta was published in 1854. Graves described thyrotoxicosis in 1835, and his book *System of Clinical Medicine* was published in 1843. In more recent times, this fine tradition was carried on by Brian Mayne. Brian was appointed clinical assistant to the physicians of the Meath in June 1947, and physician to the hospital in October 1948. Brian was an astute physician, acerbic at times, but with a profound compassion behind his shyness. He was a talented physiologist and teacher, and early on developed a substantial and well structured coronary care unit at the Meath. His contribution to Irish cardiology has probably been seriously underestimated. Perhaps one might allow one anecdote to illustrate his personality. This comes from oral tradition and I do not vouch for its accuracy. On one occasion, Brian Mayne was examining with an external examiner whose marks appeared to be inversely proportional to the shortness of the candidate's skirts. Brian grew steadily more irritated as the prettiest students were awarded the highest marks. Eventually he dealt with the problem in a characteristic way by saying, 'Look, I do not mind giving them ten for tits, but I refuse to give them ten for each tit!' This anecdote should not distract one from stressing Brian's intense care, compassion, incisive mind and meticulous attention to detail.

Undoubtedly the greatest contributor to modern cardiology over the past quarter century in the Federated Hospitals was Gerard Gearty. He introduced cardiac catheterisation and coronary arteriography to our hospitals, and went on to pioneer the development of angioplasty and stenting. While new 'hawks' perform astounding feats, Gerry exhibited the pure bravery to 'have the courage to fail' which marks out surgeons and cardiologists involved in practical procedures who have the faith in themselves and their techniques to proceed through adversity to success. Gerry is also a legendary and gifted teacher. He brought clarity and youthful enthusiasm to his teaching throughout his clinical career. Such courage exacts a price. One felt that perhaps he sometimes suffered while always fighting to maintain the highest standards.

In 1924 Willem Einthoven was awarded a Nobel Prize for elucidating the principles of electro-cardiography. An electro-cardiograph was purchased for about £300 and installed in the Adelaide in 1929. In 1935, Dr D. M. Mitchell was appointed assistant in the electro-cardiographic department. He replaced the original Einthoven machine with a portable electro-cardiogram machine with valve amplification in 1936.

Richard (Dick) S. W. Baker was appointed to the Adelaide in 1954. He took a particular interest in cardiology, developing especially the methodical reporting and filing of electro-cardiograms; he also introduced phono-cardiography. As with all physicians at this time, he was required to undertake many other tasks; I particularly remember him, for example, performing liver biopsies with the Vim-Silverman needle. One of Dick Baker's great strengths was his 'nose' for trouble. He had an uncanny ability to identify a sick patient and channel him or her in the right direction.

I was appointed to the Adelaide in 1982 and also took over the department of cardiology in the Meath the following year. The first task was to establish a coronary care unit at the Adelaide for which there was much support. Next followed the establishment of echocardiography and cardiac catheterisation services, initially through the generosity of Baggot Street. A cardiac rehabilitation service was established, and a comprehensive research programme initiated. The latter focused on an understanding of the predictors of risk of heart attack, and the elucidation of the role of new risk factors such as homocysteine. The department became heavily involved in the affairs of the European Society of Cardiology, and the development of preventive strategies at European level. The appointment of new consultants at this time was extremely difficult, and an old tradition of appointing 'physicians to the outpatients' department' was invoked to secure the services of a talented clinician and echocardiographer, David Moore. Dr Moore became established as an international leader in echocardiography and consultant cardiologist at the new hospital at Tallaght. He is now perhaps the country's leading authority on both transthoracic and transoesophageal echocardiography. Dr Moore was joined by Vincent Maher who had worked with Gregg Browne in Seattle and was involved in seminal work on understanding of atherogenesis. He majored in preventive cardiology at the Adelaide and subsequently at the Adelaide and Meath at Tallaght.

In 1995 David Mulcahy was appointed as consultant cardiologist with a special interest in coronary arteriography and interventional techniques. He proved to be a dynamo, and secured a large referral base from hospitals all around the country seeking coronary arteriography and interventions such as angioplasty and stenting.

While these developments were occurring, the Royal City of Dublin Hospital, Baggot Street moved to St James's. There, Gerry Gearty, in partnership with Professor Michael Walsh and Peter Crean, later joined by Brendan Foley, established a formidable reputation particularly with regard to interventional cardiology. Their efforts helped in the establishment of the St James's cardiac surgery unit with Eilis McGovern and Vincent Young.

Medical politics

Comhairle na nÓspidéal's second report of 1976–8 stated: 'The Federated Dublin Voluntary Hospitals—comprising Sir Patrick Dun's, Mercer's, the Royal City of Dublin, Dr Steevens', the Adelaide, the Meath and the National Children's Hospital—agreed to enter into a partnership with the Eastern Health Board to develop a major general hospital on the site of St Kevin's Hospital to replace the services of the seven hospitals named.'

In the event, this did not happen. Sir Patrick Dun's, Mercer's, Baggot Street and Dr Steevens' all closed. The orthopaedic services from Dr Steevens' moved to the Adelaide but otherwise services were transferred to St Kevin's, renamed St James's. By 1976, it was agreed that the Adelaide, the Meath and later the National Children's Hospital would move to a new 'first-rate teaching hospital' at Tallaght, Co. Dublin. Mercer's closed in 1983. Sir Patrick Dun's was closed quite abruptly by the governors in 1986. This was followed by the closure of Baggot Street with transfer of cardiac, cardio-thoracic and pulmonary care to St James's. The board of Baggot Street made a strong case for maintaining their premises as a community general hospital for secondary care. Dr Steevens' found itself in financial difficulties, and withdrew its accident and emergency services in an attempt to draw attention to its plight. The result was that it was closed within months.

The Adelaide, faced with similar pressures, did not withdraw services even though it was eventually funded only on a week to week basis. It took the view that there should or must be a place within the state for minority participation in health care. From being within weeks of closure, the situation gradually changed. Within England and Northern Ireland there was a concern that, if Belfast could sustain its Mater, why could not the Republic permit the continuation of voluntary, minority participation in health care? Ultimately, strong support came from the silent majority of the Catholic population of Ireland. Gradually, the political climate changed until closure of the Adelaide became impossible.

Next came the negotiations to secure the amalgamation and move to Tallaght of the Adelaide, the Meath and the National Children's Hospital. Tensions ran high. The Meath felt with complete justification that they were the largest hospital in the group, with an accident and emergency department. The Adelaide felt passionately that minority participation in health care should be sustained. The National Children's Hospital was justifiably intent on maintaining its independent national status.

A review body under David Kingston of Irish Life was established to address these issues, later shared with David Kennedy as the Kennedy/Kingston Committee. This committee met 39 times. Success might not have been achieved but for the vision of two Ministers for Health—Brendan Howlin and Michael Noonan. Both possessed the determination to facilitate the resolution of the issues, and this was eventually achieved with modification of the original Adelaide Charter to accommodate the positions of the Meath and National Children's Hospital. It is likely that this arduous, painful process prevented some of the conflicts experienced by other hospitals which have been the product of mergers, and has led to the establishment of an integrated cohesive institution in Tallaaght.

17. Clinical Medicine at Trinity

Donald G. Weir

It may seem extraordinary by the standards required for the teaching of clinical medicine today, but the fact remains that until 1960 there was no department of clinical medicine in Trinity College or indeed in any other medical school in Ireland. A series of illustrious people had held the chair of Regius Professor of Physic; they had been responsible for the delivery and organisation of clinical medical education since the inception of this chair by John Stearne in 1662. Such teaching was in the main carried out at the bedsides of Dublin hospitals, such as Sir Patrick Dun's and the Meath; it was the method of clinical instruction for which Dublin medicine was justly internationally renowned, since its introduction by Robert Graves and William Stokes at the Meath Hospital in the early 1800s. However, there had never been a department of clinical medicine as such.

The inception of the Department of Clinical Medicine

The Department of Clinical Medicine started with the appointment of Peter B. B. Gatenby to the Chair of Clinical Medicine in 1960, at the instigation and motivation of Jerry Jessop, the dean of the medical school and one of the architects not only of the department but also of the Federated Dublin Voluntary Hospitals (FDVH).

At a time when there had been a marked dearth of academic endeavour in the field of clinical medicine in Ireland, Gatenby and Eddie Lillie (as a result of their clinical experiences in the Rotunda Hospital), had published original work on the pathogenesis, epidemiology and management of the megaloblastic anaemia of pregnancy. Although Gatenby was a full-time professor, the university still required him to make the majority of his stipend by continuing his clinical duties as a consultant to Dr Steevens', the Meath and the Rotunda, and at the same time significantly curtailed his rights to private practice. At first his department consisted of a secretary and the use of the ENT outpatient rooms at the Meath for three afternoons a week. These rooms had initially been constructed for Oliver St John Gogarty, who, apart from being an ENT surgeon of repute, was a well-known writer and Dublin celebrity of the last century.

However appropriate the rooms had been for Gogarty, they were totally inadequate for a modern department of clinical medicine. Indeed, when representatives of the UK General Medical Council visited the School of Physic in 1961, the group asked to inspect the department and concluded that Gatenby was 'the most fortunate of men because whatever he did it could only be an improvement'! It is difficult at this stage to realise the enormity of the task that Gatenby took on, and the debt of gratitude owed to him by Trinity and its future generations of both under- and postgraduate students.

From such meagre origins, however, great things can evolve. The first development was the appointment of a series of research fellows to the department, usually medical graduates who had often already worked as registrars in the Federated Hospitals, had obtained their MRCPI from the College of Physicians and wished to obtain their MD from their relevant medical school. This they did by undertaking a clinically orientated research project, which was usually funded by grants obtained from the then Medical Research Council of Ireland.

The second development was the construction of a 'wooden hut' at the rear of the Meath to house the Department of Clinical Medicine. The facilities this building housed were minimal, including two offices, space for a secretary and a very modest sized laboratory. The first lecturer was appointed in 1963.

Meanwhile Gatenby, apart from running the department, teaching the medical students and performing his duties as a consultant physician, was very much involved with the development of the FDVH as an entity. In particular, this meant the creation of specialist units within the Federation as follows: (1) in Baggot Street: cardiology under Rory Childers and subsequently Gerry Gearty, respiratory medicine under Terry Chapman and subsequently Luke Clancy; (2) in the Adelaide: neurology under Eddie Martin and subsequently Michael Hutchinson and Raymond Murphy, diabetes under Gerald Tomkin, dermatology under Dorothy and David Mitchell and subsequently Marjorie Young; (3) in the Meath: nephrology under Eddie Bourke and subsequently Brian Keogh, endocrinology under Michael Cullen; (4) in Mercer's: oncology under Peter Daly; (5) in Dr Steevens': rheumatology under Eoin Casey; and (6) in Sir Patrick Dun's gastroenterology under myself. Increasingly, these units became responsible for the teaching of clinical medicine in their specialty to the under- and postgraduate students of the university, a duty which they undertook with an enthusiasm and dedication which was all the more exemplary as the financial rewards from the university were minimal.

The research fellows who were appointed to the original Department of Clinical Medicine, between 1961 and 1975 when Gatenby resigned, became known as the ' wooden hut graduates'. I was the first; my MD was on the post-gastrectomy anaemias. I subsequently obtained a Wellcome Fellowship to study gastroenterology in Edinburgh. On returning to Dublin I became the first lecturer of the department. In this post I introduced flexible gastrointestinal endoscopy to Ireland. In 1967 I moved to Sir Patrick Dun's, where I set up the FDVH gastroenterology unit, which included the first Irish endoscopic day ward facility.

Ian Temperley, who had trained as a postgraduate at the Radcliffe Infirmary in Oxford, was appointed as consultant haematologist to the FDVH. He always maintained close links with the department, and initially continued the work on the pathogenesis of the megaloblastic anaemia of pregnancy, showing that maternal serum folate levels fell progressively throughout pregnancy. Subsequently he and I worked on intrinsic factor secretion from the stomach. He went on to develop the National Haemophilia Unit, which eventually was transferred to St James's. He was a founder member of the Bone Marrow for Leukaemia Trust, which has promoted one of the most active and productive academic research units in Ireland.

Initially, a series of research fellows worked on the pathogenesis of the anaemia that characterises coeliac disease, and in particular mal-absorption of iron. These included Connolly Norman, who emigrated to Canada, where he became a consultant haematologist; Marcus Webb, who went on to join Norman Moore in the Department of Psychiatry at St Patrick's Hospital and, following Moore's retirement, became the TCD Professor of Psychiatry; Mervyn Taylor, who was a senior lecturer in the Department of Paediatrics in the National Children's Hospital before transferring to Tallaght; he became an expert in paediatric pulmonary disease. Other research fellows included Dean Sharma, who studied intrinsic factor secretion in the stomach and became a consultant surgeon in the West Indies; Owen Morgan who studied gastroferrin secretion in the stomach, and became Dean of the Medical School in the West Indies; George McDonald who studied intestinal lactase deficiency and became a senior lecturer in the TCD Department of Histopathology at St James's, and an internationally renowned expert in liver histology; Gerald Tomkin, who studied indicanuria following gastric surgery, became a consultant physician and associate professor at Tallaght and is internationally renowned for his work on diabetes, on which he has published extensively; Des Sheridan, who worked on an assay of erythropoetin in rabbits and subsequently became Professor of

Cardiology, at St Mary's Hospital, London; and Michael Cullen, who had studied in Boston before returning to the department where he developed his specialty of endocrinology; he subsequently became a consultant and associate professor in this specialty at St James's.

The next lecturer to be appointed in 1970 was Eddie Bourke who took the Department, the Meath and Dublin medicine by storm! He was a nephrologist with a mercurial personality. He was responsible for redefining and contributing to the pathogenesis of the clinical manifestations of a specific renal tubular defect (Bartters syndrome). He was the first person in the south of Dublin to develop a dialysis service for renal failure, and in doing so got into financial problems with the Department of Health. Following Gatenby's retirement in 1974, Bourke became the locum head of the department until the appointment of Graham Neale as Gatenby's successor in 1976. He then emigrated to Saudi Arabia and subsequently to America where he became a professor and head of his department.

The Department of Clinical Medicine moves to St James's

Graham Neale came to Dublin with an already well established reputation as a consultant physician, gastroenterologist and nutritionist. He was appointed to work at St James's and Dr Steevens', and he also had an attachment to the gastroenterology unit in Sir Patrick Dun's. He was dedicated to relieving the suffering of his patients, and to the development of the highest standards of clinical medical practice. With his appointment the department moved to the St James's campus and into more so-called 'temporary huts' which nevertheless remained *in situ* until 1993, the only accommodation available for all of the TCD medical faculty clinical schools. He worked tirelessly to promote the devolution of the designated FDVH hospitals to St James's. This antagonised some of his FDVH colleagues who feared for their private practice if they moved to St James's, which had formerly been 'the Union', or 'the Workhouse'. At the critical moment when, for economic reasons, the designated hospitals (Sir Patrick Dun's, Mercer's and Baggot Street) were being closed down and relocated to St James's by the Department of Health, he bailed out and returned to England and Cambridge where he continued his highly successful career in the management of the diseases and nutritional problems affecting Third World countries.

During Neale's tenure the university agreed to appoint a senior lecturer to the department. This resulted in the arrival of John Prichard, an Oxford scholar, and an expert of international standing in respiratory medicine. His appointment was as a research scientist, and as such he only had a three session clinical commitment. This, in an Irish context, he considered to be inadequate, and for the remainder of his career strove to increase his clinical sessions in order to have parity with his fellow consultant colleagues. This resulted in long and tedious battles that were never satisfactorily resolved. He was, however, an excellent and dedicated teacher, never happier than when instructing a group of students, whom he taught in a wide variety of disciplines. His tragic death in 1996 deprived the department of a significant intellect, and he was never replaced by the university, his salary being used to finance the evolving branch of the department in Tallaght, contrary to specific undertakings given by TCD at the time.

Having been appointed to the Regius Chair in 1978, I was appointed to the full-time chair and became head of the department in 1982. As a consequence, my main clinical base moved to St James's, although I maintained my association with Sir Patrick Dun's until its closure as an acute front-line hospital in 1988. This allowed me to play a pivotal role in the transfer of the resources obtained from the sale of the Sir Patrick Dun's buildings to the new academic centre at St James's.

One of the terms of my appointment was that John Scott, Professor of Experimental Nutrition in the Department of Biochemistry, would be assigned to work in the Department of Clinical Medicine. Scott and I had worked together in the field of folate and cobalamin interrelationships since his return from Berkeley, California in 1968. Indeed, this association between us remained intact until my retirement in 1999. A further boost to our research was the appointment of Ann Molloy and Joe McPartlin as scientific officers in the department. This proved to be a highly productive team producing a paper each year in the *Lancet* throughout the 1990s, as well as obtaining three large grants from the National Institutes of Health, in America. Throughout this time and beyond, Scott has remained a guiding influence in many of the academic activities of the department, especially in its relations with Trinity, in the political manoeuvres necessary to move the Sir Patrick Dun's resources to St James's and the subsequent planning and *modus operandi* of the resulting buildings. Scott has been the Trinity representative on the St James's Board from 1988 to the present, and has had an enormous influence on the relationship between Trinity and St James's, and its continuing development on the hospital campus. He is now the internationally accepted expert on folic acid metabolism, and in particular its relationship to neural tube defects (NTD).

The other event at this time was the appointment of Napoleon Keeling as Senior Lecturer in Gastroenterology within the department; he became the leading national authority in the use of the ERCP technique for the assessment of biliary and pancreatic disease. He and Ted Dinnan (Senior Lecturer in the Department of Psychiatry) also performed some ground breaking work on the influence of brain hormones on gut motility, and their relationship to the irritable bowel syndrome. He subsequently became Medical Director of the GEMS Directorate at St James's.

The Sir Patrick Dun's Research Laboratories

The first transfer of funds from Dun's to St James's came from the sale of the nurses' home of Sir Patrick Dun's on Lower Mount Street. The financial resources thus obtained enabled the construction of the Sir Patrick Dun Research Laboratories on the Central Pathology Laboratory buildings at St James's. Provost W. A. Watts officially opened these laboratories in 1982. Professors of clinical medicine from the United Kingdom, including representatives of the Wellcome Trust, attended the scientific symposium that accompanied the event. The laboratories were run by a committee set up by Trinity, consisting of the heads of the clinical academic departments, of which I was the chairman until my retirement in 1999. The laboratory sites were allocated on the basis of the technology required by the specific research project. In other words, if a member of a clinical department had an appropriate research project and the necessary resources to fund it, he/she was allocated a bench slot in the relevant laboratory with the appropriate equipment and technical assistance. These research laboratories were the first to be sited on a hospital campus in Ireland at a time when clinically based research was at its nadir in this country.

Almost immediately the success of this venture was demonstrated by the number of grants obtained by the personnel attached to the laboratories, and the flow of papers published in prestigious international peer reviewed journals. Examples of such papers include: 'Pathogenesis of vitamin B12 deficient neuropathy'; 'Chimerism occurring in transplanted bone marrow'; 'Prevalence and significance of methicillin resistant staphylococci in an acute hospital setting'; 'Serological diagnosis of, and the genetic predisposition to, coeliac disease'; 'Successful treatment of duodenal ulceration by the eradication of helicobacter pylori'; 'Discovery of a vaccine to prevent helicobacter-pylori infection in the stomach' and 'Evidence that the maternal blood level of both folic acid and vitamin B12 related to the pathogenesis of neural tube defects(NTDs)'; subsequently it was shown that genetic polymorphisms affecting certain folic acid dependent enzymes predisposed to NTDs, inflammatory bowel disease, and affected the incidence of colon bowel cancer.

The Trinity Medical Centre and Postgraduate Medical School

The second financial transfer followed the sale of Sir Patrick Dun's itself in 1988. This, along with the Chester Beatty Fund in Trinity, produced the necessary resource for the construction of the Trinity Centre for Health Science at St James's, which was to house the facilities required for the teaching of both the medical and the nursing courses. The building contained a branch of the Trinity Library, and a large lecture theatre. The latter produced a suitable forum for the weekly hospital grand rounds, and for the formal lectures given to the medical students in their clinical years. The Minister for Health officially opened this building in 1993. Once again there was a large medical symposium to mark the event which was attended by many very eminent people including the deans of Oxford and Harvard. This building, along with a similar centre at the Regional Hospital in Galway, were the first such medical schools to be built on a hospital campus in Ireland. Its presence added enormously to the prestige of the whole campus, to the relationship between the hospital and the university, and the general *esprit de corps* of the staff.

The third building constructed was the Postgraduate Medical School. This was funded from some of the resources that derived from the sale of Dr Steevens' Hospital, the board of Baggot Street, and monies raised by Con Feighery (who was at that time the director of postgraduate studies), from some of his consultant colleagues and grants from pharmaceutical companies. This building was deliberately constructed cheek by jowl with the Trinity Centre, in the hope that the two buildings would be able to interrelate; however, the administrative powers-that-be decided that the doors between the two buildings should be closed and alarmed thus effectively separating the functions of the two buildings. Nevertheless, the Postgraduate Medical School remains a necessary facility for the maintenance of close relations between the primary medical care services in the community and the hospital staff, as well as for research and postgraduate teaching seminars and meetings.

Postgraduate degrees associated with the Department

On the educational side a series of developments occurred. The first was the creation of the degree of BSc in clinical nutrition, by co-ordinating the resources of the Dublin Institute of Technology (DIT) and Trinity in 1982. The first two years of the course were run in the DIT, while in the latter two years nutrition and dietetics were taught in the Trinity Centre at St James's. To this end Michael Gibney and Nicholas Kennedy were appointed by Trinity, and Mary Moloney by DIT to run the latter half of the course. The course was controlled by a co-ordinating committee, comprising representatives from both colleges, which I chaired until my retirement in 1999. It has been an outstanding success as demonstrated by the reports of a series of external assessors. It remains unique in the UK and Ireland as being the only such course that is based in a clinical department of medicine and in a hospital setting.

The second development was the MSc in bioengineering run by Jim Malone and Barry McMahon. Both developed international reputations in their own areas. This also remains the only such course in Ireland.

The third was the start in 1997 of the MSc course in molecular medicine. This is only the second such degree course within the UK and Ireland. It was initiated by Dermot Kelleher and backed by Mark Lawlor, Ross McManus and Aideen Long. This course has since developed an international reputation, to the extent that applicants apply to attend the course from all over the world, selection for which has become highly competitive.

The evolution of postgraduate medical training at St James's was a feature of the 1980s and 1990s. The Department of Clinical Medicine led the way at that time by the promotion of a two-year course in general medicine at the senior house officer level which was mainly aimed at the acquisition of the Membership of the RCPI. The basis of the course was a 3–6 month rotation around all the specialist groups in St James's and the Adelaide and the Meath (as they were then); it was implemented and developed by the directors of postgraduate medicine at that time, who included Luke Clancy, Davis Coakley, and Con Feighery.

Following the construction of the Trinity Medical Centre (1993), additional buildings were added on to house and facilitate the teaching of the associated clinical departments of speech therapy, physiotherapy and occupational therapy. This was achieved under the direction and guidance of the then Dean, Davis Coakley. These buildings were completed in 2000. As Dean, Coakley was also instrumental in developing an association between Trinity and the other historic medical schools in Europe called EUROLIFE—Network of European Universities in Life Sciences. The schools include Edinburgh, Oxford, Maastricht, Leiden, Gottingen, Karolinska, Montpellier, Strasburg and Innsbruck. This continues to be a highly successful partnership in transeuropean research projects.

*The Institute of Molecular Medicine and the Durkan Foundation
Laboratories*

In 1999 I retired from Trinity and was succeeded as head of department
by Dermot Kelleher. Kelleher, who was already internationally renowned
for his work on inflammatory bowel disease, had also set up the
Hepatology Centre at St James's for the management of hepatitis, a disease which required very delicate handling at the time due to the infection of mothers with rhesus incompatible babies in the late 1970s and
early 1990s with hepatitis C infected plasma. Having set up the course
in molecular medicine he has subsequently gone on to study this subject as his main research theme.

At about this time two major events occurred which dramatically enhanced the international standing of the Department of Clinical Medicine
and will continue to do so. The first was the donation by the Durkan
family of the resources required to build research laboratories with the
specific objective of enhancing our knowledge of, and therapeutic
endeavours in, the field of leukaemia. Shaun McCann, who had succeeded Ian Temperley as head of the Department of Haematology, became the first director of these laboratories. In collaboration with Mark
Lawlor, McCann had already built up an enviable reputation in this
field of medical research.

The second event has been the formation of the Dublin Institute of
Molecular Medicine which is a collaborative venture between Trinity, University College Dublin and the College of Surgeons, the objective of which
is 'to study the underlying mechanisms of disease' with the ultimate aim of
improving their management.

The proposal was submitted to the HEA by Kelleher (Trinity) and Hugh
Brady (UCD), and subsequently Des Fitzgerald (RCSI); this produced
a £14 million grant. The result from the Trinity perspective has been the
construction of the Institute of Molecular Medicine at St James's, which is
a unique clinical research facility on a hospital campus in these islands. The
Minister for Education opened the Institute in 2003, on the occasion of
the Fifth Annual Symposium on Molecular Medicine

The Department of Clinical Medicine also moves to Tallaght

The construction of the AMNCH hospital in Tallaght allowed the relocation of the Adelaide, the Meath and the National Children's Hospital
to this site in 1997. Subsequently the Trinity Centre for Medical Science
was constructed on this campus, and was formally opened in 2000. The

funding for this was largely acquired through the inspirational efforts of the then Dean of Health Sciences, Davis Coakley who, at a time of academic penury in Trinity, increased the size of the undergraduate year by bringing in more fee-paying non-EU students. This section of the Department of Clinical Medicine was headed from its inception by Colm O'Morain, who has been a prolific author on gastroenterological subjects, and in particular in recent years on the pathogenesis and treatment of helicobacter pylori infection in the stomach. O'Morain was formally appointed as Professor of Clinical Medicine and Head of the AMNCH section of the department in 2002.

Other internationally recognised clinical medicine departments set up in AMNCH include: cardiology by Ian Graham, who showed the association of hyperhomocystinuria to coronary artery disease; diabetes by Gerald Tomkin, who demonstrated the association of dyslipidaemia in diabetics to coronary artery disease; geriatrics by Des O'Neill, who studied the effects of motility disorders in the elderly on such functions as driving; nephrology by Brian Keogh, who subsequently became President of the RCPI; and metabolic diseases by John Barragry.

Thus, in a period of less than half a century, the Department of Clinical Medicine has grown from a minimal position in 1960, to its present state which is comparable, at least academically, both in terms of courses offered and in publications in internationally accredited medical journals, with the majority of similar departments in the UK, although receiving less than a tithe of the funding they receive per medical student. There can be little doubt that the recent events as described above, have ensured a bright and exciting future for the department, which at the very least, will make it the equal of the best academic departments of clinical medicine in Europe and America.

18. Clinical microbiology

Conor Keane

The development of the clinical microbiology laboratory in the Adelaide Hospital (as part of the Federated Dublin Voluntary Hospitals) was closely linked with Trinity College. In the 1950s laboratory services were provided by departments on the college campus: biochemistry by Professor W. J. E. Jessop, pathology by Professor R. A. Q. O'Meara, and microbiology (or bacteriology as it was called) by Professor Stanley Stewart. The future development of the laboratory services in these islands was profoundly influenced by the formation of the Royal College of Pathologists in 1961 in London. This sounded the death knell of the general pathologist who covered all disciplines and accelerated the establishment of separate departments for each discipline. As a result, a reorganisation took place in the Trinity hospitals. The Central Microbiology Laboratory was established in the Adelaide and provided a service to all the seven Federated Hospitals. A service was also provided for St Ultan's.

The location of the clinical microbiology service away from the academic centre in the Moyne Institute in Trinity was less than ideal, but it was efficient and the only possible way forward at the time, prior to the move to St James's and subsequently Tallaght. However, strong and productive research links were established with the Moyne Institute and the service laboratory developed its own strong research programme. The service continued in the Adelaide until May 1981 when it was relocated to St James's. In June 1999 AMNCH was opened in Tallaght and developed its own laboratory service there.

During this period of expansion, great changes in the field of infectious diseases were taking place to which the service responded. Antibiotic-resistant bacteria became increasingly prevalent and restricted the choice of antibiotic therapy. Old diseases, such as tuberculosis, were still spreading in many parts of the world. New infectious agents were being discovered such as the Human Immunodeficiency Virus (HIV), Legionella, Helicobacter pylori, and the agent of the new variant Creutzfeldt-Jakob Disease (Mad Cow Disease).

Development of the clinical microbiology laboratory

The general laboratories of the FDVH were located in four different hospitals, except for histopathology which was on the Trinity campus. The clinical microbiology laboratory was established in the Adelaide in 1967. A subsection, serology, was located in Mercer's. The consultant microbiologist in charge was Betty Wallace and in the Adelaide laboratory the senior laboratory technician was Arthur Ogilvie and the chief technologist John Ryan. Tom Scott was appointed to the serology laboratory in mid 1967, but he resigned shortly afterwards and joined the teaching staff of the Dublin Institute of Technology where he had a distinguished academic career. Mr Ryan left for a post in industry and was replaced by Alex Whelan.

In 1970 Dr Wallace left for an appointment as consultant microbiologist in the Royal Sussex Hospital. At that time I was Medical Research Council Fellow in the Institute for Child Health and the Hospital for Sick Children, Great Ormond Street, London; I took up the headship of the department in 1971. At this time it was clear that serology was developing into a new discipline—immunology. Mr Whelan resigned from microbiology and became chief technologist in the immunology department which later moved to the School of Pathology on the Trinity campus. John Greally was appointed head of the discipline, a post now held by Professor Con Feighery.

In 1972 Liam English was appointed chief technologist to the Central Microbiology Laboratory. He brought the great gifts of leadership and ability to the post. He became a major influence on the development of diagnostic microbiology in Ireland and its academic advance. His efforts were recognised by the creation of an annual award in his honour for the person who has made a major contribution to the development of clinical microbiology.

The staff of the Central Microbiology Laboratory included medical consultants, non-consultant hospital doctors, phlebotomists, infection control nurses, secretaries, porters and laboratory technicians. On the medical side, Professor Bill Gillespie, a Trinity graduate and formerly the distinguished holder of the Chair in Clinical Microbiology in Bristol, joined the staff from 1978 to 1981. Eric Mulvihill joined the service in 1981 bringing an extra clinical dimension. There was a strong commitment to staff education and development and facilities were provided for staff to undertake the training requirements for the MRCPath exams, MD, MSc, and PhD degrees and other qualifications. Over the years many successes were achieved. Marie-Thérèse Clancy was the first person in Ireland to obtain the new membership qualification of the Royal College of Pathologists (MRCPath) in any discipline. An important advance in the academic standing of laboratory medicine was the change introduced for technical personnel in 1993 when their qualification was raised from diploma status to a five year BSc degree course validated by Trinity College.

The elements of the service were of necessity dictated by the requirements of the specialists in various hospitals. The National Children's Hospital had a particular need for expertise in the diagnosis of meningitis, septicaemia and gastroenteritis. Such specialties as orthopaedics, burns, oncology, and gastroenterology each had specific requirements. Thus it became necessary to develop a centralised service which could engage in all aspects of clinical microbiology. With the moves to St James's and Tallaght, the corresponding clinical specialties followed accordingly. In Tallaght a new consultant microbiologist was appointed—Phillip Murphy who, together with chief technologist, Margaret Lynch, has developed a sophisticated laboratory service to serve the needs of that hospital and indeed of Naas Hospital.

Infection control

Hospital acquired infection has become a plague in hospitals and beyond. The reasons are quite clear. Compared to, say, 20 years ago, the patients under our care in hospitals are increasingly at the extremes of age—periods when they are very susceptible to infection. More adventurous surgery is being performed and the increased use of cytotoxic and immunosuppressive drugs increases the susceptibility to infection. Added to this is the wholesale use of antibiotics which has led to a Darwinian type of selection for resistant micro-organisms.

The Federated Hospitals were pioneers in Ireland in infection control. In the early 1970s, infection control committees were established in all the Federated Hospitals. These reported to a central infection control committee based in the Federation offices on Ranelagh Road. Each hospital committee was chaired by a hospital appointee. This was sometimes a contentious and difficult task. Some chairmen come immediately to mind: Eric Fenelon (Adelaide) firmly controlling a meeting, a box of Senior Service 20s in front of him, conducting the proceedings in a cloud of blue cigarette smoke; Derek Robinson (Meath) quietly making sure business was completed; and David Lane, a distinguished oboeist as well as a distinguished surgeon, the epitome of tact and efficiency.

Some areas of infection control became extremely important; for instance, the sterilisation of surgical instruments. Standard procedures were introduced into all the hospitals. The wisdom of this policy can now be seen with the advent of new variant Creutzfeldt-Jakob Disease. This is very resistant to heat and so the cleaning and sterilisation of surgical instruments is crucial. Fred Falkiner introduced another important control infection technique—fingerprinting of bacteria. This made possible the tracing of rogue bacteria and their sources in the hospitals. The first infection control nurse in the Republic of Ireland was Sister I. M. Kerrison, an Adelaide nurse who was appointed in 1972. Since then, similar appointments have been made in all the major hospitals in Ireland.

Genitourinary medicine

In any history of Irish medicine the establishment of the genitourinary medicine (previously venereal disease) service in St James's must be a major landmark. As clinical microbiology is intimately associated with this department and has been involved in its development, a brief account of the development of the role of the laboratories in FDVH and then St James's is appropriate.

Up until the early 1980s venereal disease (VD) clinics were held regularly in two of the Federated Hospitals—Dr Steevens' and Sir Patrick Dun's. Patients for these clinics attended in the evening, in contrast to all other outpatient services which were held at normal hours. It was therefore obvious to hospital staff and the public that these clinics were somehow different or 'special' as they became known. In the 1970s it became clear that a whole range of infectious diseases could be transmitted by sexual contact so the wider term 'genitourinary medicine' was coined which also embraced other parts of the service. It was also apparent that these clinics should be held at the same time as other clinics to encourage attendance. In the 1970s an on-site microbiological service was established for rapid diagnosis. However, the service was under-funded and needed complete re-organisation.

In 1973 Professor Hourihane (principal pathologist) and I visited the genitourinary medicine department in the Middlesex Hospital in London—a department of international standing. The head of the department, Duncan Catterall, recommended that it would be appropriate to establish a consultant post in genitourinary medicine and to amalgamate the two existing clinics to form one reasonably resourced clinic in Dublin. A successful application was made to the Department of Health for a consultant post and a single clinic was established in St James's. Fiona Mulcahy was appointed the first consultant in genitourinary medicine in Ireland despite interviewers' worries about the appropriateness of a woman examining male genitalia! Dr Mulcahy, together with consultants Colm Bergin and Ceppi Merry, established a service of international standing particularly in the management of HIV/AIDS patients.

Research

Continuing research is essential for the development of any discipline and microbiology is no exception. After the retirement of Professor F S. Stewart, Professor of Microbiology, in 1975, John Peebles Arbuthnott was appointed to the chair. This was an inspired choice. He brought to the post great attributes of intellect and leadership, as well as linking the clinical and scientific branches of microbiology in research. Professor John Arbuthnott and I made a joint application to the Medical Research Council for a substantial grant to study hospital-acquired infection. This was successful and research of international standing resulted. One of the main areas of investigation was Methicillin Resistant Staphylococcus Aureus (MRSA). These bacteria were first isolated in the Republic of Ireland in the Central Microbiology Laboratory in the Adelaide.

From the research group, and arising from its establishment, distinguished research was performed by former FDVH employees Rosemary Hone (consultant microbiologist, Mater Hospital), Mary Cafferkey (consultant, Rotunda and Temple Street), Lynda Fenelon (consultant microbiologist, St Vincent's), Professor Hilary Humphreys (RCSI and consultant microbiologist, Beaumont) and Niamh O'Sullivan (consultant microbiologist, Our Lady's, Crumlin and the Coombe). Professor David Coleman gave superb support on molecular studies. Professor Arbuthnott left Trinity to become Vice Chancellor of Strathclyde University and subsequently received a knighthood.

Professor Colm O'Moráin is one of the leading world authorities on H. pylori infection. In the 1980s the clinical microbiology department was privileged to be involved in research on these infections with him. A highlight was a joint paper in the *Lancet* on the response of peptic ulceration to chemotherapy. Other important joint research projects were performed with Professor Donald Weir and Professor Rory O'Moore on the Blind Loop Syndrome, Barry O'Connell on Serratia Marcescens, Professor Luke Clancy on tuberculosis, and David FitzPatrick investigating the management of acute haematogenous osteomyelitis. Over many years studies on surgical infections of the urinary tract were undertaken with Dermot O'Flynn, Victor Lane, Michael Butler and Denis Murphy.

There has always been a close association between clinical microbiology and the haematology and oncology services: firstly with Professor Ian Temperley and subsequently with Professor Shaun McCann and Professor Peter Daly with whom research into different aspects of immunosuppressed patients has been performed and published. A major study was also undertaken with Professor Davis Coakley, Bernard Walsh and Professor Des O'Neill on respiratory tract and Cl. difficile infections in the elderly. These studies were published in prestigious journals and presented at international meetings. The laboratory work could not have been performed without the facilities of the Sir Patrick Dun's Research Laboratories which were established in St James's after the closure of Dun's.

Clinical microbiology—the future

The transfer of the clinical microbiology laboratories to St James's and Tallaght from the old Central Microbiology Laboratory and their development there have been entirely successful. There are crucial elements in the clinical service which are of local, national and international importance. These will have a major bearing on the future development of microbiology in St James's. The bone marrow transplantation service will make increasing demands on the supporting clinical microbiology laboratory service, as will the department of genitourinary medicine. The National MRSA Reference Laboratory, which was opened in January 2002 by the Minister for Health and Children, Mícheál Martin, on the St James's campus, has already made important contributions to the development of the service and in research.

The Department of Health and Children has also designated St James's campus as the site for the new Tuberculosis Reference Laboratory. This initiative is timely, as the Tubercle bacillus has become resistant to many first and second line anti-tuberculosis drugs. There is therefore an opportunity to make an impact on control of this disease not only in Ireland but in those areas of the world where poverty, AIDS and tuberculosis are causing devastation. Underpinning these initiatives has been the appointment to three new consultant microbiologist posts in St James's of Brian O'Connell, Eleanor McNamara and Brendan Crowley. These appointments will add vigour and thrust to the service and research elements of the service.

On the Tallaght site Phillip Murphy has led rapid and exciting developments in the clinical microbiology service. He has instituted important initiatives on reference work on the microbiology of cystic fibrosis. A plan to combat bio-terrorism is being developed. This increased workload has highlighted the need for an additional consultant microbiologist there.

Finally, there are two elements that are essential for the successful development of the discipline on both sites. Firstly, there is the need for increased resources to provide more laboratory space and personnel to support the expanding service. Secondly, to ensure the continued academic development of the service at all levels, strong links must be maintained with the science departments on the Trinity campus.

19. Dermatology

Marjorie M. Young

My association with dermatology and the Adelaide began in 1972 as registrar to Drs David and Dorothy Mitchell. David held the position of consultant physician and dermatologist to the hospital and his wife Dorothy was assistant in the dermatology department. When they retired in 1974 I succeeded Dr Mitchell as consultant dermatologist, and Professor Gerald Tomkin was appointed consultant physician.

David Mitchell's appointment to the Adelaide in 1945 followed a long line of dermatology tradition and service to the local community. It originated with the appointment of Wallace Beatty in 1905; he was succeeded in 1935 by Geoffrey Harvey. There was also a lady dermatologist, Augusta 'Gussie' Young, who was attached to the Meath from 1925 until 1957. She died in 1964. In later years I was frequently asked by patients whether I was her daughter. Such questions were answered with a polite 'no' as, by all accounts, Dr Augusta was a prim, unbending spinster.

David Mitchell's appointment at the Adelaide as both physician and dermatologist would be considered highly unusual today. However, such combined appointments were not unusual at that time. He was a very highly respected physician and dermatologist and had been President of the Royal College of Physicians of Ireland. He had a strong academic instinct and encouraged research. His clinical cases at dermatology meetings such as the annual meeting of the Irish Association of Dermatologists were of the highest standard, frequently provoking discussion.

When I joined the department I was the first registrar in dermatology. By 1976 the workload had increased so much that an additional SHO post was created, a post first held by the late Liam Diskin. Over the years the Adelaide continued to prove a very popular place for dermatology meetings. There were expressions of regret when the nurses' highly individual and distinctive uniform was changed when the Adelaide moved to the new hospital in Tallaght. In 1983 we held a meeting with several British dermatologists and the sherry reception before lunch gave our visitors an opportunity to enjoy the garden which had been developed from nothing by Dr Sheila Kenny and her helpers.

Dermatology, being an outpatient rather than inpatient service, revolved around clinics and on reflection the Federated Hospitals' patients were well served. With the exception of Baggot Street all of them held clinics and all were provided with an inpatient consultation service. For many years there were two consultant dermatologists within the Federated Group, Dr Mitchell in the Adelaide, and Norman Jackson, who held appointments to Dr Steevens' and Sir Patrick Dun's where he held twice weekly clinics.

The principal dermatology workload was at the Adelaide where three clinics were held each week and inpatient facilities were also available. The Meath held a weekly clinic supervised by Dr David, and Dr Dorothy supervised a weekly paediatric clinic at the National Children's Hospital. David and Dorothy Mitchell complemented each other very well. David's academic approach was balanced by Dorothy's practical, down to earth dealings with patients. Occasionally patients were puzzled when David explained how treatments were carried out. Instructions which to him seemed simple and straightforward could be perplexing to them. On the other hand Dorothy, being a mother of three children herself, was very adept at dealing with the mothers of babies who had nappy rashes. She also had the capacity to develop an instant rapport when talking to children.

Whereas David Mitchell was cautious and slow, Norman Jackson was quick and able to see numerous patients in a clinic, dispensing advice between puffing away at a cigarette and writing prescriptions for antihistamines, antibiotics or creams—whatever was required—amidst a cloud of smoke. All patients were quickly dealt with so that the clinic had frequently finished by mid-morning before the all-important adjournment for coffee in the consultant staff room of Sir Patrick Dun's. Consultants would sit around a large table on which many of their predecessors had carved their names (see photograph on page 135) and would discuss medical politics and exchange stories and anecdotes.

Whilst the dermatology clinic would be a hive of activity and flurry the waiting area outside was a place of calm and organisation. Patients came well prepared for the long wait for medical and surgical clinics and for some it seemed to be an enjoyable experience and one not to be missed. After checking in, often hours before the appointed time, they would settle down and out would come the sandwiches and flasks of tea. This would be followed by long pieces of knitting drawn from a large bag and the sound of knitting needles clicking away seemed to provide some comfort whilst they whiled away the hours. The waiting also provided an opportunity to meet old friends, to exchange details of illnesses and complaints with others who would have a sympathetic ear.

At the Adelaide the most colourful part of the week, and for many patients the high point of their existence, was the leg ulcer clinic on Friday mornings. Three clinic rooms would be filled with patients, invariably ladies, to have their ulcers dressed. When one opened the door one was met by an array of legs of various shapes and sizes and in varying states of undress. Some of the legs would be immersed in buckets containing an antiseptic—the pink solution of potassium permanganate. Then the legs would be covered in bandages of various hues—beige for icthopaste, grey for tarbands, pink for calibands and yellow for quinobands. All of this would be conducted over gossip, tea and biscuits. Many patients would arrive by ambulance from various parts of Dublin and beyond. For some this would be their main outing of the week. They would comment on each other's progress and the fact that improvement was frequently slow did not seem to bother them. There was little time to address the underlying problems of anaemia due to poor diet, obesity and failure to rest. All these procedures were conducted under the experienced eye of Sister Amy Kenny. The more severe and persistent cases were admitted for bed rest and an inpatient stay of two or three weeks was often very beneficial in the healing process.

Later, many of these patient were taken over by Mary Henry who, having trained with and assisted Professor George Fegan, was an expert in the management of varicose veins and varicose ulcers.

One of the advances in dermatology has been the increasing awareness among the general public of the devastating effects that skin diseases such as psoriasis and eczema can have on one's life. The spread of such knowledge has been due in part to the activities of support groups such as the Eczema Association and the Psoriasis Association. In the 1970s and 1980s skin disease was still stigmatised and many patients were reluctant to talk about their problems. Such knowledge was also limited among my colleagues some of whom would delight in telling me of their teaching in dermatology as medical students which could be summarised in one sentence: 'if it is wet, dry it and if it is dry, wet it'.

When I first admitted patients with severe skin disease to the wards there was initially some surprise and criticism by senior colleagues. Not having an allocation of beds in my own right I was dependent upon the generosity of my medical colleagues. To them it seemed inappropriate that hospital beds should be made available for such patients. I hoped that in time they would become aware of the benefits of such treatment. It is well proven that bed rest alone for patients with eczema where they are away from stress, a triggering factor, will lead to an improvement. Equally important, the lack of carpets, and the clean surfaces in hospitals, reduced exposure to house dust mite, another triggering factor. Among the first patients that I admitted was a middle-aged man who had suffered from severe eczema since infancy. He was unable to keep a full-time job and his life was miserable through a combination of continuous itching leading to scratching and loss of sleep. In acute phases the skin would weep and become secondarily infected. Another patient was a middle-aged woman who had such extensive psoriasis that most of her skin was permanently red, inflamed, and scaling. It was gratifying to try a new drug, Methotrexate, an immunosuppressive drug which cleared her skin for the first time in many years and made life tolerable again.

Besides trying to cope with the distress and discomfort of the skin disease some of my patients were subjected to discrimination. I recall one woman with psoriasis and several members of her family similarly affected who, on joining a swimming class, was ordered by the instructor in front of the group to leave because of the unsightliness of her skin. Many patients like her were often refused treatments in hairdressing salons. Sadly, the discrimination did not only apply to adults. For children it was often worse and possibly more psychologically damaging. I remember a boy of seven being made to sit in a corner of the classroom away from the other children and treated like a leper because of his psoriasis. A little girl of six who had the same condition was asked by her friends if she had AIDS. The mother of another little six-year-old girl decided that the most effective way of dealing with her daughter's scalp psoriasis was to have her head shaved.

Although patients undoubtedly benefited from inpatient treatment it nevertheless intruded into their home and work life and, in the case of children, disrupted their schooling. Moreover, patients were well aware that diseases like eczema and psoriasis were incurable and unpredictable and whilst the aim of treatment was to induce a long remission in some cases the disease quickly relapsed.

The introduction of day care treatments from the 1980s onwards whereby patients came daily for care at a time convenient to them was a major development. It allowed adults and children to continue with work, home duties and school and was in line with dermatology practice in the UK and Europe. Patients were exposed to small, safe doses of UVB light followed by the application of whatever cream or ointment was necessary, then covered by tube gauze to prevent the preparations sticking to the patient's clothing. It was discovered that small increments of UVA light combined with a tablet—Psoralen—taken before exposure were effective in clearing psoriasis and, to an extent, eczema in adults; this was a highly popular treatment with patients as it obviated the necessity of creams, ointments etc. Moreover, such patients were only required to attend two to three times per week. In 1986 the Adelaide purchased a PUVA machine which was situated in the physiotherapy department and run by the physiotherapists. Under the direction of Julia Stevenson they provided a superb service and without their expertise and input it would not have been possible.

Until the 1970s there was a children's ward within the Adelaide, where from time to time I admitted babies and children. Then, in line with the recognition that all children up to the age of 14 years should be referred to and admitted to children's hospitals, it closed and all children were referred to the National Children's Hospital. There, I was fortunate to have the support and enthusiasm of the medical and nursing staff who were always receptive to new ideas. The expertise and organisational skills of Matron Maura Connolly and staff nurses Karen Keegan and Dorothy Rohio were of immense value.

In Harcourt Street day care and inpatient treatments were administered by the physiotherapist Diane Boylan. She had a great rapport with children and their parents. She fully understood the necessity of minimising the disruption to schooling and would treat children after they had finished school for the day. She always provided a listening ear for anxious parents. Treating children was always rewarding as, with few exceptions, they settled in well to hospital routine and responded well to treatments; as a result many children would remain in remission for months.

Dermatology is a specialty very dependent indeed upon nurses—not only do they carry out treatments and dressings but in doing so they act as listeners and counsellors. Patients very often pour out their problems while receiving treatment and this for many of them is a safety valve. Such tales of woe had to be listened to, for stress was and is a precipitating or aggravating factor in skin disease. We were particularly fortunate at the Adelaide in having a long history of caring and responsible nurses who over the years provided terrific support for patients. For many years Sister Amy Kenny had been the lynchpin of the weekly leg ulcer clinic and later all aspects of the dermatology service were supervised by Sister Denise Barkman. The staff nurses who from time to time ran the many outpatient clinics included Felicity King, Jenny Payne, Anita Goodbody, Valerie Houlden, Daphne Henley and Anna McCarthy.

Another saying quoted to me by my colleagues was that 'patients with skin disease are never cured and never die'—this too was untrue. Whilst obviously dermatology is a disease more concerned with morbidity than mortality and emergencies are uncommon, the death of two sisters with a rare inherited skin blistering disease gave an insight into the kindness and care given to them by the nursing staff throughout their lifetime. They were cared for initially as babies by Raymond Rees in the National Children's Hospital and then when older were transferred to the Adelaide where they continued to attend until their deaths in early adult life. The nuns who cared for them in the orphanage and carried out the daily dressings for many years relied upon the support they received from the nurses and particularly so in the months prior to the girls' deaths. Indeed, Matron Yvonne Seville became like a mother to them often buying them presents and staff nurse Anna McCarthy invited the younger sister to spend Christmas with her at her home.

A number of registrars spent a year or more in the dermatology department after completing training in general medicine in order to gain an insight into the specialty. Their interest flourished and they continued their training in prestigious centres in the UK and North America and later were appointed to consultant posts. They included Patrick Kenny, a consultant dermatologist in Ontario, Canada, Frank Powell at the Mater Hospital, Dublin, Bart Ramsey at Limerick Regional Hospital, Pauline Marron at University College Galway, Marion McEvoy at the Mayo Clinic, USA, Brigid O'Connell at the Bons Secours in Dublin, John Bourke at the South Infirmary, Cork, and Julie Prendiville in Vancouver, Canada. Edel O'Toole holds an academic post in dermatology at the Royal London Hospital and Dermot McKenna has recently accepted a consultant post in Cavan/Monaghan. In later years, when meeting them they would frequently enquire of the Adelaide and the nursing staff. Others, like Liam Diskin, went into general practice where their knowledge of dermatology proved invaluable.

No account of the Adelaide would be complete without mention of Arthur Ogilvie who was regarded as part of the fabric of the place. When slides and photographs were needed for case presentations and teaching, invariably at the last minute, Arthur could always be relied upon and never once did he let us down. In addition he gave me help and support in establishing laboratory research into psoriasis which later continued and developed with the help of a grant from the Adelaide Hospital Research Foundation and was presented at meetings in the UK and USA.

As in other branches of medicine, patterns of skin disease changed over the years. Acute infections like impetigo became less common and the referrals and workload began to reflect the recognition of and concern about the adverse effects of sun exposure and consequent development of skin cancers. This was a particularly acute problem at the Meath and Adelaide where there was a cohort of renal transplant recipients. These patients, because of their immuno-suppression, were particularly prone to develop aggressive skin cancers. Effective management was only made possible by dermatologist and surgeon co-operating and combining their expertise. A group of small hospitals such as the FDVH encouraged communication and co-operation between colleagues and we were always conscious that our role was to care for patients. These qualities proved invaluable when we moved to the combined Adelaide, Meath and National Children's Hospital site at Tallaght in 1998.

20. *Diabetes and Endocrinology*

Gerald Tomkin

The choice of career within medicine is never an easy one, but for me the goalposts were set following residency and then internship with Professor Robert Micks in Sir Patrick Dun's. Professor Micks was quite an exceptional person, highly educated, highly intelligent and a little eccentric. As King's Professor in Pharmacology he published a textbook on the subject which had enormous success, being translated into more than 11 languages and used by medical students all over the world. As a clinical researcher he was also outstanding and is credited with bringing to this side of the Atlantic the concept of the dangers of potassium fluxes in diabetic ketoacidosis, thereby saving many lives.

The other reason I chose diabetes and endocrinology was the fact that there was no diabetologist and no endocrinologist consultant in the Trinity group of hospitals at the time when I was looking for a post and therefore had no hesitation in being delighted to choose the specialty as a career. I was appointed to the Adelaide and the Meath in 1974 within a year of my starting work as a consultant in Birmingham. I came back to Dublin in 1975 to the Adelaide, a small well-run intimate hospital where responsibility could not be shirked, team spirit being very much in evidence.

I was most fortunate in that staff nurse Valerie Houlden was the nurse detailed to my outpatients. Together we started a diabetic clinic, and became involved in diabetes education. Valerie Houlden had a wonderfully dynamic personality and forged the diabetes department. She had a marvellous ability to get people to work with her to achieve common goals. I think it was a registrar, John Stinson, now a medical director of Leo Laboratories who first gave her the name 'she who must be obeyed'. The diabetes practice flourished but with no premises.

Many requests to the hospital for a diabetes unit finally resulted in a disposable hut being built for it. It still seems incredible to me how much effort it took to obtain a hut and it was only when I moved to Tallaght that I realised that the effort was nothing compared to that required to get a hut built in the new hospital, but more of that later.

However, the value of a hut should never be underestimated!

When I came back to the Adelaide I was enthusiastic and determined to progress research and was rather taken aback when I was taken aside one day by a senior member of staff whose claims to fame included the naming of her father in James Joyce's *Ulysses*. This lady told me that I should really stop the research as patients did not like it and it would be bad for my private practice. She encouraged me to pay much more attention to the private practice and leave the research alone. I had thought that on returning to Dublin I would perfect my golf but found that it was actually more enjoyable to do research whilst waiting for the private patients to emerge from the undergrowth. In the absence of the flood of patients to Fitzwilliam Square I was able to devote a considerable amount of time to research and gradually built up expertise in the field of lipoproteins and diabetes. Laboratory space was a problem and initially I was delighted to be given space in Professor John Scott's lab in Trinity. Professor Scott was happy to give me the space but under no circumstances was he prepared to be associated with my research, explaining to me that it would be of great disadvantage to him if he strayed outside the narrow field of folic acid metabolism!—a useful lesson for me to have learnt. Later I moved to the department of biochemistry in the College of Surgeons by kind invitation of Professors Patrick Collins and Alan Johnson. This became a very rewarding co-operative experience. The proximity of the College of Surgeons to the Adelaide meant that the PhD students could come on ward rounds and the MD students could carry out laboratory work without being too far away from the hospital.

We had many excitements and successes. Perhaps the most memorable is an International Diabetes and Atherosclerosis meeting which we ran in the RCPI in 1991 prior to the annual meeting of the European Association for the Study of Diabetes (EASD). (In 1985 I had been successful in my bid to have the meeting held in Dublin.) Professor George Alberti, who later became President of the Royal College of Physicians and of the International Diabetes Federation, gave a wonderful lecture on 'Atherosclerosis, Dementia and the fall of the Conservative Party'. The illustration that I remember most vividly is one of Margaret Thatcher, the then Prime Minister, hitting someone with her handbag!

The EASD meeting was held in the Royal Dublin Society grounds. It was the biggest medical conference ever held in Ireland with almost 3,000 delegates and 1,000 pharmaceutical industry and accompanying persons. The undertaking was not completed without difficulty and indeed my agreement to host the conference in Ireland was taken through a considerable degree of naiveté. I had many sleepless nights in the five-year period between accepting the conference and 1991. A major hazard arose in 1988 when the accountants advising the RDS decided that it would be of economic benefit to sell the grounds and invest the money. Suddenly I had no conference venue!

Carrying out research in a hospital that had little in the way of ongoing research and no research laboratories was obviously going to prove difficult. I started research with enthusiasm and little in the way of expectations. My primary goal was to encourage registrars to get involved in research and perhaps in time one of them would become really famous. Although I may not have encouraged many registrars to become enthusiastic in research I did encourage one to go and have singing lessons. In 1991 Ronan Tynan was helping me with the EASD conference. At the final gala evening in the RDS we had a jazz band that turned out to be not very exciting. Very few people were listening, being more interested in The Dubliners in another room and a ceili band with dancing in the third entertainment area. It was therefore with surprise that a few minutes after I had passed by the band my daughter came to me to suggest I go to see what was happening. When I went back there was a huge crowd around the performers. It turned out that the band had disappeared and instead Ronan Tynan and a cleaning lady were singing—it was an extraordinary sight. I persuaded Ronan that he should have lessons and his career took off under Veronica Dunne. By the time he became my intern he had already won major competitions and had become a television personality. My ward round used to consist of Ronan leading the way to the acclaim of the patients and after they had congratulated him on whatever concert he had given the day before that had been televised I would then perhaps get a chance to speak to the patients. Even then I used to feel that actually the patients would rather prefer if I went away and they could just continue their conversation with Ronan.

The funding of research was always going to be difficult but I had three pieces of luck. The first was that new theatres were to be built in the Adelaide and as part of the project fundraising was set up. This consisted of the seeking of direct donations and deeds of covenant. It was discovered after a considerable amount of money had been raised that deeds of covenant monies could not be used for buildings and perhaps with some embarrassment the board of the hospital decided to put these monies to research. I was fortunate in being able to utilise some of these monies to support a couple of PhD students.

The second piece of luck came with the EASD meeting in 1991. Due to the All Ireland finals being held on the weekend following the conference we had no difficulty in selling back to the hotels all the rooms which were not used on the weekend. As numerous rooms had been booked but not released by the various companies prior to the start of the conference the companies forfeited this money which came to us. Thus we made a profit on the conference and this was handed back to the EASD central office. We were delighted when the EASD gave us back a very considerable proportion of this money for our research department.

The success of the fundraising for the Adelaide theatres and perhaps also that of a concert held in aid of multiple sclerosis when Daniel Barenboim, at that time one of the two greatest pianists in the world, came to Dublin to play in the National Concert Hall stimulated me to have our Diabetes Research Foundation registered as a charity and funded by donations. Very quickly I realised that to get donations you actually have to ask for them and thus we set up fundraising activities with a target of £150,000. With the very exceptional help of Eleanor Herron, later chairman of the Ladies Committee of the hospital, we organised a series of concerts, tennis tournaments and, with the help of the expertise of the late Ted Figgis, an art auction. These were indeed exciting times and it was really a delight to be involved in concerts given by Louis Kentner who came to Dublin at the end of his career to play for us. He was a guest whom I fear we tried to poison by a very rich dinner the night before the concert. The concert was magnificent but we became a little anxious as he came back to the stage to play an encore. Obviously very tired by this time (he was in his 80s) he tottered and only just made it to the piano stool. Other performers included Julian Lloyd Webber, brother of the composer, who gave a cello recital and Edward Beckett, nephew of Samuel Beckett and a professional flautist in London. Another memorable concert was given by John O'Conor, the pianist who raised Irish music to new international fame and importance through the Dublin International Piano Competition.

Fundraising is certainly very hard work but very exciting and the opportunity to meet so many people outside medicine during the fundraising events added a new dimension to my experiences. My goal was to continue research until I was 50 and then leave research and concentrate on patient care and (of course) private practice. This forecast of how my life would develop did not materialise, mostly due to the amazing good luck I had in raising just enough money to continue the research from year to year to year. It is really hard when you have money for research not to spend it first before giving up research! At least this is what I found. Secondly, I had the good fortune to meet Daphne Owens, a biochemist who came in 1984 to work for six months after a career break of some years. The six months extended to a PhD and then a position as honorary research lecturer with all the insecurity of wondering when the next grant might come, the next clinical drugs trial or successful fundraising event. It would not have been possible to succeed in research and to tutor successfully PhD students, MD students and MSc students without Daphne Owens. Without her enthusiasm and drive my efforts in research would surely have evaporated.

Our research has always been related to cholesterol, lipids and diabetes, looking for the reason why patients with diabetes develop so much vascular disease. We started with low density lipoprotein, the major cholesterol carrying protein, in the blood and gradually went backwards with little forays forwards. The forays forward were into HDL 'the good cholesterol' and backwards to the very low-density lipoproteins and the chylomicrons. These particles come mostly from the food we eat. Our original observations were translated into papers in various journals and invitations to speak at international meetings around Europe as an invited speaker.

The planning of the new hospital in Tallaght provided many years of excitement. I was on the first planning board and used to attend meetings regularly in the offices in Harcourt Street and before that in the hospital boardroom. It was perhaps a little disturbing to have the assistant architect of the Department of Health explaining that any of our suggestions that seemed original, interesting or innovative would not be considered feasible or possible by the department. Mostly this was based on a tour that he had done of English hospitals some seven years before. However, I did not lose heart and continued my term on the planning board. I had the wonderful opportunity to design a metabolic ward and a diabetes centre for outpatients. It was only later that we found out that the new hospital had been downsized by a third without any discussion and, of course, the final blow came to my dreams when just before we moved to Tallaght it was announced that the diabetes unit would be transferred to make way for other specialties such as gerontology, dermatology and urology.

The prospect of moving to the new hospital which had been downsized with no diabetes centre was so appalling that I considered various options such as suicide or murder but decided I would instead get a PR company to represent people with diabetes. It was a particular blow because at the time I was Chairman of the Irish Diabetes Federation and Vice President of the EASD. The irony of the situation I fear was lost on the hospital. After much publicity I was partially appeased by being given space in the geriatric unit. After considerably more time-consuming negotiations we were finally given two disposable huts between the geriatric and psychiatric units. A third hut, which could have housed our research unit, alas was denied us.

The move took place with the amalgamation of the Adelaide and Meath diabetes services under the direction of John Barragry and his diabetes nurse specialist Helen O'Reilly. The amalgamation of the unit into a two physician unit was achieved smoothly, without any difficulty, and we continue to get on well as one unit. The appointment of chemical pathologist Gerard Boran has added a third consultant physician who takes part in the metabolic and diabetes clinic. We now have an application for a fourth consultant physician with interest in diabetes to make the team into a more homogenous unit ready to cope with the increased workload. We have a successful co-operation with Professor Hilary Hoey and her paediatric diabetes unit and there is now a smooth transition of adolescents with diabetes into the adult diabetes service. We have good social work support but unfortunately psychologist and psychiatrist support has not yet been forthcoming due to staff shortage.

The diabetes unit has, in spite of the difficulties, expanded enormously under the nursing guidance of Fiona Daly and now Helen O'Reilly. We have a nursing establishment of 4.5 wholetime equivalents, 2 secretaries, 1 receptionist, 3 clerks and 1 clinical supervisor, 3 sessions for the chiropodist/podiatrist, 1 full-time dietician and 1 part-time dietician. It is a happy unit with an excellent team spirit. The population in Tallaght has increased enormously and the number of people with diabetes is also increasing at an alarming rate. This has put the service under very great strain but in spite of that we seem to be able to give a reasonable service. We have excellent chiropody/podiatry and ophthalmology services attached to the unit. We have close integration with the nephrologists with whom we hold a joint clinic once a week and we work closely with our cardiology colleagues, between us looking after risk factors for heart disease. Our research efforts have intensified since the opening of the Trinity laboratories on site and we have now moved up from the College of Surgeons to the new laboratories. The move has, of course, been traumatic. A simple matter of furnishing a room with some desks and shelves was too much for the hospital which denied our request and I therefore had to go to the Board of Works to borrow furniture to furnish our research room; even the change of name on one of the doors to the clinical room was beyond the budget of the hospital, the paper label having to remain!

Two disposable huts in a brand new hospital might seem to some a legacy to diabetes and to the people in Tallaght with diabetes that one should be ashamed of but I remind myself that it is the work within the unit that matters not the building and certainly it is not the attitude of the board and its administrators that matters. I am proud to have developed diabetes in the Adelaide and later in the Adelaide and Meath and I leave behind me a team of people who are committed to the best care of people with diabetes. I have also left behind an ethos of research and investigation since it is through these efforts that we have attracted the best people to work in the department raising the standard of care of diabetes.

21. *Gastroenterology*

Colm O'Morain

Gastroenterology is one of the major sub-specialties of medicine. It is a relatively new specialty as it only came of age with the development of endoscopy in the late 1960s. This historic revolution, as it was called, was a major breakthrough as it allowed visualisation of the gastrointestinal tract, and the ability to take biopsies under direct vision.

The British Society of Gastroenterology, which also included Ireland, was founded in 1937. Its annual meeting was held in Dublin on two occasions. Professor Oliver FitzGerald, from St Vincent's, was the local organiser in 1968 and Professor Donald Weir, of Sir Patrick Dun's and St James's, organised the meeting in 1992; both of these meetings were deemed a huge success not only scientifically but also socially. The first world organisation meeting of gastroenterology was held in Washington, USA, in 1956.

The Irish Society of Gastroenterology was founded in 1964. Professor Peter Gatenby, the emeritus Professor of Physic at Trinity College and the Meath, was a founder member and was subsequently elected its president. The society has grown in the interim and now has its own offices in Dawson Street and more than 200 members. Professor Donald Weir and Professor Tom Hennessy from Baggot Street and St James's have been previous presidents. I am the current president.

Personalities

Gastroenterology has contributed enormously to academic medicine in Ireland. The chairs of medicine in three of the five universities in the Republic were occupied by gastroenterologists in the 1980s. The chair of Queen's University Belfast, Professor Garry Love, was also a gastroenterologist. The appeal of the specialty as a career has attracted the brightest graduates as it combines general medicine with procedures and opportunities for research.

The Federated Dublin Voluntary Hospitals, in conjunction with Trinity, played their part in allowing gastroenterology to thrive. Professor Graham Neale, a gastroenterologist, was appointed as the Regius Professor of Physic to Trinity in 1973. He came with an established international reputation for his research in absorption from the gastrointestinal tract and was a respected senior consultant at the Hammersmith Hospital, London. Professor Neale's task was particularly difficult as he had to provide a clinical service to all the small hospitals of the Federation. He also had a major teaching portfolio. He was often to be seen in Dublin on his moped travelling between his many outpatient clinics.

Professor Neale was committed to clinical research and set the foundation for this to flourish in St James's, but he was frustrated by the medical system that existed in Dublin. Private practice expanded to the detriment of research. This led to the 'Dublin syndrome' where consultants were appointed with enviable track records in research obtained in centres of excellence abroad but did not produce any research on taking a definitive post in Dublin. This might be explained by the demands of clinical practice and the fact that the arduous prolonged training abroad postponed their ability to command a reasonable salary. The same problem exists today in that some consider a consultant appointment as a lap of honour after a difficult, competitive race to achieve it. Despite these reservations, Professor Neale enjoyed his post with the Federated Dublin Voluntary Hospitals.

On Professor Neale's return to Cambridge he was replaced by Professor Donald Weir, another gastroenterologist. Professor Weir has an exemplary track record in research. He has published in excess of 200 peer-reviewed papers. What is the more significant is that all of his research was carried out in Dublin at a time when there were no funds for research. He and Professor John Scott were successful in obtaining major funding from the National Institute of Health in the US for research into folate metabolism. He also formed a dynamic partnership in research on coeliac disease with Professor Con Feighery, Alex Whelan and Cliona O'Farrelly. Professor Weir trained many doctors who are successful consultants all over the world. His recent Festschrift was attended by over 400 former students. Professor Weir was also visionary in the provision of clinical gastroenterology, founding the first endoscopy unit in Ireland with provision for day care beds in Sir Patrick Dun's. He was joined by Dr Nap Keeling as a senior lecturer and they subsequently transferred their unit to St James's. This gastroenterology unit is the busiest in Europe, offering a wide range of diagnostic and therapeutic endoscopy.

Dr Nap Keeling has been a pioneer in developing new endoscopic techniques and as a result has an international reputation in this field. He has perfected the use of stents to relieve blockage of bile ducts caused by malignant growths; this is now accepted as the best practice treatment for this condition.

Professor Dermot Kelleher joined the team in St James's. He had worked previously as registrar and lecturer in Sir Patrick Dun's having had a brilliant undergraduate career in Trinity, graduating with a first class honours degree and an equally sterling postgraduate career. He was first in Ireland to be funded by the Wellcome Trust as senior lecturer in medicine and gastroenterology. He attracted major funding for a diverse number of projects relating to gastroenterology as well as publishing widely and in peer review journals, and setting up many postgraduate courses. He succeeded Donald Weir as head of the Department of Clinical Medicine in Trinity. His crowning glory was the creation of the Dublin Molecular Medicine Institute, a multi-million-euro project that has attracted many international researchers to Ireland.

Adelaide/Meath

In 1984 I was appointed as a consultant physician with an interest in gastroenterology to the Meath and the Adelaide. I replaced Bryan Mayne—in fact, it is said it that took two physicians to replace him, myself and Professor Ian Graham, and there is a certain truth in this as his dedication to his work was legendary. There were no endoscopy facilities present in the hospital at this time. Endoscopy was carried out in the operating theatres at the end of a long surgical list. Patients were admitted as day cases to a bed occupied by an inpatient who would be asked to stay in a day room. Although there was a tremendous need for the service it took several years to establish a practice and then it became impossible to contain.

I was first to perform an endoscopic retrograde cholangio pancreatography (ERCP) in Ireland having learned the technique from Japanese endoscopists while working in France, in Nice. It was first described in 1973 by Japanese gastroenterologists. A specially designed endoscope with a lateral view allows the endoscopist to view the opening of the bilary and pancreatic duct in the second part of the duodenum (ampula of the Vater). Dye can be injected through a catheter inserted through the endoscope into the bile duct to verify the presence of bile duct stones. If stones are present the patient will be jaundiced and by making a hole (a sphincterotomy) by passing a current through the catheter, which is attached to a diathermy machine, the stone will fall into the duodenum through the opening created.

Although single handed in gastroenterology for a long period, eventually a second post was approved in 1997. Martin Buckley who had worked with me as a senior house officer, registrar and lecturer was appointed. I had been impressed with his ability, particularly his rapport with patients. He further developed his endoscopy skills at my old alma mater in Nice, skills much needed after the move to Tallaght. He also introduced endoscopic ultrasound, a new technique that allows staging of cancer in the upper intestine. Endoscopy was the stimulus to create a day ward in each hospital. The endoscopic revolution was based on fibreoptic bundles, which allowed light to be deflected and endoscopy to be developed. The fibreoptic bundles were subsequently replaced by microchip technology. The Meath was the first hospital in Europe to purchase this new technology.

The gastroenterology service could not have developed without the support of my surgical colleagues, Bill Beesley, Professor Frank Keane and Professor Arthur Tanner. An endoscopy room was created in the old ENT theatre on the ground floor in the Meath. The demand for the service was so enormous that another endoscopy room was necessary in the Adelaide. Outpatient clinics were conducted in both hospitals. It was possible to integrate the service as the same medical personnel staffed both units and this paved the way for a smooth transfer to the new site in Tallaght. However, the unit's division between two hospitals of course led to duplication. It also created the added burden of additional committee meetings for both individual hospitals, the combined hospitals and planning meetings for Tallaght.

When appointed I had been advised that the move to Tallaght was imminent. This made it difficult to develop the service in the base hospitals, as the promise was that the new hospital would provide all the necessary facilities. The great advantage of working in the base hospitals was the collegiality of the staff and their ability to get on with one another. There was a resistance to the amalgamation by some of the senior staff but most saw a new hospital in Tallaght as our only future. As Chairman of the Meath/Adelaide Medical Board in 1989–92 I regarded my position as a conduit to pave the move to Tallaght. I was on the Meath Hospital Board, elected by the governors of the hospital, and as such I was nominated to the Federated Dublin Voluntary Hospitals Central Council and am still a member.

The management skills of the secretary-managers, John Colfer and Alan Burns, were most impressive. They had visionary plans to unite both hospitals but were too *avant garde* to be accepted. Eddie Thornhill and Nicky Jermyn succeeded John Colfer in the Meath in the 1990s and Des Rogan and Tim Delaney succeeded Alan Burns in the Adelaide. They were extremely hard working and diligent. The commitment of the lay members of the hospital boards in terms of enthusiasm and true voluntary spirit was exceptional, and it is pleasing that this is retained in the new hospital.

I was also appointed to the Board of Tallaght Hospital, chaired by Professor Richard Conroy. This led to further meetings and my introduction to members of the Departments of Finance and Health. There was excitement that the new hospital would soon be a reality. However a major blow was the report of the Kennedy Committee that resulted in a reduction of the number of beds in the new hospital.

The secretary-manager of the National Children's Hospital, Des Rogan, was concerned with the expenditure on the Crosby capsule. This was a method used to obtain biopsies from the small intestine, in order to confirm or rule out coeliac disease, sensitivity to wheat, affecting over 1 in 200 people in Ireland. The capsule is swallowed the night before and is attached to a fine tube so that it can be retrieved the following day. The capsules were frequently lost and did not obtain samples as they disintegrated in the intestine. At meetings of the NCH Medical Advisory Committee it was made clear that endoscopy is the preferred method of obtaining intestinal tissue and making the diagnosis. We continue to provide an endoscopy service for children in Tallaght.

The appointment of Dr David McCutcheon as Chief Executive Officer for the new hospital in Tallaght was imaginative. He was in many ways ahead of his time and his vision was impressive, especially for academic endeavours such as research at the new hospital.

The major problem with the move to Tallaght was that the number of beds planned was less than in the base hospitals. We in the base hospitals had already experienced a loss of beds when Dr Steevens' closed and the orthopaedic service moved to the Adelaide. The medical as well as the general surgical complement of beds had been reduced. Working in the 1980s was stressful, as there were severe budget constraints and a reduction in the number of beds. In an effort to cope with this, patients admitted through accident and emergency in the Meath were transferred to the Adelaide. This worked reasonably well in some specialties but not in all as some consultants did not have joint appointments. In the Meath we began to experience the problem of patients requiring medical admission having to stay overnight in casualty. This was always an item at the hospital board meetings. Unfortunately, this situation persists and now presents an even greater problem, as there has been no increase in the number of hospital beds. There is very limited ability to discharge patients with long term disability which is one of the root causes of the problem. Another local cause is the lack of manpower. There has been very little expansion of the number of consultant physicians, which makes frequent ward rounds impossible. There is a greater expectation from the public that patients should be treated by specialists in the field of their illness, which requires transfer of patients. They now expect to be cured—years ago they were glad to get out alive!

More committees

As chairman of the physicians' subgroup (Division of Medicine) of both hospitals, acting academic head of department (until appointed to full post in Tallaght in 2002) and dean of undergraduate studies I was asked to make a major review of the curriculum and visited many other universities to incorporate new ideas. The Meath and Adelaide were under-represented at university meetings due to lack of academic appointments and to redress the balance I attended all the faculty meetings. The teaching of under-graduates was excellent, due mostly to the enthusiasm of the part-time staff and the acceptance by everyone that the hospitals, despite their size, were major teaching hospitals.

Further energy was expended in negotiating a teaching agreement with Trinity. The major difficulty was the exclusivity clause with the university which stipulated that undergraduates from other schools could not attend the hospital for tuition.

I was not involved in negotiating the Charter that governs the new hospital. Professor Brian Keogh, Dr John Barragry and Professor Ian Graham must be complimented for all the time and work they put into this, ensuring that the Charter will guarantee the voluntary aspect of the new hospital.

As a member of various committees I have gained considerable experience which has stood to me both nationally and internationally. These positions include all the executive posts of the Irish Society of Gastroenterology, election to the Council of the Royal College of Physicians of Ireland, Royal Academy of Medicine and the Irish Medical Organisation. As a founder member of the European Board of Gastroenterology, a committee founded to harmonise gastroenterology training throughout the European Union, I had the opportunity to visit and accredit different hospitals and to incorporate the services which impressed in the new hospital in Tallaght. This included one-stop clinics, where a patient with gastrointestinal symptoms would be assessed, endoscopy performed and reviewed and treatment given, all at one session. X-ray facilities are provided in the endoscopy suites. A patient-centred service, with outpatient clinics with a specialty interest in coeliac disease, inflammatory bowel disease and haemochromatosis, as well as family cancer-screening clinics, was established. I was also a founder member of the European Helicobacter Study Group in 1987, a multidisciplinary group that promotes research into this organism that causes peptic ulcer and is associated with gastric cancer. It holds an annual scientific meeting and the 1992 meeting was held in conjunction with the quatrocentenary celebration in Trinity College Dublin. Despite a postal strike in the preceding six weeks, the attendance was greater than 1000 compared to several hundred the previous years and the meeting was regarded as a tremendous success—particularly gratifying to my wife and staff who had organised it.

My training in France proved useful on European committees as I acted as the translator at the union of monospecalists. In addition, my training in the US and the UK allowed me to be elected to the council of the British Society of Gastroenterology, the nominating and education committees of Organisation Mondiale de Gastroenterolgie and the international liaison committee of the American Gastroenterology Association.

Being President of ASNEMGE, Association des Sociétés Nationales Européennes et Méditerranéennes de Gastroentérologie, an umbrella society for 38 national societies of gastroenterology, was the most arduous stint on these international committees. Subsequently elected on to the council of the United European Gastroenterology Federation I am the current vice-Chairman of the Public Affairs Committee whose mission statement is: 'The UEGF PAC aims to raise the awareness of gastrointestinal disease by prevention, early detection and treatment thereby contributing to the development of an effective health policy for the citizens of Europe.' Part of my remit is briefing politicians at European level with the Commissioner and the European Parliament.

Sister societies, such as the American Society of Gastroenterology, which employs 72 staff members to organise its affairs and lobby politically, and the European Heart Foundation, both of which are well in advance of the other specialties in terms of organisation, haave much to offer by their example.

Research

An important aspect of the workings of the Federated Dublin Voluntary Hospitals was the Ethics Committee, which included lay, medical and legal representatives. The committee reviewed research projects, particularly clinical trials. The Department of Gastroenterology had many studies approved for both national and international trials. During a ten-year period clinical trials approved by this committee saw the eradication rate of Helicobacter pylori and duodenal ulcer cure improve from 15 to 90 per cent. This committee has now been replaced by a similar body functioning jointly for Tallaght and St James's.

The environment of the hospitals helped me to develop and research two major areas, inflammatory bowel disease and Helicobacter pylori. I was able to focus on these topics due to huge clinical demand.

In 1983 there was little money for medical research. I decided to host an international conference in gastroenterology in order to generate funds and a very successful meeting on inflammatory bowel disease was held enabling me to recruit my first PhD student and to access a network of European researchers. Through these contacts an Erasmus exchange programme was inaugurated in which Trinity students spend a year in France and French medical students are welcomed here in return.

Research into Helicobacter pylori led to the cure of duodenal ulcer; this was due to a multidisciplinary approach with Professor Conor Keane in microbiology and Professor Eamonn Sweeney in pathology in St James's and Trinity.

The original letters to the editor from Barry Marshall and Robert Warren about finding Helicobacter pylori in the presence of acute gastritis were published in the *Lancet* in 1982. There can be no doubt that a Nobel Prize would be a just reward for the work carried out by these doctors. The severity of pain that patients experience if they have a duodenal ulcer is impressive. This could be explained in that an ulcer is accompanied by widespread gastritis. A study was designed in which patients with duodenal ulcer diagnosed at endoscopy were treated randomly with Cimetidine (the market leader at the time) which reduces acid secretion, or bismuth, which has antibacterial properties that heal ulcers.

Ulcer treatment was effective, but invariably the ulcer relapsed with treatment aimed at reducing acid secretion and once the medication was discontinued the acid secretion would return. The profit for the pharmaceutical companies increased, as the patient required long term acid suppression treatment. The only other effective treatment was surgery, which was aimed at cutting the nerve that secreted acid, but this resulted in considerable morbidity.

The patients who were treated with antibacterial medication had a much lower relapse rate than the patients with acid suppression and this was due to eradication of the bacteria.

This study was difficult to complete, as it was necessary to convince patients who were well of the need to have an endoscopy to confirm ulcer healing. Dr Gerry Coghlan, my registrar at the time, had to go to their homes to convince them. The unsuspecting patients thought the caller at the door was the milkman looking for arrears as their consumption of milk had reduced dramatically as the patient's ulcer was cured.

In the 1990s the bacteria was classified by WHO as a Class 1 carcinogen. More recently the Department of Gastroenterology has researched the link between bacteria and gastric cancer.

We are the first in Europe to have an open access urea breath test, a simple non-invasive method to diagnose Helicobacter pylori which my wife helped to set up in order to reduce the demand for endoscopy.

Our current research project is to promote colon cancer screening with the aim of reducing cancer mortality by 300 deaths per year in ten years. The Department of Gastroenterology has been very fortunate over the years to have had very energetic and enthusiastic junior medical and research staff and a very capable and committed group of nursing staff without which it would not have been able to thrive.

I am grateful to the Federated Dublin Voluntary Hospitals which have supported and encouraged the development of gastroenterology not only in Ireland but also internationally.

22. General surgery

Thomas P. Hennessy

The establishment of the Federated Dublin Voluntary Hospitals in 1961 was simply the formal and legal recognition of a situation which had existed for decades whereby a particular group of Dublin hospitals maintained close links with Trinity College Dublin. The hospitals were the Adelaide, the Meath, Mercer's, Baggot Street (Royal City of Dublin), Dr Steevens', Sir Patrick Dun's, the National Children's Hospital, (better known as Harcourt Street Hospital) and the Rotunda (which did not become part of the Federation).

Undergraduates from Trinity attended these hospitals for clinical instruction. Graduates of the Trinity College medical school worked as interns and often did part of their specialist training there and the majority of consultant appointments at these hospitals were graduates of Trinity. The clinical departments of Trinity medical school were located at these hospitals and Trinity's clinical professors had been established there since the latter part of the 18th century.

The intention behind the Federation was to integrate and unite a group of hospitals under central direction and management in order to provide a full range of hospital services to the population of Dublin and the Eastern Health Board area and, in the area of tertiary referral, to the entire Republic; to provide a wide range of specialist training; and finally, to promote laboratory and clinical research.

How well the hospitals attained these objectives can be seen from their achievements in the fields of cardiac surgery, vascular surgery, urology, plastic surgery and orthopaedics. In medicine, they were to the forefront in haematology, neurology, endocrinology, nephrology and cardiology.

At the time the Federation was established, one of its primary surgical strengths was in urology where T. J. D. Lane had created a self-contained urological department, well staffed both at senior and junior level and well equipped. In addition, a pioneer vascular department was established at the Adelaide by Nigel Kinnear who was President of the Royal College of Surgeons in Ireland from 1962 to 1964 and later was appointed Regius Professor of Surgery at Trinity College Dublin.

At Baggot Street, Keith Shaw single-handedly expanded his thoracic surgery work to lay the foundations of a cardiac surgery department which later joined forces with its sister unit at the Mater, established by Eoin O'Malley; it subsequently became the national cardiac surgery unit with a full complement. Eventually the Federation component of the national unit branched off as a separate unit at St James's.

The national plastic surgery unit was located at Dr Steevens' under the leadership of Brendan Prendiville. This unit also incorporated a burns unit, which acted as a tertiary referral centre.

Orthopaedics as a specialty had been established by Arthur Chance and J. C. Cherry at Dr Steevens' and subsequently by John Boyd Dunlop. John Sugars headed the orthopaedic department at the Adelaide. It was subsequently expanded to a six-man group established throughout the Federation with units located at Dr Steevens', the Meath and the Adelaide and subsequently at St James's.

General surgery was well represented throughout the Federation. In those days most general surgeons were largely engaged in gastroenterology of which gastric surgery took up a large part. Thus we had David Lane at the Meath, Jack Coolican at Mercer's, Tom O'Neill at Sir Patrick Dun's and Paddy Logan and Dick Brenan at Baggot Street doing a lot of general surgery including gastroenterology. Brandon Stephens at the Meath took endocrinology as a special interest, as did Stanley McCollum at the Adelaide. So, despite the fact that general surgery was still very 'general', most special interest areas in this discipline were covered by the surgeons of the Federation.

Some general surgeons strayed even further from their 'general' practice, for example, Jack Henry who also did thoracic surgery, as did the senior J. Coolican, although he became exclusively thoracic in time, and George Fegan achieved an international reputation for his work on varicose veins. In contrast, Seton Pringle and Douglas Montgomery remained general surgeons.

Otolaryngology was always strong in the Federation with Robert Woods and Walter Doyle Kelly in Sir Patrick Dun's and Eric Fenelon in the Adelaide.

In ophthalmology there was Frank McAuley in Baggot Street. Most of the others were concentrated in the Eye and Ear Hospital.

Casualty departments at this time were staffed by junior doctors, usually at SHO level. The Meath was one of the first to appoint an accident and emergency consultant, Derek Robinson, thus effectively setting up an A&E department.

Professors of surgery at that time were part-time and possessed only the barest nucleus of a department and no support staff. When George Fegan was appointed Clinical Professor of Surgery in 1965, he had already achieved a worldwide reputation for his pioneering work on the physiology and pathology of varicose veins and for his use of sclerotherapy in the treatment of this condition.

Although continuing as a part-time professor, George quickly expanded the department of surgery, appointing lecturers, research fellows and technicians. When TCD suggested he become a full-time professor he told them they couldn't afford him.

When I returned from the US in 1967, I joined the Trinity department of surgery as a lecturer. I had worked with Dr Owen Wangensteen at the University of Minnesota and was at this stage committed to surgical gastroenterology as a career. Fegan, greatly to his credit, allowed me to continue in this field rather than involving me in the expanding varicose veins programme.

After three years as a lecturer in the department. of surgery working at Sir Patrick Dun's, a post which was very rewarding and which I hugely enjoyed, I was appointed to UCC as a senior lecturer. I spent almost five years in Cork after which I returned to Trinity and the Federation as Professor of Surgery, succeeding George Fegan who had retired early on health grounds.

Already the transfer of part of the Federated Dublin Voluntary Hospitals to St James's was being mooted. I recall being asked at my interview for the chair how I would propose to effect the transfer. I cannot recall my full answer, but I remember saying the hospitals would have to be moved one at a time.

During the three years in Sir Patrick Dun's and my subsequent five years in Cork, very significant changes had taken place within the Federation and the department of surgery in Trinity. The cardiac surgery department in Baggot Street, under the leadership of Keith Shaw, had developed its open heart surgery programme and transferred to the national heart unit at the Mater, retaining thoracic surgery work in Baggot Street. This amalgamation of high technology surgery into a single national unit was effective from the economic point of view.

The urological unit at the Meath, led by Dermot O'Flynn, Victor Lane and Michael Butler, continued to provide a high quality clinical service to the public, a first-class training to aspiring urologists and a very significant body of research. Fortunately, the urology department was complemented by a progressive and productive nephrology department. The plastic surgery unit at Dr Steevens' continued its role as a national plastic and burns unit. Vascular surgery was still active at the Adelaide, and J. C. Milliken ran a single-handed vascular unit at Sir Patrick Dun's with Mary Henry looking after the varicose veins section.

Many of the older surgeons, for instance, Douglas Montgomery and Seton Pringle, had retired and Paddy Logan had died around the time of my return. David Lane had transferred to Dun's to support Tom O'Neill in gastroenterological surgery. Nigel Kinnear had retired and Stanley McCollum had succeeded to the Regius Chair of Surgery.

When I started as professor of surgery in 1975, a secretary, a few offices and a teaching centre were provided in the basement of Sir Patrick Dun's but no beds. Robert Quill, with whom I had previously worked in Dun's, was senior lecturer in Surgery. We decided to work as a team with shared junior staff. This worked very well in Baggot Street where we had an adequate complement of beds and operating times and the system eventually worked out satisfactorily at St James's although initially our clinical access was limited. There were insufficient facilities at Dr Steevens' to allow for two-man teams, so I did a few sessions there alone.

So I began with an administration and teaching unit at one hospital and beds and clinical responsibilities at three others, which appeared a rather unsustainable situation. However, most surgeons had multiple appointments in those days so it didn't seem very strange but I spent a lot of time driving from one place to another.

The first thing Bob Quill and I decided was that we needed another lecturer. George Fegan had appointed lecturers in the Adelaide, the Meath, Sir Patrick Dun's and Dr Steevens' and some of these were still in post but they had their own duties and we needed someone who would work with us exclusively. We appointed Peter Delaney.

Most senior surgeons in the Federation were very experienced teachers and were fortunately still active in clinical bedside teaching. More recently-appointed surgeons, like Bill Beesley, David FitzPatrick and Michael Pegum, had been full-time lecturers and were experienced in all aspects of teaching and we knew that we could rely on their help, but we needed someone who would help us organise the teaching, get the research programme going and help with the clinical work and Peter was ideal.

It was clear that we had the facilities and personnel to provide excellent teaching programmes both at undergraduate and postgraduate level. Developing the clinical services at St James's was a somewhat more daunting prospect. While St James's had enormous potential there was no doubt that clinical services were underdeveloped. There were only two general surgeons, Hugh McCarthy and Frank Ward, to look after 120 surgical beds. There was one part-time visiting urologist, no vascular surgeon and no orthopaedic surgeon. There was no A&E department and consequently emergency admissions were rare.

There were two obvious priorities: first the establishment of an A&E department and second a department of vascular surgery. Despite some initial reluctance on the part of the older staff, an A&E department was opened quite quickly. Within a matter of weeks this revolutionised the entire atmosphere of the hospital. From being a medical and surgical backwater, the place suddenly came to life with an enormous increase in acute admissions and a greatly increased attendance at all outpatient departments. Soon we were pressing for increased operating theatre facilities and we converted an old store room in the operating theatre block in Hospital 7 to serve as an extra theatre.

There was some delay in getting our vascular surgeon, probably because of the expense of setting up such a high-tech unit, but before long we were able to appoint Greg Shanik. Our next priority was to establish an orthopaedic department. Because of the A&E need at St James's, the department was principally involved in the treatment of orthopaedic trauma but, like all appointments to St James's at that time, some sessions were allocated to a Federation hospital. The new appointees were Gary Fenelon and Hugh Smyth who also were assigned to Dr Steevens' for their elective work..

Because of the high-tech nature of vascular surgery, there is a need to concentrate the service in one unit. As a consequence, James Milliken transferred some of his sessions from Sir Patrick Dun's to the vascular unit at St James's and a third surgeon, Dermot Moore, was appointed within a few years.

The increased clinical activity at St James's called for increased urological services. This service was initially provided by Michael Butler, working part time between St James's and the Meath. Eventually he transferred full time to the Meath and two new urological appointees to the Federation, Ron Grainger and Ted McDermott, provided services at St James's and the Meath.

Meanwhile, maxillo-facial surgery services had been developed at Dr Steevens' by Frank Brady who also provided services at St James's.

Although open-heart surgery had moved from Baggot Street to the Mater, thoracic surgery continued to expand there with the appointment of David Luke and, later, Eilis McGovern. By this time virtually all the senior surgical staff of the Meath and Adelaide had retired; they had been replaced by Frank Keane and Arthur Tanner who joined Bill Beesley in general surgery and by Martin Feely in vascular surgery. David Lane had transferred to Sir Patrick Dun's where Tom O'Neill was still in post. Robert Quill and I continued to provide general surgical services at Baggot Street along with Dick Brenan.

At this time the surgeons of the Federation were providing a high level surgical service to the local community as well as regional and national referral services in a variety of surgical disciplines including surgical gastroenterology, surgical oncology, breast and endocrine surgery, cardiac surgery, thoracic surgery, vascular surgery, plastic surgery, orthopaedics, urology and maxillo-facial surgery. They looked after the educational needs of 250 medical students each year and were active in both clinical and laboratory research. But although consultant appointments continued to be made in the Federation they were all either linked to St James's or structured in such a way that they could be transferred to the new Tallaght Hospital which in due course would replace the Meath, the Adelaide and the National Children's Hospital.

The closure of the Federated Dublin Voluntary Hospitals was done in two phases. The first hospitals to close were Mercer's, Baggot Street, Dun's and Steevens'. The arrangements were that as each hospital closed the medical and some nursing staff would transfer to St James's. In the case of Mercer's, which was the first to close, most of the medical and surgical staff were close to retirement and there were no transfers to St James's. Next to go was Baggot Street. Since Robert Quill and I were already on the St James's staff we automatically became full-time staff there. By this time Dick Brenan, a marvellous clinical teacher, regrettably, had died. When Sir Patrick Dun's closed a few years later only one surgeon, J. C. Milliken, transferred to St James's. Both Tom O'Neill and David Lane retired.

The closure of each of these hospitals was a poignant moment deeply felt by the staff. In the case of Baggot Street this small but active hospital had provided sterling service to the citizens of Dublin and the wider Irish community over its 150-year history and had given no fewer than eleven presidents to the Royal College of Surgeons in Ireland during that time.

Sir Patrick Dun's had a distinguished history and the chair of surgery was located there for many generations with such distinguished occupants as Edward Hallaran Bennett.

Dr Steevens' was the last of the group to close with the transfer of the departments of plastic surgery and maxillo-facial surgery, headed by Matt McHugh and Frank Brady respectively, to St James's and orthopaedics and trauma to the Adelaide and Meath.

The second closure phase took place in 1998 with the transfer to Tallaght of the Adelaide, the Meath and the National Children's Hospital.

The Federated Dublin Voluntary Hospitals represented a laudable attempt at creating an integrated and co-operative hospital group and while there were inevitably tensions and stresses in the system, it was, on the whole, highly successful.

The Federation served the people of Dublin and the people of Ireland well and played a major role in the development of urology, vascular surgery, cardiac surgery, orthopaedics and plastic and maxillo-facial surgery in Ireland. These developments were brought about by men of vision like T. J. Lane, Keith Shaw, Nigel Kinnear, Arthur Chance, George Fegan and Brendan Prendiville among others.

I remember with great affection the older surgeons of the Federation, many of whom were my mentors and advisers not only in my young days but also after I became Professor of Surgery.

Arthur Chance had the endearing habit of rapping you on the knuckles with a forceps or needle holder if he didn't like what you were doing while assisting him in the operating theatre.

Nigel Kinnear, a man of impeccable decorum and correctness, really startled me when speaking to the Biological Society on the occasion of my inauguration as President of the Society. Referring to the term 'borborygmi' he announced that in his young days it was defined as 'the frustrated rumbles of a baffled fart'.

There were innumerable stories about Tom O'Neill. The one I like best is unrepeatable. The one I like second best refers to an occasion when he missed an easy putt. Having ground his teeth, thrown his putter on the ground and the rest of his clubs into a nearby pool he turned to his partner and snarled, 'Barry, isn't it fortunate that I have a sunny disposition!'

George Fegan's restless energy and drive often unsettled his colleagues at Dun's. Jackie Wallace once told him he was too much of an entrepreneur. 'What do you mean?' asked George. Joe Kirker, who was always ready with a *bon mot*, said, 'He means you're a spiv, George!'

Following their pioneer work and developments during the years of Federation, the departments of surgery fully achieved that most difficult of feats, a transition that through self dissolution arrived at a new and more integrated state with enormous potential. The dissolution of the Federation, while marking the end of an era, also heralded the beginning of a new chapter in a long and noble history of service to medicine and to the community. St James's and Tallaght face the future with a confidence born of a sound pedigree and a unique ethos.

23. *Gynaecology*

John Bonnar

When I took up my post in September 1995 in Trinity as professor and head of the department of obstetrics and gynaecology, my consultant appointment had six sessions in obstetrics and gynaecology in the Rotunda and three sessions in the Adelaide. The Trinity department of obstetrics and gynaecology included the Rotunda and all the Federated Hospitals. Each of the hospitals had some gynaecological beds and consultant services. Overall 35–40 beds were allocated to gynaecology.

Consultant gynaecologists

The most senior gynaecologist was Rory O'Hanlon who provided consultant services in the Meath and Mercer's and between them 12 to 14 beds were allocated to gynaecology. Rory O'Hanlon was a great character, widely known for his sailing skills and love of the sea. He claimed to have trained all of the masters of the Rotunda from Alan Browne onwards in both gynaecology and obstetrics.

Another well-known gynaecologist in Dublin was Ninian Falkiner who was assistant master in the Rotunda Hospital from 1923 to 1926 and subsequently gynaecologist in Baggot Street. In the 1930s he had an outstanding record of scientific research in reproductive medicine. In his work he had the help of Bronte Gatenby, Professor of Zoology, Trinity College Dublin. The areas of research included menstrual bleeding, biology of implantation and the placental circulation. In the years 1940–7 he was Master of the Rotunda and was among the first to extend the use of caesarean section to the management of severe pre-eclampsia. In these years he worked with Jay Fleming, consultant anaesthetist, who introduced spinal anaesthesia. Ninian Falkiner was an accomplished yachtsman and in the 1960s he was accompanied often by Peter Denham, the gynaecologist in Sir Patrick Dun's, in long cruises and as far north as the Arctic Circle. Some years after Peter Denham retired I recall visiting the harbour in Copenhagen where I noticed a ship flying the Tricolour. This was the *Asgard*, the Irish sailing ship for training young people. On the foredeck dressed as chef was the familiar figure of Peter Denham who was the ship's cook. He was enjoying life cooking for a crew of at least 20 young people.

Michael Solomons was the gynaecologist at Baggot Street. He was meticulous in his work and was a courageous captain in the stormy sea of the development of family planning services in Ireland. In a recent book, *Maternity in Ireland,* sociologist Patricia Kennedy paid tribute to Michael Solomons and referred to his book *Pro Life?* (1992) in which he concluded that Church and State had colluded with the medical profession in controlling women's fertility through not allowing contraception:

> When it came to the prevention of conception and unwanted pregnancy the Church and the State had the Irish people in a moral and legal stranglehold . . . Meanwhile, the health of women coping with successive pregnancies frequently suffered. When these women looked to the medical establishment for help it was not there.

In Dr Steevens' the gynaecology services were provided by Hugo McVey who was also the lecturer in obstetrics and gynaecology in the TCD department. He had come to Dublin from Glasgow to do his medical training in Trinity College. In the late 1960s, Sandy McVey, as he was known, had represented the Fellows of the Royal College of Obstetricians and Gynaecologists on the Council during the presidency of Sir John Peel. Sir John Peel had apparently remarked, 'Who is this new Fellow on the Council, he looks like a Jew, speaks with a Scottish accent and talks of the Irish as "we"'! Sandy McVey and his wife Nuala became close friends and I had the feeling that I had almost been adopted into the McVey family as a refugee from Scotland. They were a delightful and charming couple devoted to their family. Nuala McVey in her younger years had appeared on the front of *Time Magazine* representing Ireland as one of the twelve most beautiful women in the world.

Background

I had graduated from Glasgow University and had my specialist training in Glasgow where I was senior registrar with Sir Hector McLennan. In 1969 I was appointed first assistant to Sir John Stallworthy in Oxford. Gynaecology was highly developed in Oxford with 40 beds in the Churchill. Six consultants provided the service in obstetrics and gynaecology and each had two major gynaecological lists each week. Sub-specialisation had its early shoots in Oxford, which had a gynaecological/oncology referral service and a specialised clinic for infertility. In the gynaecology/oncology service consultant radiotherapists worked with the gynaecologists in deciding the appropriate treatment for cervical carcinoma and carcinoma of the endometrium. Patients with cancer of the cervix were referred from a wide area to Oxford and 15–20 Wertheim's operations were performed annually for stage 1B and stage 2A cervical cancer following pre-operative radiation. In Oxford my eyes were opened as to what was needed to provide high quality gynaecological care and I was heavily influenced there as to how gynaecology should be developing.

Gynaecology

A review of gynaecological services in the British Isles by the Royal College of Obstetricians and Gynaecologists in the early 1970s revealed that a gynaecologist in England did twice the gynaecological surgery of a gynaecologist in Scotland and a gynaecologist in Scotland did twice the gynaecological surgery of a gynaecologist in Ireland. One reason for this was that the consultants in Ireland tended to be Fellows of the College of Physicians whereas those in the UK became Fellows of one of the Royal Colleges of Surgeons. In Ireland they devoted most of their practice to obstetrics and the main part of the private income of a consultant was from obstetrics. With the deficit in gynaecological services in Ireland prior to the 1970s it was accepted that Irish graduates had to go England or the United States to have gynaecological training. Since 40 per cent of the population in Ireland has private health insurance which covers obstetrics there is a high demand for private obstetric care in Ireland. This has been one of the factors which has delayed the development of the sub-specialties in obstetrics and gynaecology. Another factor which undoubtedly influenced development of gynaecological oncology was the relatively low incidence of cervical cancer compared to the United Kingdom.

Federated Hospital gynaecolocical sub-group

During the years 1975–80 the consultant gynaecologists in the Federated Hospitals endeavoured to create a single gynaecological unit in the group. In each of the Federated Hospitals the gynaecologist had a 50 per cent share of an intern who usually changed every three months. In the Adelaide I had a lecturer/registrar who was partly funded by Trinity and this post was shared with the Rotunda. This post did provide good training opportunities in gynaecological surgery and most of the individuals went on to be consultant obstetricians and gynaecologists in Ireland. These include Eamon McGuinness, Peter McKenna, Noreen Gleeson and Julian Dockery.

The consultant gynaecologists in the Federated Hospitals all recognised that the specialty was unlikely to develop by the perpetuation of small single-handed consultant units spread throughout the six hospitals. A gynaecology unit in the Meath was the nearest we came to establishing a gynae-cology department. The moving force behind this was Rory O'Hanlon. An added attraction was that the Meath had pioneered urology and had an established national centre for urological surgery. We felt that the two specialties would complement each other in the Meath. At this time the Meath/Adelaide Hospital group had been established and a gynacology unit of 25 beds in the Meath with 10 in the Adelaide was proposed. To establish this it was proposed that orthopaedics should be transferred from the Meath and Adelaide to Dr Steevens' where a large elective orthopaedic unit would be established. The development was discussed with the Department of Health who were positive about providing funds which would establish the gynaecology unit in the Meath and the orthopaedic unit in Dr Steevens'. In the event, both the Meath and the Adelaide were reluctant to agree the transfer of orthopaedics and the status quo was preferred.

Professor Ian Howie, Vice-Provost of Trinity, had a major role in the planning of the new St James's which was originally intended to replace the six Federated Hospitals with a large modern teaching hospital within one mile of the existing hospitals. From 1983 to 1987 I was Dean of the Faculty of Health Sciences in Trinity. The clinical professors of Trinity all recog-nised the urgent need for a new teaching hospital or hospitals to replace the Federated Hospitals which had been built in the 18th and 19th centuries. The developments in hospital medicine required high-cost capital equip-ment which could only be justified in acute hospitals of 5–600 beds and such high-cost hospital development and intensive training of specialised staff could not be provided in six small hospitals.

The professors of the clinical departments and laboratory medicine were committed to the establishment of a new teaching hospital on the St James's site. Professor Graham Neale, Professor of Clinical Medicine, and Professor Tom Hennessy, Professor of Surgery, began the move to St James's. In 1985 I followed, with Professor Harrison moving from the Rotunda to expand the gynaecological service in St James's which had been provided by Tom Hanratty with the help of Donal O'Brien from the Coombe.

In St James's there was also a maternity unit with approximately 3,000 births per annum. We had difficulty in St James's maternity unit in estab-lishing a tertiary care neonatal service and had to rely on the Coombe for the care of very low birth weight babies. At this time the number of babies being delivered in the Coombe had decreased and it was possible for the Coombe with its large neonatal unit to accommodate the deliveries of St James's. The proposal was that if we transferred the St James's maternity unit to the Coombe, Dr Steevens' could be closed ahead of schedule and transferred to St James's with ENT and plastic surgery and a gynaecological unit could then be established in the maternity unit.

Within the Federated Hospitals my understanding of the situation in the mid 1980s was that there was a reluctance in the Meath and the Adelaide to commit to the transfer to St James's. In the event, two new major teaching hospitals were developed with Mercer's, Dr Steevens', Sir Patrick Dun's and Baggot Street transferring to St James's. The Meath/Adelaide with the National Children's Hospital were to continue for the time being on their existing sites with a view to subsequent transfer to Tallaght as the second teaching hospital of Trinity. I recall when, as Dean of the faculty, with Provost Bill Watts I had a meeting with consultants of the Meath and Adelaide who were concerned that Tallaght could end up being the poor relation of Trinity as the academic units might be concentrated in the Trinity Centre for Health Sciences in St James's. Bill Watts gave the commitment of Trinity to the academic development of Tallaght and the building of facilities there comparable to those at St James's. After the meeting I expressed my concern to him that finances were already over committed at St James's. His reply was that funding would be the problem for the people coming after us and they would have to deliver on this commitment given by Trinity. Trinity has delivered and continues to do so!

Gynaecology therefore followed the hospital groupings with the gynaecological services of Dr Steevens', Mercer's, Sir Patrick Dun's and Baggot Street developing as a single gynaecological unit in St James's where the gynaecological service is provided by five consultants with two specialising in gynaecological oncology. It is planned that Trinity will shortly appoint two professors, a professor of gynaecology based in St James's with sessions in the Rotunda Hospital and a professor of obstetrics based in the Coombe, probably specialising in maternal and foetal medicine. The gynaecology units of the Meath/Adelaide subsequently transferred to Tallaght Hospital where it is planned that four gynaecologists will provide the service.

Conclusion

Trinity now has two modern teaching hospitals. These are the finest teaching hospitals in Ireland with well-trained, highly specialised medical and nursing staff. The Trinity Faculty of Health Sciences with the School of Physic, and Schools of Speech and Language Therapy, Physiotherapy and Occupational Therapy all have a major presence in both hospitals. Perhaps the future will see the Coombe relocating on the site of either St James's or Tallaght following the example of Holles Street which, it is proposed, will move to St Vincent's. There seems no doubt that, to provide the best quality service, a maternity hospital should have the security of an adjacent general hospital to allow specialised medical care and facilities to be immediately available.

I would like to end by paying tribute to the substantial input of the non-medical senior academics at Trinity in the development of St James's and Tallaght. In particular I wish to thank Ian Howie, Vice-Provost, Bill Watts, Provost, Tom Mitchell, Provost and John Scott, Bursar, who all devoted enormous skill, energy and time to the development of the Trinity teaching hospitals and in no small way played their part in the successful move to these new institutions.

24 Haematology

Ian Temperley

In 1958, when I was appointed junior pathologist, the school of pathology was responsible, under Professor R. A. Q. O'Meara, for morbid anatomy and histopathology of all the hospitals which formed the Federated Dublin Voluntary Hospitals (FDVH) in 1961. At this time the School supplied a limited haematology and biochemistry service for these hospitals.

Following a visit from the GMC a ruling was made that each hospital should have its own laboratory which would take care of 'general' pathology. Dr Celsus McCrea was appointed pathologist to Baggot Street, Dr Niall Gallagher to Dun's, Dr Nick Jaswon to Dr Steevens' and the National Children's Hospital, Dr Betty Wallace to the Adelaide and Dr Mullaney (senior lecturer in pathology) to the Meath. All would have been responsible to a varying degree for haematology in their laboratories.

By the late 1950s, haematology in Ireland was very much in its infancy. Dr Liam O'Connell had arrived back in Dublin at or around this time. He was trained in haematology in the US and ultimately was appointed to St Vincent's. Dr Douglas Mellon was identified with haematology in Dr Steevens' and more specifically in the Rotunda. In 1959 the Trinity lecturer in pathology (later professor of pathology UCD), Dr Noel Clarke, began to introduce more sophisticated coagulation tests.

Professor Peter Gatenby was concerned that haematology should be developed in Trinity and its associated hospitals and with R. A. Q. O'Meara recommended me for the Adrian Stokes Memorial Fellowship. It was arranged in 1960–61 that I should train in the Radcliffe and Churchill Hospitals, Oxford, under Professor L. Witts, Dr Sheila Callender, Professor R. MacFarlane and Dr Rosemary Biggs. It would have been difficult to find a more expeditious way of learning the trade of haematology in so short a time.

Laboratory haematology

In 1962 I was appointed lecturer in haematology and in the same year set up vitamin B12 and later folic acid assays in the laboratory of the school of pathology. These eventually provided a service for doctors throughout the country and became the focus of an important sub-unit of haematology. This unit supported research undertaken by Professors Donald Weir and John Scott and in 1970 Sean O'Broin became its technical head. In the early 1960s a small radioactive isotope laboratory was set up in the Meath carrying out red cell volumes, red cell survival tests, Schilling tests and ferrokinetic studies. The investigation of coagulation disorders, started by Noel Clarke, was expanded in the Meath laboratory during the mid-1960s to include the estimation of coagulation factors VIII and IX essential for the diagnosis and management of haemophilia. By 1970 the Federated Hospitals were in advance of all the other hospitals in the Republic in the investigation of haematological disorders. Invaluable contributions were made during the 1960s by many technologists and scientists including Kathleen O'Mahony, Tom Driver, Nuala Horner, Daphne Colleary and Marie Meehan.

The management of laboratory medicine in the Federation took a further turn in 1966 following a visit from the Royal College of Pathologists. Specialisation became the order of the day; biochemistry was centred in Dun's, microbiology in the Adelaide, haematology in the Meath and morbid anatomy and histopathology in the school of pathology. In 1968 the Federation gave all senior pathologists consultant grading.

I was appointed consultant in haematology centred in the Meath and a year later became associate professor and fellow of TCD. In 1971 the first Coulter S automatic blood cell counter in Ireland was added to the equipment in the central haematology laboratory in the Meath. All branches of haematological investigation were expanded and more complex tests introduced. A caravan, to be replaced by a small building, was put up against the surrounding hospital wall to house the 'cutting edge' investigations of coagulation abnormalities!

In 1982 laboratory haematology, like all the other centralised Federated laboratories, moved from the Meath to the Central Pathology Laboratory (CPL) in St James's Hospital, a new purpose-built laboratory beside the TCD temporary teaching block. For the first time all the scattered sub-units of the FDVH haematology laboratory came together. They joined with the St James's in situ haematology laboratory of which Dr Kim Ryder was the haematologist in charge. The Federated Hospitals, apart from the Meath, the Adelaide and the National Children's Hospital, were gradually incorporated into St James's. Laboratory centralisation was, in general, a success but transportation of samples from, and reporting of results to, the remaining hospitals were on-going challenges.

During the 1980s the new St James's haematology laboratory concentrated on expanding the diagnostic service for coagulation defects and leukaemia and allied disorders. One of the important laboratory advances was the development of a leukaemia/lymphoma cell marker immuno-phenotyping service by Dr Emer Lawlor. Emer first joined the Federation haematology laboratory in 1972. In 1985 she was appointed lecturer and in 1992 senior lecturer in haematology. She is now deputy medical director of the IBTS and consultant in charge of the department of transfusion medicine in St James's.

Clinical haematology: the National Children's Hospital

With the encouragement and support of Nick Jaswon and Dr Raymond Rees a small clinical haematology unit was established in the National Children's Hospital from 1965 onwards. The unit was serviced by the NCH laboratory and the larger haematology unit in the Meath. Raymond Rees provided beds and essential paediatric back-up. In 1965, a systematic therapy programme was established in the NCH for the treatment of childhood leukaemia. In 1970 the UK Medical Research Council's children's leukaemia protocol was introduced. The vital difference was the introduction of CNS prophylaxis using radiotherapy and intrathecal chemotherapy. With this began the close co-operation between St Luke's Hospital and clinical haematology in the Federation and St James's. A review undertaken in 1980 revealed a 47 per cent complete remission rate for childhood leukaemia treated between 1970 and 1975 using the MRC protocol.

By 1971 the clinical haematology unit in the NCH, with its leukaemia and haemophilia base, began its career as a referral centre. A weekly outpatients' clinic was already in operation. During the 1970s co-operation grew with the clinicians of Our Lady's Hospital for Sick Children, Crumlin. In 1983, I was appointed haematologist to Our Lady's. Eventually the more complex haematological cases were referred to the NCH. By 1995, as judged by admissions, haematology was the largest unit in the hospital.

Despite this development, the NCH was never comfortable with the concept of becoming a national leader in the specialty of haematology. From 1987 Dr Fred Jackson, lecturer in haematology, and Dr Joan O'Riordan, St James's haematology registrar, played substantial roles in the management of patients in the NCH in addition to their roles in St James's. In 1992 Fred Jackson was appointed consultant haematologist to Waterford Regional Hospital. He was followed as lecturer in haematology by Dr Joan Fitzgerald who continued to provide the same support. Joan is now a consultant haematologist in the Irish Blood Transfusion Service (IBTS).

A determined effort in the 1990s was made by Professor Hilary Hoey and Catherine McDaid, NCH secretary-manager, to support haematology as a front-line NCH unit. A specialist haemophilia nurse was appointed for the first time. Dr Owen Smith, appointed my successor in the haematology sub-units of paediatrics and haemophilia in 1995, advanced the cause of the specialised unit following the hospital's move to Tallaght with the Adelaide and Meath, in 1998. However, towards the early 2000s, rationalisation and politics ruled the day; St James's and Our Lady's became the centres for adult and paediatric haematology incorporating general haematology, leukaemia, bone marrow transplantation and haemophilia. In 2002, Owen Smith was appointed professor of haematology by Trinity, relinquishing the directorship of the National Centre for Hereditary Coagulation Disorders, (incorporating the National Haemophilia Centre). In 2003, he agreed to move, together with the NCH paediatric haematology unit, to a new haematology centre in Our Lady's, joining the incumbent haematologist, Dr Aengus O'Marcaigh. More recently they have been joined by a third newly appointed haematology consultant and the unit now shares a further consultant with the National Centre for Hereditary Coagulation Disorders.

Haemophilia

In 1969 the Irish Haemophilia Society was formed mainly due to the efforts of Mrs Eithne Scallan of Wexford and Dr Jack O'Riordan of the Blood Transfusion Service Board. Because the Central Haematology Laboratory had a coagulation unit developed to required standards I was asked by the Society and by Dr Cyril Joyce of the Department of Health to establish a haemophilia centre. The Meath allotted four beds in the west wing and the National Children's Hospital agreed to provide an 'adequate number of beds'. In 1971 the Minister for Health, Erskine Childers, formally established the National Haemophilia Centre at a ceremony in the Meath. The division of the centre, necessitated by the need for paediatric back-up, remained a source of weakness. The centre was charged with forming a register of all patients with an inherited coagulation factor deficiency and providing guidance on request for the diagnosis and management of these disorders.

The average life span of 110 severe haemophilia patients registered in 1971 was 15 years; only 11 were over the age of 30. Initially the majority of severe patients had serious arthropathy. During the early 1970s the emphasis was on bed rest, physiotherapy and orthopaedic surveillance. A weekly haemophilia outpatients' clinic was established. In the Meath a patient could see a dentist (Dr Gerry Owens), an orthopaedic surgeon (John Sugars), a social worker (Mary Lahiffe) and a haematologist in the course of one visit. Dr Adrian Cowan, David FitzPatrick and Laurette Kiernan were their counterparts in the National Children's Hospital. Patients were encouraged to come to the wards of both hospitals to receive prophylactic infusions of factor VIII or IX concentrates if they felt a bleed coming on—an early form of 'day care centre'.

In 1976 the adult section of the centre moved to St James's together with the remainder of the clinical haematology unit originally centred in the Meath. An important advance was made when, in the late 1970s, Margaret King SRN was appointed by St James's to care solely for patients with haemophilia. In 1977 a major programme of 'home therapy' was initiated. Patients were trained to give themselves their concentrates intravenously at home. This was made easier by the introduction of more refined concentrates allowing large doses to be given in a small amount of fluid.

Orthopaedic surgeons were an integral part of the service for patients with haemophilia. About 1975 they began to correct a backlog of deformities and by the late 1970s elective knee synovectomies were being carried out. During the early 1980s hip and knee prostheses were introduced. John Sugars retired in 1981 and was replaced by Hugh Smyth. In the period 1972–2001 David FitzPatrick provided orthopaedic care for haemophilia children in the National Children's Hospital. Before the advent of the National Haemophilia Centre dental care was limited. The backlog of extractions was undertaken in the Meath and National Children's Hospital under the cover of concentrates. During the early 1980s Drs Barry Harrington and Liam Convery of the Dental Hospital took over the pioneering work of Gerry Owens and Adrian Cowan. The Dental Hospital provided a comprehensive service in advance of most haemophilia centres in other countries.

The emerging spectre of AIDS, associated with concentrate therapy, did not spare Irish haemophilia patients and in November 1984 the first case was noted in the National Haemophilia Centre. Anti-HIV results became available by April 1985; 68 per cent of severe haemophilia A patients were positive. It is important to record the service given by Drs Peter Daly, Helene Daly and Fred Jackson to the centre during the second half of 1985 in my absence on sabbatical. A total of 104 patients with both types of haemophilia were infected in the Republic; about 80 were associated with the National Centre. From 1985 a continuing number of patients developed the manifestations of AIDS and unfortunately by 1999 52 of the 104 patients were dead. These sad events engendered great stress among the staff of the haematology units of both the National Children's Hospital and St James's.

Hepatitis was observed in the mid-1970s as a side-effect of plasma product (concentrate) treatment. While a few cases were diagnosed as being due to hepatitis B the majority could not be serologically typed and were referred to as having non-A, non-B hepatitis (NANBH). It was not until 1991 that these patients were confirmed as having hepatitis C. The hepatitis C serological test revealed that 81 per cent of patients with haemophilia B and 35 per cent of patients with mild haemophilia A and B were infected; 200 patients attached to the National Haemophilia Centre were involved. NANBH was regarded for a decade as being a relatively modest problem. NANBH/hepatitis C is a slowly progressing condition and it was not until the second half of the 1980s that clinical manifestations of chronic hepatitis and hepatic failure were noted by the centre. Patients were referred at first to Professor Donald Weir, from 1992 to Dr Anne Tobin, lecturer in gastro-enterology, and in late1994 to Professor Dermot Kelleher, head of the newly formed department of hepatology in St James's.

The consequences of HIV and hepatitis C blighted the major advances made in the management of haemophilia during the 1970s and early 1980s. In 1999–2001 a tribunal of inquiry into the 'infection with HIV and hepatitis C of persons with haemophilia and related diseases' was held under Judge Alison Lindsay. The tribunal report illustrates the difficulties and perils faced by doctors providing care at times of medical uncertainty and in the face of limited resources.

Despite these serious problems the centre continued to expand. By 1990 over 400 patients were registered with an inherited coagulation factor disorder. By this date concentrates free of HIV, HCV and hepatitis B had been introduced and during the 1990s great strides were made in the management of HIV and HCV. In 1988 Sister King, the haemophilia sister, retired and was replaced by Sister Aideen O'Shea and in 1992 the space allocated by St James's to the haemophilia centre was increased to accommodate a separate day-care centre and a dental surgery. The centre started to register patients with thrombophilia. This expansion was fully supported by the coagulation laboratory in St James's under the able guidance of Sophia Kelleher and later Mary Byrne.

By 2000, Dr Owen Smith, who took charge of the National Haemophilia Centre in 1995, had organised funds to build a separate haemophilia unit, including a 'state of the art' laboratory in the St James's compound near the Rialto gate. This unit, incorporating the National Haemophilia Centre, was renamed the National Centre for Hereditary Coagulation Disorders. At last, the wishes of the Irish Haemophilia Society were realised after 25 years of representation to the Meath and St James's and the Department of Health. Owen continued to develop molecular biological technology for the diagnosis of both thrombophilia and coagulation deficiency syndromes, an endeavour which was only completed recently. In 2001, he was replaced by Dr Barry White as director of the centre. Barry has been joined by two fellow consultants, Drs Beatrice Nolan and James O'Donnell, specialising in bleeding disorders. The former is also responsible for patients with haemophilia in Our Lady's. Aideen O'Shea's position has been filled by 10 specialised nursing staff!

Clinical haematology in the Meath and St James's

Gradually during the late 1960s and early 1970s a clinical haematology unit grew in the Meath under the wing of Peter Gatenby. The unit incorporated the adult section of the service for haemophilia. A separate weekly outpatients for non-haemophilia patients was established. By 1978–9 over 70 patients with acute leukaemia were treated in the Meath/St James's using the latest UK MRC protocols. In November 1974 Peter Gatenby resigned hospital and university posts to take up a position in the United Nations, New York. This was to have an unexpected beneficial effect. I did not have clinical consultant status in the Meath and it was felt by the hospital that I was using resources which could be better employed elsewhere. I appealed to Graham Neale, the new TCD professor of medicine, who offered me 15 beds in Top Floor, Hospital One, St James's for the treatment of general haematological and haemophilia patients. This great advance in 1976 established the future of the major haematology unit in St James's.

With a rapidly advancing specialty and only one consultant, non-consultant medical appointments took on a more significant role than usual. Dr Gordon Mullins was appointed lecturer in haematology in 1974. Dr Shaun McCann was appointed haematology registrar in 1976 and then lecturer in 1978 following the departure of Gordon Mullins to the Bon Secours Hospital, Cork, as consultant oncologist. Dr Peter Daly was appointed consultant to the FDVH in 1979. He was allocated three St James's oncology sessions. Following the retirement of Professor Neale (1980) 15 oncology beds became available in the same ward area as haematology. Peter Daly's medical expertise was of much importance in the management of patients with leukaemia and haemophilia and of those undergoing marrow transplantation. He was appointed associate professor by Trinity in 1996. Haematology and oncology still share facilities as evidenced by the new St James's 2005 day care centre

By 1978 it became clear that any unit with pretensions of providing a referral service for leukaemia would require bone marrow transplantation as an essential arm of its service. It was evident that substantial extra funding would be required to provide facilities, new technology and trained staff. Furthermore, it was necessary to convince St James's, the Department of Health and the interested medical community that this was a significant advance.

Funding and influence were tackled by a controlled appeal to the public and the authorities. The Bone Marrow for Leukaemia Trust (BMLT) was officially launched in the Thomas Prior Hall, RDS, in November 1980. The Trust was the concept of Eugene Murray, a patient with treated CML, and supported by his professional business advisors. Fundraising was started forthwith and shortly the trust was in a position to guarantee St James's £115,000 per annum for marrow transplantation. By its 25th anniversary the Trust had given St James's, in one form or another, over €14 million.

In January 1981, Shaun McCann, now senior lecturer in haematology, was funded to visit the Fred Hutchinson Centre marrow transplant centre in Seattle for three months. Nurses were sent for training to the Royal Marsden, London. Structural changes to the haematology/oncology ward took place in 1982–3 to accommodate specialised rooms. In 1983 Shaun was appointed haematology consultant and in 1984 the first transplant was carried out.

Under the direction of Shaun McCann the leukaemia/bone marrow transplant section of the St James's haematology centre became the National Centre for Adult Bone Marrow Transplantation developing at the same time an international reputation. Dr Joan O'Riordan became marrow transplant co-ordinator. In 1995 she was appointed haematology consultant, IBTS and St James's, continuing to follow up long term effects of bone marrow transplantation in recipients. Marrow transplants increased from 12 in 1985 to 50 in 1990. The first unrelated transplant was undertaken in 1994. This initiative is supported by the setting up by IBTS of the Irish Unrelated Bone Marrow Registry. In 1996 a second consultant, Dr Paul Browne, was appointed to the clinical haematology unit. Under his guidance the autologous stem cell transplant service was expanded. Drs Eibhlin Conneally and Elizabeth Vandenberghe were subsequently appointed consultants in 2001 bringing the number in general haematology/leukaemia/transplantation to four.

In 1985 I was appointed to a personal chair in haematology. Shaun McCann became associate professor of haematology in 1991 and, succeeding me, the George Gabriel Stokes -rofessor of haematology in 1995. In 1996 the haematology ward moved from its St James's birthplace in Top Floor, Hospital One to the new custom-built Denis Burkitt Ward in the main hospital building.

In the late 1980s Shaun McCann introduced Mark Lawlor to haematology. During the next decade Mark developed molecular biological technology in the Sir Patrick Dun's laboratory as a tool for research in bone marrow transplantation and leukaemia. He now plays a substantial role in the Institute of Molecular Medicine, a combined TCD/UCD research unit, and in the John Durkan Leukaemia Laboratory (founded in 2003). In 2003 Mark was appointed associate professor by TCD.

The Adelaide and Meath Hospital, incorporating the National Children's Hospital (AMNCH)

The St James's Central Pathology Laboratory served the remaining three Federation hospitals up to 1998 when they moved to Tallaght. Dr Helen Enright was appointed haematologist in 1997. A complete and comprehensive laboratory service was in operation within a short period of time and the first haematology test was carried out in June 1998. A clinical unit was simultaneously formed and there is now a busy unit with an average of 25 inpatients. All branches of haematology are now investigated and treated except for haemophilia and marrow and stem cell transplantation. With regard to the latter there is close co-operation with the transplant service in St James's. In 2004 a second haematologist was appointed, Dr Niamh O'Connell. The unit has taken a special interest in the myelodysplastic syndrome for which it has established a national registry.

Overview

In 1960 red cell and white cell counts were estimated by microscopically counting individual cells in Neubauer chambers. Up to 1965 leukaemia was treated with palliative measures by the Irish medical profession. Until 1968 there was no concentrate therapy available to staunch bleeding in haemophiliacs.

Those serving haematology in the FDVH and later St James's have led the country in developing the laboratory, clinical and research aspects of the specialty. No similar Irish haematology unit can equal the number of its publications. It has been the training ground for a large number of consultants in haematology and blood transfusion and to a lesser extent in oncology. The combined tradition is now being carried forward in Tallaght and Our Lady's. The process has seen a major increase in the number of full-time consultant staff. In 1982 there was one Federation haematology consultant (none in Our Lady's). By 1983 there were three in the Federation/St James's. In 2004 there were seven in St James's, two in Tallaght.

There are now four in Our Lady's.

I must apologise to the literally hundreds of nurses, technologists, scientists, social workers, physiotherapists, administrators, doctors and other staff (particularly the ward cleaners who contribute so much to patient morale) who have not received an individual mention but who worked so hard to develop and improve the haematology service from 1960 to 2005. I can only plead that the burden of numbers and an ageing memory prevent me from giving due recognition to all concerned.

The author would like to thank Dr Emer Lawlor for her assistance in the preparation of this contribution.

25. Neurology

E. A. Martin

Neurology, like most specialties in these islands, had no permanent establishment until after the Second World War (1939–45). True, there were three hospitals in London, one of which—the National Hospital for Nervous Diseases, Queen's Square, which began as the National Hospital for Paralysis and Epilepsy—was founded in 1860 and still survives. The earliest British neurological journal, *Brain,* was first published in 1878.

In 1959 there were 50-60 neurologists in England, about half in London and the rest irregularly placed; for example, there were two in Newcastle and none in Liverpool. United Kingdom neurologists formed the Association of British Neurologists and decided (against the wishes of some of the most distinguished senior members, one of whom appealed under the slogan '*Tria Juncta in Uno*'[1] for the continuation together of neurology with neurosurgery and psychiatry) that the future lay in pursuing a closed-shop specialty, excluding also those who claimed only an *interest* in neurology. It was decided, too, that neurologists would not participate in non-neurological emergency medicine.

By and large this satisfied neurologists but in any case their students and successors have had to bear with it. The wisdom of this policy has been questioned; it may have contributed to the downward slide of psychiatry. Sparsely distributed multi-consultant neurological centres left considerable intervening neglected areas. General medical colleagues resented the sparing of neurologists from the swamping and stressful general medical take; academics disliked the independence neurologists gained. Efforts were made to persuade neurologists to be more moderate.

In 1946 Sydney Allison (b. 1899) came back from the Navy to Belfast and undertook the task of setting up a neurology service. He went to London to train and persuaded his older colleague Hilton Stewart (b. 1900), primarily a psychiatrist, to go over to neurology. In time Harold Millar replaced Stewart and thereafter neurology prospered in the integrated hospital and university and administrative system which prevailed in the National Health Service in Northern Ireland. Consultants travelled to peripheral hospitals, taking an outpatient clinic in the morning and ward consultations in the afternoon. Cecil Calvert came back from the war—he had worked at the services' head injury unit at Oxford—and started up a parallel and equally successful department of neurosurgery. Pearse O'Malley practised neuro-psychiatry at the Mater. In Dublin Adams McConnell, who started his career as a general surgeon at the Richmond, specialised in neurosurgery—one of the pioneers in these islands.

For a couple of generations a tradition of interest in the neurosciences had been maintained at the Richmond and the nearby Richmond Asylum where research and neuropathology were active. Robert William Smith's great work on multiple neurofibromatosis, *A Treatise on the Pathology, Diagnosis and Treatment of Neuroma,* was published in 1849. There were early operations for cerebral tumour and abscess. Gordon Holmes (1876–1965), who had done his first house job at the asylum after student days at Sir Patrick Dun's, and Robert Foster-Kennedy (1884–1952) of Belfast, aspired to consultant posts at the Richmond but none were available. They made their names in London and New York. Frank Purser (1877–1934) was McConnell's neurological colleague. He was co-author of a textbook of medicine with William Boxwell of the Meath. He had studied at the National Hospital for Nervous Diseases. He became Professor of Neurology at TCD and later Regius Professor of Medicine.

On Purser's death McConnell persuaded Harry Parker, a Dublin graduate, a very able and experienced neurologist and a dramatic teacher at the Mayo Clinic, to come back to take over Purser's appointments. Parker's brilliance was offset by personality problems. He was very restless, tactless and sometimes aggressive. He had an American wife who was unhappy in Dublin. He needed to do psychiatry on the side to make a living. Physicians and psychiatrists felt that they could do most of their own neurology and that their primary need was somebody to exclude or take over neurosurgical conditions. Neurosurgeons undertook neurological consultations. Parker's teaching classes lasted for 40 minutes, which he considered the limit of human concentration. The first ten minutes were on psychiatry. When he returned to the Mayo Clinic he published a unique book *Clinical Studies in Neurology* (1956) on his teaching sessions in Dublin. He laced the clinical detail with descriptions of the city and very good anecdotes. His assistant, Brendan McEntee, succeeded him. Brendan preferred to be regarded as a general physician with an interest in neurology. He had permanent disabilities from poliomyelitis.

In my early postgraduate days Alan Thompson, physician to the Richmond and a model of commonsense, advised me not to take up neurology. He said that there wasn't a living in it. David Mitchell, an Adelaide physician, quoted a senior colleague on neurologists: 'They go to all this trouble

. . . and no treatment comes out of it. Unless they are dishonest enough to give liver injections the patients won't feel any obligation to pay.'

Dublin hospitals were weak on camaraderie and strong on competition. Fergus Donovan returned from the Mayo Clinic and set up a department of neurosurgery at St Vincent's. Edward L. Murphy, who had been at Johns Hopkins in Baltimore, covered neurology although handicapped by continuing poor health.

At the Mater, Gerald FitzGerald (1913–45), brother of Oliver and Paddy FitzGerald of St Vincent's, was commissioned by the Medical Board in 1939 to go to Queen's Square in London to train in neurology and psychiatry. Brilliant of intellect and personality, he did memorable research there with Cawthorne and Hallpike. They standardised the caloric tests used in the diagnosis of vestibular disease. He then spent a year studying psychiatry at Edinburgh with Sir David Henderson. He returned to Dublin but had developed malignant disease, was unable to practice and died within a year. The Mater Medical Board then selected Sean Malone who practised neurology and psychiatry and later went over fully to psychiatry and became professor at UCD.

In the Federated Hospitals, John Kirker was a product of Sir Patrick Dun's. With the help of R. H. Micks, Professor of Pharmacology and Therapeutics, he went to Boston to study with the specialists in epilepsy, Lennox and Gibbs. When he got there the Gibbses had gone to Chicago. He went on to work in Chicago and also in Montreal with Jasper, another epilepsy specialist. When he came back to Dublin he soon replaced Clement Dempsey who had initiated EEG work at the Richmond. For many years he provided the major part of EEG services all over Dublin, the remainder being covered by Fergus Donovan at St Vincent's and Niall O'Donohoe in paediatric circles (O'Donohoe's *Epilepsies of Childhood* appeared in 1974).

J. B. Lyons, who was consultant at Mercer's and St Michael's, Dún Laoghaire, had trained at Manchester in neurology. He and John Kirker maintained their special interest in neurology and were major contributors to the Irish Epilepsy Association. Among J. B.'s numerous publications in clinical and historical medicine is *A Primer in Neurology* (1974).

I was appointed assistant physician, and then physician with a special interest in neurology, at the Adelaide in 1951 and at the same time director of research at St Patrick's where Norman Moore gave me strong support. Later I was invited to be neurologist to St Vincent's (with specific exclusion of general medicine). I shared my time equally between the two hospitals as did Michael Hutchinson who joined me in 1978. There was no shortage of beds and waiting times in the outpatient department were not long. Around this time discussions on the question of sessional visits to county hospitals came to nothing.

At the Richmond, Hugh Staunton joined Brendan McEntee and Sean Murphy succeeded Brendan to set up a strong secure department. The last normal year was 1986. From then on bed numbers were reduced and out-patient attendances pruned. Waiting times lengthened and patients de-faulted. There was a great increase in junior doctors who had previously travelled, usually to England, for their intern posts and then often further afield. General practitioners were bypassed and attendances in casualty mounted.

From the 1960s neurology developed steadily. Doing electrical tests in a corner of a maid's bedroom or in the laundry gave way to working in a dedicated room. Endless begging letters were necessary. A senior house of-ficer post was recognised and then a joint registrar post between St Vin-cent's and the Adelaide. Teaching for undergraduates and postgraduates was provided in both hospitals. Research was keenly pursued but no revo-lutionary results or breakthroughs were achieved. John Kirker established an EEG service. Elizabeth Hicks was the first technician; she was followed by Deirdre Glynn and Cindy Augustine. I practised electromyography and nerve conduction studies and in time these passed to Michael Hutchinson and eventually to Sean Connolly, a new consultant in electrophysiology. Ophthalmodynamometry was practised in cerebrovascular cases and proved a waste of time. A skull table was purchased. Shan Henderson and then Max Ryan and David McInerney undertook carotid angiography. I did my own air encephalograms. John Dinn worked between the department of pathology in Trinity and St Vincent's and provided a first-class service in neuropathology. At one time two in seven new neurological outpatients in the Republic were seen at the Adelaide and St Vincent's.

Michael Swallow in Belfast and I set up the Irish Neurological Associa-tion which was keenly supported from the beginning by all who worked in the neurosciences, north and south. It meets annually still. The Section of Neurological Sciences of the Royal Academy of Medicine was created as a forum for local supra-departmental meetings. It makes a surprise appear-ance occasionally still. Research prospered under Michael Hutchinson, es-pecially in multiple sclerosis and immunology. Radiology and department presentations were held at St Vincent's. Some who passed through the de-partment went on to become neurologists. Consultations were undertaken all over the city. I saw private patients in the traditional way at my home while Michael elected to have rooms at St Vincent's Private.

When I retired there was the usual administrative delay before Raymond

Murphy joined Michael. Janice Redmond came as a new appointment largely to St James's which had been impatiently waiting for neurological expertise for a long time. So the department over these years quadrupled in consultant strength and it seems not unlikely that numbers will double again.

From the 1960s the increase was driven by specialisation in medicine. Other departments felt diffident about carrying out a neurological examination or making neurological diagnoses. Small queues of consultants formed outside the door each with a problem patient. Psychiatrists, too, began to feel they either did not know how to examine a patient or that it was not their job to examine them. Psychologists appeared on the scene and found reduced mental functioning in the psychiatric population, notoriously prone to poor concentration and medication-induced sluggishness. Investigations and referrals spiralled.

Another factor in the increase in patient numbers was the falling tolerance in the population for discomfort and pain, however temporary. Pressures from drug companies with new products emerging from their pipelines probably contributed. Neurology had tended to be regarded as largely diagnostic, solitary and difficult, accompanied for some by unpleasant invasive investigation. Patient expectations have increased to such a degree that it appears that a symptomless, perfectly functioning human being can be aimed at. Investigations have become more complex and, although hardcore major neurological disease will remain, the numbers in the care of an individual neurologist will fall.

In the 1960s there was a competitive element in conversations about numbers of new patients attending outpatient clinics. We laughed at stories of patients in Greece making appointments with two neurologists on the same day when they went to Athens for an opinion and wondered at the way everything closed down at lunchtime on Friday in Scandinavia.

Routine, often accompanied by frustration, was part of my neurological life and probably that of everyone in Irish medical life, since and now. Painful decisions had to be made about how much time would be given to altering commitments, to teaching, to committees. My files show that in 1971 I asked the Medical Board of the Adelaide to release me from any commitment to general medical patients other than acute admissions on my duty days. I must have amazed or amused the Department of Health by proposing a neurosurgical department at the Adelaide. I used my own money to insulate the electrophysiology room. When the skull table was installed in 1967 and Max Ryan came, regulations for neuro-radiology were required and were submitted and approved by the Medical Board. Among the trivia in 1977 Fannin's quoted £60 + 20 per cent VAT for one only human vertebral column, articulated on nylon. When Michael Hutchinson came his requests were pleasantly small—a Juler Scotometer and a Goldmann Perimeter and Farnsworth-Mansell Hue Test materials.

In 1977 I made moves to give investigation rights at the Adelaide and St Vincent's to Dr Kirker and Professor Lyons. Proposals that the department at the Adelaide would accept for admission all head injuries and all stroke patients were resisted. At St Vincent's participation in general medical emergency take was resisted vigorously on the basis that it had been specifically excluded on appointment and on current skills and experience. This was countered by the remark, 'But we are all doctors, aren't we?'

Negotiations to establish a neurology registrar appointment started about 1972 and were still going on in 1977. A computerised axial tomographic scanner began to be sought from 1975. I stored many documents prepared by neurologists elsewhere on their workload, situations, predicaments and needs, the better to be able in my turn to prepare appeals and requests for my department. I still have the statistics maintained by the Department of Health on the disposition and activity in neurology in the city in those years. In one Adelaide *Annual Report* I complained that for neurologists the hospital's motto *Labor omnia vincit* had been replaced by *Modicum laboris sufficit*.

Perhaps I am painting a depressing picture of neurological life, as one of never ending struggle. Indeed I was happy to retire at 62 but I had always been stimulated by the struggle. Now, 14 years, later I note that my former colleagues and my successors are still faced with the same problems in their professional lives. My experience of medical history tells me that it was always the same in the medical profession and I think it is likely always to be the same in the future.

Note

[1] This was the title of the Hugh Cairns Memorial Lecture delivered by Sir Charles Symond to the Society of British Neurological Surgeons 1970.

26. Nursing services

Sibéal Carolan, Mary T. Moore and Anna Dolan

The Meath Hospital

Sibéal Carolan

The Meath Hospital on Heytesbury Street was founded in 1753; situated in the 'liberty' of the Earl of Meath, it was opened to serve the sick and poor in the crowded area of the Liberties. At this time there was a high incidence of infectious diseases and a special wing of the hospital was devoted to the treatment and care of patients suffering with infectious diseases. The Meath School of Nursing played a very important part in nurse education in Ireland. It was established in 1884.

The first course for tutors was inaugurated at University College Dublin in 1960. Angela Hoey, who qualified in 1957, was nominated for the course by the Matron, Miss Magee. Miss Hoey completed the course in 1962 and was the first qualified tutor in the School of Nursing. On the death of Eileen Forde in 1968, Angela Hoey was appointed principal tutor, a post she held until her retirement in 1994.

The nursing educational system was organised in block format. Students were allocated to various 'blocks' for a number of weeks at a time. The curriculum was delivered in a sequential way. This replaced the older system, which involved attendance at lectures which were of one hour's duration and were delivered by medical staff and ward sisters. This system was incorporated into the nursing shift.

Each year approximately 60 nurses qualified from the school with a certificate in general nursing. There were two intakes per year, autumn and spring. A course in urological nursing was developed in the Meath. Post-registration programmes and operating theatre courses were also available. A partnership with Kevin Street College was developed and a course in physics, social science and chemistry for nurses was provided. This was an additional module to the certificate programme which proved very beneficial to nurses at that time looking for work opportunities in countries such as the USA and Australia. Miss O'Dwyer and Miss Hoey certainly demonstrated great foresight in developing this link with a third level institute.

During this time there were many changes in nurse education at both local and national levels. The Diploma in Nursing, followed by registration on the General Register with An Bord Altranais, was established in partnership with Trinity College. The Meath offered a number of prizes including the Georgina Wade Award, the Lucy Dimond Award and the Nora Lyons Award. Margaret McCarthy, who was a past student of the Meath School of Nursing, was the first co-ordinator of the diploma programme in TCD. In 2002 nurse education was fully integrated nationally into third level institutions. Cecily Begley, who also undertook general nurse training at the Meath, is the director of the School of Nursing and Midwifery Studies.

On the opening of the new genitourinary unit in 1953, Elizabeth Cunningham was the first nurse to be trained in urological nursing. When the new department was opened in 1955, she was appointed sister in charge of the unit, a post equivalent to that of assistant matron. Miss Cunningham demanded high standards in urological nursing and this contributed to the international recognition of the unit. Nursing personnel at the time included Elizabeth Hoey, assistant matron, and ward sisters Nora Lyons, Mary Duffy, Evelyn Doherty, Josephine Mullen, Mena Lambert, Rose McCarron, Rosaleen Hearty, Maureen Fallon, and Roslyn Casey, affectionately known as 'Pinky'.

During the period of Federation Elizabeth O'Dwyer was the matron. Under her leadership many nursing initiatives and services were developed; these included the replacement of Nightingale wards with smaller units for ease of management and patient comfort, the recruitment of men for postgraduate general training, significant uniform changes, structural improvements within the hospital, policy changes, advances in clinical practice and appointment of support staff—ward clerks and ward attendants. Miss O'Dwyer also ensured that staff of the Meath School of Nursing participated in the early discussions on the development of nurse education at local and at national level.

Mary McCarthy was appointed Matron in 1996 and took up the position of Director of Nursing at the Meath and transferred to Tallaght Hospital in June 1998. Her success continued with her appointment as Chief Nurse in the Department of Health and Children. It is worth noting that the title 'Matron' is now returning to nursing services with a slight change; the term 'Modern Matron' is currently widely used in the United Kingdom. The Modern Matron is a strong clinical leader with clear authority at ward level, who is highly visible, accessible and easily identifiable by patients and has real authority to ensure that the basics of care are correct.

The Adelaide Hospital

Sibéal Carolan

The Adelaide School of Nursing was established in 1859 under the direction of Miss Bramwell. She was given permission to recruit one probationer nurse for training but there is no evidence that one ever arrived. Miss Bramwell was occupied in getting the hospital started as a new organisation. Mrs Ruttle replaced Miss Bramwell and in 1861 she spent one month at Kaiserwerth, which had gained international recognition, to promote the development of a nurse training department in the hospital. She introduced a one-year training course for females of good character between 25 and 35 years of age. The system prospered but still lacked formal structure.

A booklet, *The Adelaide Hospital Dublin—Nursing Department Rules and Regulations 1879*, provided for an organised training with a nursing structure of 'A lady Superintendent, 4 Divisional Lady Nurses, Ward Nurses attending to patients under their direction, probationers learning to be nurses who acted as assistants'. At this stage Miss Reynolds, the Matron, went to St Bartholomew's Hospital in London for a course in nurse training and management.

In 1888 the hospital rules stated that the duties of the Matron included arranging for the admission and overall care of the patients including their diets. The standard of food seemed to be a big issue at that time and the Matron had to ensure that it was of good quality, and was properly cooked. She also had to ensure that the servants received proper meals.

The uniform dress adopted at the Adelaide, navy with white spots, was a copy of that worn by the sisters at St Thomas' Hospital where Miss Bramwell trained. During the 1900s nurse grades were distinguished by the colour of belt worn; students wore white belts, newly qualified nurses black belts, and senior staff nurses red belts. The nurses were called by the colour of their belts. In the mid 20th century, the wearing of stripes on the arm by students was introduced to distinguish between junior and senior students. The wearing of the 'shower of hail' dresses and the 'Sister Dora' caps continued until the hospital closed, to transfer to Tallaght, in 1998.

By this time, up to 40 students per year entered nursing for the three-year certificate course. The superintendent of the nursing department was responsible for the probationers and nurses and held the title of 'Home Sister'. The probationers and nurses were required to live in the nurses' home. The practice of living in continued until modern times. Up to the 1980s the student nurses had to live in for their three-year training course; the period of living in was then decreased to one year.

While male nurses had been training for some time in other hospitals it was not until 1989 that the first two males commenced training in the Adelaide.

The National Children's Hospital, Harcourt Street

Sibéal Carolan

The National Children's Hospital was founded as a hospital for sick children in 1821 by three of Dublin's most distinguished doctors, Henry Marsh (later Sir Henry Marsh), Philip Crampton (later Sir Philip Crampton) and Charles Johnson. It was the first hospital in Great Britain and Ireland to be devoted exclusively to the care and treatment of sick children and was called the Institution for Sick Children, on Pitt Street, now Balfe Street. The main purpose of the hospital was to treat the sick children in the Liberties area of the city, where there was a large number of deprived children. The hospital had three objectives: to afford free medical and surgical aid to sick children, to give medical students the opportunity to learn about infantile diseases, and to extend information to mothers and nurses regarding the proper management of children, both in health and illness.

Many renowned physicians and surgeons worked at the hospital. Charles West trained there and later founded the Hospital for Sick Children, Great Ormond Street, London, in 1852.

The National Orthopaedic and Children's Hospital, which was located on Upper Kevin Street, was formally joined with the Institution for Sick Children in 1884. In 1887 both these institutions moved to 87–8 Harcourt Street and the National Children's Hospital was opened.

The first Matron at the National Children's Hospital was Bessie Lyons. She retained that post until 1908 when Geraldine Matthews became Matron until 1921. Miss Matthews was awarded the Order of the British Empire for her work at the hospital during the 1916 Easter Rising. In more recent years Matrons at the National Children's Hospital included Anne Quigley, Betty Brady, Ann Taylor, Aileen Hendricks, Catherine McDaid and currently Maura Connolly.

In 1998 the National Children's Hospital closed its doors for the last time and joined with the Meath and the Adelaide to form the new hospital in Tallaght. There are 513 beds at this new state-of-the-art facility, 67 of which are children's beds. Tallaght is a suburb at the west of the city with an estimated population of 320,000, 40 per cent being children under the age of 14 years. The vision for the hospital is to develop a centre of excellence which will provide healthcare for the entire lifespan, from cradle to grave.

Clinical specialties at the hospital include endocrinology, cystic fibrosis, respiration, neurology, ear, nose and throat and dermatology. Until 2003 haematology was a specialty service at the hospital; it has now transferred to Our Lady's Hospital for Sick Children at Crumlin.

The clinical areas within the hospital include Oak Ward where children with medical conditions are treated and cared for. Within Oak Ward there is a three-bedded high dependency unit where children requiring more intensive nursing care and medical intervention are admitted. On Beech Ward, children requiring in-patient surgical management are admitted. Adjacent to this ward there is a six-bedded day unit caring for children requiring day care specialist services including diagnostic tests and minor surgical procedures. On Maple Ward, sick infants under three years of age are managed. Departments dedicated to children include operating theatre, accident and emergency, outpatient and radiology.

School of Nursing

In 1884 Lambert Ormsby, a senior surgeon at the Institution for Sick Children, founded the Dublin Red Cross Nursing School for nurses in the National Orthopaedic and Children's Hospital in association with the Meath Hospital and County Dublin Infirmary. This nursing school moved to Harcourt Street in 1887. It was the first nursing school exclusively devoted to the training of women to become hospital nurses for children.

In the early years the training was of three years' duration. After the first year students sat an examination which had to be passed before proceeding on to the second year. The final examination was taken at the end of three years and led to registration as a sick children's nurse on the register now held by An Bord Altranais. The hospital continued to accept students for this course twice a year until 1986. In 1984 the school began a post-registration sick children's nursing education programme, run over 18 months with twice-yearly intakes. This course continues to be available today as a postgraduate Diploma in Sick Children's Nursing and is co-ordinated in association with Trinity College since 1996.

A more recent proposal includes the development of a four and a half year undergraduate degree programme integrating the education of sick children's and adult nursing leading to the award of BSc Nursing (Children's and General) and dual registration as a Registered Children's Nurse (RCN) and Registered General Nurse (RGN). This course is in the advanced stages of development; it is envisaged that it will proceed through the Central Applications Office in the autumn of 2006.

The nursing tutors of the School of Nursing at the National Children's Hospital over the years included Kathleen Keane, Do Do McGovern, Peg Hogan, Brigid Wall and Carole King. Elizabeth Fahey-McCarthy was based in the School of Nursing before transferring to Trinity College where she continues to be involved with developments in children's nursing education.

Visiting children in hospital

Up to the late 1960s sick children often remained in hospital for many weeks with minimal contact, if any, with their family. Until then, visiting children in hospital was viewed as a contentious issue. Visiting by parents was discouraged as it was thought to upset the child! Visiting by siblings was not even considered. For some, the presence of parents in the ward was seen as a threat. Research published during the late 1960s and early 1970s[1] clearly indicated the benefits of parental involvement in care during hospitalisation of a child. As a result, visiting restrictions were relaxed in the late 1960s when 'open' visiting was introduced at the National Children's Hospital. Since then, parents, and indeed siblings, have been encouraged to visit the sick child freely while in hospital. It was then accepted that a parent/guardian might wish to stay in hospital overnight with their sick child and a demand for parent accommodation appeared. In the late 1970s a dedicated parents' accommodation area became available.

Family-centred care

A natural progression from parents visiting and staying overnight with their sick child is the concept of family-centred care. In family-centred care the family is considered a partner in the child's care, contributing to all clinical decisions made regarding the child. The National Children's Hospital promotes this concept which considers the entire healthcare team to be partners with the parents/guardians in delivering holistic care to the child.

Sir Patrick Dun's Hospital 1713–1986

Sibéal Carolan

There is no record governing nursing in the early years of the hospital although Moorhead in his history of the hospital[2] does record some of the nursing arrangements in the earlier days. He notes that the Institute of Nursing was established in Dublin about 1855 and in 1866 a nurse training school was formed with the Institute, Sir Patrick Dun's and Dr Steevens' also playing a role.

Lady Superintendents had entire control of the nursing department under the direction of the attending physician and surgeon and had the power of engaging and discharging nurses. Miss Probyn was Lady Superintendent from 1867 to 1870, Miss Harrison from 1870 to 1871, Miss Greenstreet and others from 1871 to 1884. Miss Huxley combined the matron and lady superintendent posts in 1884. Matrons engaged and controlled the servants, and were accountable for the furniture and linen supplies.

Initially there were three ward areas consisting of a male medical acute, a female medical acute and a surgical ward. At the time of the hospital closure the following ward areas were in place: acute male and female medical, male and female surgical, children's, ear/nose/throat, gastroenterology, intensive care, A&E, outpatients, theatres.

Miss Huxley was a pioneer of modern nursing in Dublin, establishing courses in elementary anatomy for nurses, these lectures being added to the duties of the house surgeon in 1886. In subsequent years courses of lectures were added in many other subjects. The Metropolitan School of Nursing was founded largely on Miss Huxley's initiative. The matrons of the voluntary hospitals drew up and put into practice the first nursing science course for nurses, assisted by the Royal College of Surgeons and the Royal College of Physicians. Nurses from at least nine voluntary hospitals attended this school. At first the period of training was for 12 months only, before nurses were sent out to private cases. In 1892 this period was extended to 18 months and in 1895 to two years. In 1900 the school became known as the Metropolitan Technical School for Nurses.

In 1905 the first preliminary training school in Ireland was opened in Sir Patrick Dun's where all probationers spent a period of 12 weeks before entering the wards. During this period lectures were given in anatomy, physiology, first aid, bandaging, cookery and practical skills.

Miss Haughton suggested that nurse training should be extended to three years because nurses trained for two years were not eligible for the navy, army or other services. The Board readily agreed.

In the mid 1980s Sir Patrick Dun's and Baggot Street combined schools to provide nurse education in allocated blocks. Students from each hospital spent time on certain wards in the other hospital. Baggot Street students spent time in ENT and children's wards at Sir Patrick Dun's while Dun's students spent time on cardiothoracic wards at Baggot Street.

The uniforms for Sir Patrick Dun's initially consisted of pink dresses, white aprons, Dun's cap, black stockings and shoes. In 1962 white dresses with the hospital crest appliquéd on the left lapel, a modern style hat, brown stockings and white shoes replaced the older uniform.

It is not possible to ascertain the original student numbers; however, from the 1970s the hospital took approximately 10–18 students twice a year in February and September.

The Royal City of Dublin Hospital, Baggot Street

Sibéal Carolan

Throughout the 20th century there were numerous attempts to amalgamate the smaller Dublin voluntary hospitals. These have been fully described in other chapters of the book. So far as Baggot Street is concerned the result of Federation was the closure of the hospital as an acute institution in 1987 when its services transferred to St Kevin's, renamed St James's. The hospital was integrated into the community care services and currently it provides facilities for elderly patients and a wide range of public health services

Miss I. Corbet, Matron of the hospital, reflected in 1982: 'I am proud of the nursing tradition of this hospital. It is a tradition which embodies all that is best in nursing and which has been and is being carried throughout the world by the nurses who have passed through the school.' The school at one stage was receiving 1,000 applications for a total of 30 places.

Miss Peta Taaffe, Matron of the hospital, remembered her last day in the hospital:

A final walk around the hospital—empty of patients, and all but a few staff, staying on either because no appropriate position was available or because they were remaining in the hospital to work for the Health Board. My memories particularly focus on the ICU—all the high tech equipment gone—a few chairs and bed tables—dust gathering. I remembered some of the people who had fought for life there—some who won, some for whom it was the final battle. The x-ray department with most of the 'machinery' gone, a half cup of tea on the window-sill—magazines in the waiting area—no-one to read them now. The nurse's home was a fine 19th-century building, but inconveniently 'bitty' inside—it served as residence and school of nursing, full of the bustle of students, and the comings and goings of teachers, catering staff and other visitors, the 'home' was alive! On that last day the debris of old gas masks, ancient hockey sticks, discarded cloaks and the like had taken over, and the building seemed old and tired. (Quoted in Davis Coakley *Baggot Street—A Short History of the Royal City of Dublin Hospital* Dublin, 1995.)

Mercer's Hospital

Mary T. Moore

The strength and uniqueness of nursing lies in the extent to which nurses share the everyday living experience of the patients. For the past 249 years the nurses of Mercer's have shared these experiences and cared for the sick. It is a sad occasion when the first small, personal hospital closes. Time will tell whether this closure is for the better.

In the year 1220 the original building on this site was a chapel called St Stephen's. Ellen Morton, an affluent lady, endowed the chapel in 1394 for the reception and maintenance of the poor of Dublin suffering from leprosy, without charge. The general care of the patients was in the hands of women of low character, as sickness was regarded as a humiliating condition. This was not a hospital in the modern sense of providing medical treatment of the sick. In 1703 the church was demolished and all that remained was a churchyard.

The date of birth of our foundress Mary Mercer is unknown. After her parents' death Mary was a lady with considerable wealth. She built a stone house on the old site of St Stephen's churchyard in 1724 for the maintenance of poor girls. Later she transferred the deeds of the stone house together with the land to a group of trustees for the purpose of converting it into a hospital. Mary Mercer did not endow the hospital; she made her will on 8 August 1733 and the bulk of her fortune went to her charity school (Mercer School) at Castleknock. This was for the education of 35 poor girls.

On 17 August 1734 the hospital was opened with 10 beds. Music was a major source of income for Mercer's; performances usually took place in St Andrew's Church. Handel, who came to Dublin in 1741, was a notable benefactor. His name first occurred in the hospital records on 21 November 1741. The *Messiah* was performed for the first time in the music hall, Fishamble Street, on 13 April 1742, directed and assisted by Mr Handel. The proceeds were divided between Mercer's, the charitable infirmary and the prisoners of the Marshalsea.

There does not appear to be any record of activity within the hospital between the years 1734 and 1736; the earliest minute book preserved in the hospital is dated 28 May 1736. At this time the hospital was run by a board of governors and the rules and regulations were laid down by the board for the members of staff. It is not quite certain how many nurse keepers were first appointed, but there were instructions laid down for them and approved by the board on 13 September 1736.

Some of the instructions were as follows:

Keep wards and bedding clean, light fires.
Wash clothes, bed linen, bandages.
Fill beds with fresh straw every two months.
Put clean linen on beds every month 'or oftener if the occasion arises' (of course, new sheets were put on patients' beds before surgeons' ward rounds).
Attend upon the fluxing rooms according to the direction of the surgeon in waiting.
Attend constantly upon the sick and give assistance and nourishment as directed and 'to receive for that purpose at meal times the respective allowances of food from the clerk and faithfully deliver to each patient in your ward, or under your care his one quantity'.

No patient was to have lighted candles in bed: this was one of the most important regulations adopted in 1736. Imagine such a thing as a bath was never heard of! It was suggested that a bath be installed and after use it was reported that it was such a success that a second bath was applied for.

It is clear from the minutes of 6 July 1771 that at £5 per annum nurse keepers were not excessively paid; even then work was hard and conditions were strict.

As the years passed, Mercer's gradually established a reputation, particularly in surgery. It had on its staff many outstanding men, especially in the 1860s, 1870s and 1880s. In 1863 170 medical students were enrolled there—the lectures were given by Richard Butcher. Surgeons from Mercer's had contributed to Irish medical education by acting with colleagues from Dr Steevens' and the College of Surgeons. A Mercer's man, Henry Morris, was President of the Dublin Society of Surgeons, founded in 1780, and a number of the staff were among those who, four years later, founded the Royal College of Surgeons of Ireland. At first the College occupied premises in Mercer Street adjoining the hospital and obviously would have availed of the clinical facilities. The College moved to St Stephen's Green; it then sold its premises to Mercer's for £300. To this date the College of Surgeons remains in St Stephen's Green.

Cathleen Gallagher was a student nurse at Mercer's Hospital in 1917. She informed me there were no set times of entry; there were about four intakes a year of four or five students. Those who were accepted for training were mainly gentlemen farmers' daughters. An entrance fee of 50 guineas was required. They had to provide their own uniforms. If this fee is compared with the amount the nurses were paid, it is clear how difficult it would be for the less well off to enter nursing.

Students were not allowed out after 10 p.m.; they lived in for their three years of training. In their third year they had to go to England to work in a fever hospital to complete their training. This was due to the fact that Mercer's did not have enough beds to constitute a training school.

At the end of Miss Gallagher's third year she sat her state examination. She was registered under the Nurse's Registration Act which was passed in 1919 and gave professional status to nursing. This legislation held for the Republic of Ireland until 1950, when An Bord Altranais was founded.

The nurses cared for the sick—bed bathing, wound dressing etc. They cooked special invalid meals and carried out the dusting and cleaned the brasses which I believe was their Sunday duty. There was a Linen Guild which met once a month.

Miss Gallagher spoke highly of the surgical and medical team, with particular reference to Sir William De Courcey Wheeler, orthopaedic surgeon, who was a pioneer in his field. Dr Bethel Solomons was the nurses' guardian and dealt with any problems of misconduct. He held a party at his home once a year for the nurses and hired a taxi to collect and return them to the hospital. This was one of the happy memories Miss Gallagher recalls of Mercer's.

Mercer's closed on 31 May 1983 and the building was later put on the open market for sale. Eventually it was bought by the Royal College of Surgeons as an extension of the College. In this way the constitution and tradition of this great hospital is carried on for the benefit of the community.

Nursing in Dr Steevens'—a personal recollection

Anna Dolan

In April 1972, on entering Dr Steevens' as a student nurse, I became one of 16 young girls who had chosen a nursing career. Personally, I must not have given it much thought, as on arrival at the nurses' home I was totally unprepared for the rigid restrictions and conditions inflicted on me.

As first-year students we were made to live in the dormitory-style nurses' home, reporting to a 'Home Sister' (who was to be like our mother) who enforced our curfew of 11.30 nightly. We were allowed two late night passes till 2.30 a.m. and could only stay out all night if we had written permission from our parents. We made very deep friendships during this time, something I think is lost in the new style of nursing.

We spent the first ten weeks of our career in the classroom learning the basics of nursing. After this we commenced ward duties, going back to the classroom for six weeks each year. Ward duties were difficult, as each ward had a total of 4–5 staff nurses, thus two on each day shift. Most of the 'hands-on' work was done by students.

On night duty one staff nurse covered two wards and the student nurse took on all responsibilities. This gave us great confidence, something I now appreciate as I felt capable of coping on completion of my student days.

We had to attend external visits to observe certain specialties. Here we saw that our training in Dr Steevens' was excellent; we learned through practice and this became engraved on our minds.

The social calendar revolved around the annual dress dance and the annual Christmas panto. At both of these, everybody got involved and everyone was equal on these nights.

Our serene world was rocked when we heard that the hospital was closing and we were going to be transferred to the Meath, St James's or the Adelaide. We got on with the task and eventually relocated to these hospitals. We were anxious that things would be different. However, the staff from the hospitals opened up their arms to us and welcomed us. Here we saw that life in these hospitals was similar to that in Dr Steevens'. Again our world was rocked with the move to Tallaght. We thought that in the big organisation we would lose our identity, but this in fact never happened. We moved in 1998 and have retained the same hospital atmosphere. Meeting colleagues on the corridor is similar to meeting in the coffee shop in the Meath or Adelaide or the staff dining room in Dr Steevens'.

The only great change is the nursing structure; now students are in either the diploma or the degree course. They spend most of their time in university and only get hands-on experience in their third year. This system does not instil confidence in the students as they become staff nurses.

I personally feel our old system was the best, but I am biased. Things that I learned in first year I still refer to now.

We remain a big organisation with a small friendly attitude.

Note

Sibéal Carolan writes: Anna Knightly, Mary Moore, Phil Donnelly, James Jackson, Marian Connolly, Mary Cotter, Carole King and Siobhan O'Connor gave valuable information for the sections on the Meath, the Adelaide, the National Children's Hospital, Sir Patrick Dun's and Baggot Street. I am very grateful to them for providing the information so graciously

References

[1] J. Bowlby *Child Care and the Growth of Love* (2nd edition) Harmondsworth: Penguin 1965; J. Robertson *Children in Hospital* (2nd edition) London: Harper and Row 1970; P. J. Hawthorn *Nurse—I Want My Mummy!* London: Royal College of Nursing 1974.

[2] T. G. Moorhead *A Short History of Sir Patrick Dun's Hospital* Dublin: Hodges Figgis 1942.

Bibliography

D. Coakley *Baggot Street—A Short History of the Royal City of Dublin Hospital* Dublin 1995.

P. B. B. Gatenby *Dublin's Meath Hospital* Dublin: Town House 1996.

I. Jeffries 'The National Children's Hospital of Dublin, Ireland'. *International Paediatrics* 1991, 14(1): 54-57.

A. Kelleher and E. Musgrave 'Sick Children's Nursing'. In: Robbins, J. (ed.) *Nursing and Midwifery in Ireland in the Twentieth Century*. Dublin: An Bord Altranais 2000.

J. B. Lyons *The Quality of Mercer's: The Story of Mercer's Hospital 1734–1991* Dublin: Glendale 1991.

D. Mitchell *A 'Peculiar' Place, The Adelaide Hospital, Dublin: Its Times, Places and Personalities 1839 to 1989.* Dublin: Blackwater Press 1989.

27. Orthopaedics

David FitzPatrick

In a sense orthopaedics as a specialty may be regarded as having started at least with the Greeks. For example, there is the well known illustration of the Hippocratic method of reducing dislocation of the shoulder. In the 18th century Nikolai Andrei is credited with creating the emblem which is today associated with all orthopaedics; that is the image of a crooked tree being corrected by tying it to a stout, straight support. This of course illustrates the derivation of the word orthopaedics from the Greek $O\rho\theta oo$ and $\Pi\alpha\iota\sigma$—straight children. It was about this time that Percival Pott described his tibial fracture but it was not until the 19th century that Hugh Owen Thomas, the son of an Anglesey bone-setter, who had moved to Liverpool, became medically qualified and commenced an early orthopaedic practice. His name is still associated with 'Thomas's sign' and the Thomas wrench although this has gone out of use now.

Hugh Owen Thomas's nephew was Sir Robert Jones who was appointed surgeon to the Royal Liverpool Hospital in 1901. He may well be regarded as the first general surgeon to devote most of his practice to orthopaedic problems; he is certainly one of the first to make his name as such.

During the First World War Sir Robert Jones established a number of what were termed 'Hospitals for Special Surgery'. These were hospitals used for the treatment and convalescence of troops who had been injured in the war in France. With Dame Agnes Hunt he founded the Orthopaedic Hospital in Oswestry.

It is likely that these hospitals were developed initially as TB sanitaria. Such sanatoria were also developed in Ireland, and in both Britain and Ireland many of them were used subsequently as orthopaedic hospitals.

Orthopaedic hospitals were established in many large British centres; the Royal National Orthopaedic Hospital in Stanmore, the Nuffield Hospital in Oxford, and the Princess Margaret Rose Hospital in Edinburgh are just three of a number. In Ireland, Merlin Park, Croom and Cappagh were just a few of the hospitals which, having been used for the treatment of tuberculosis, were developed subsequently as orthopaedic units.

In 1961, when the Federated Hospitals Act was passed, orthopaedics as such was very different to what is practised today. In the United States and in Britain there was a number of hospitals similar to those mentioned above in which the practice was entirely orthopaedic and specialisation within the specialty had begun to emerge. Despite the advent of antibiotics and the introduction of Streptomycin bone tuberculosis was still common. The sequelae of the polio epidemics of the late 1940s and 1950s still cried out for orthopaedic attention. In trauma cases internal fixation, while practised commonly, lacked the sophistication which was to develop with the advent of the Synthes AO system for fracture fixation.

Each of the Federated Hospitals at this time had an accident unit or 'accident room' as it was often called. Patients with fractures were admitted to each of the hospitals but the practice of elective orthopaedics as a specialty was essentially confined to the Adelaide and to Dr Steevens'. Those who practised orthopaedics in these hospitals were appointed as general surgeons in the first instance and were expected to carry out their share of general surgery.

At the establishment of the Federation Mr John Sugars was the sole orthopaedic surgeon in the Adelaide. He had succeeded Mr C. O. L. Somerville-Large in 1951. His interest at the time was the management of bone tuberculosis and he had a particular interest in the management of children's disorders, particularly congenital dislocation of the hip (CDH) and club foot. This was at a time when operative treatment of CDH was in its infancy and the management of club foot still consisted mostly of manipulative treatment, occasionally using a Thomas wrench and casting. As the 1960s passed John Sugars, who provided orthopaedic care to the Rotunda, became adept at the early diagnosis of congenital dislocation, the operative treatment of TEV (club foot deformity), the open reduction of resistant or recurrent congenital dislocations removing the limbus as advocated by Mitchell and carrying out Pemberton and Salter osteotomies.

In Dr Steevens' there were three surgeons who devoted much of their time to orthopaedics. Arthur Chance, for whom a personal chair in orthopaedics was created in Trinity College, had been among the first to treat fractured neck of femur by internal fixation. In the late 1930s he had invited a Swede to demonstrate the use of the Sven pin. In Britain the Sven pin had been overtaken by the Smith Peterson pin and the McLaughlin pin and plate. However, in Dr Steevens' in 1968, the term Sven was still used in relation to hip pinning. Arthur Chance was also surgeon to the Irish Turf Club and as such many of his patients derived from the Curragh.

J. Boyd Dunlop had been appointed to Dr Steevens' after the war. One of his interests was the management of post-polio deformities and for somebody who had not been practising during the worst periods of these problems to watch Boyd Dunlop examine and assess a patient with post-polio problems was to see a master practising his art. He was an expert in corrective tendon transplants and performed a number of Colonna procedures for post-polio hips. In addition to his interest in polio Boyd Dunlop also had enormous interest and expertise in the management of children with problems related to cerebral palsy. Part of his practice was devoted to the management of these children and with Lady Goulding he was instrumental in the successful development of the Central Remedial Clinic in Dublin.

The third surgeon in Dr Steevens' who devoted much of his time to orthopaedics was Jack Cherry. He was less involved administratively than Boyd Dunlop or Arthur Chance but in the mid-1950s he developed a prosthetic replacement of the radial head for use in cases of fracture of that bone. This was indeed in advance of his time.

Together with John Sugars, Boyd Dunlop and Jack Cherry had attachments to the Incorporated Orthopaedic Hospital which functioned with an outpatient department in Merrion Street where numerous small children were seen weekly with, for the most part, relatively minor complaints such as intoeing or flat feet. However, a number of others had more serious problems—late CDH, relapsed TEV, or Perthes' disease. These required surgical intervention which was carried out in the residential part of the hospital in Castle Avenue in Clontarf. This hospital was also used for the management of children with long-term problems. It was not unusual for two or three children to be in that hospital at any one time suffering from Perthes' disease for which the then treatment was rest in bed, often for many months or even years.

As an intern in the early 1960s it seemed to me that there was relatively little communication between these surgeons, although no doubt case discussion did take place. It was at this time that McKee and Farrar introduced a metal upon metal hip replacement in Norwich and John Charnley began to develop his low friction arthroplasty for replacement of the hip, utilising a stainless steel femoral component, and a polypropaline cup, both cemented with acrylic. These developments were to set the scene for the present environment in which hip replacement, and indeed replacement of most other joints, is carried out almost universally.

In the early 1960s osteo-arthritis of hip was treated by a variety of means—cup arthroplasty, osteotomy, hemi-arthroplasty, and arthrodesis. John Sugars was an exponent of the Britain V-type arthrodesis which proved very successful. As the 1960s passed Paul Ring developed another metal upon metal arthroplasty—without cement.

When I was appointed Lecturer in Surgery at Trinity College my time was divided between working with Professor Nigel Kinnear in the Adelaide Hospital, a general surgeon with considerable pioneering experience in vascular surgery, and Boyd Dunlop in Dr Steevens' Hospital. Dunlop had started to use the Ring arthroplasty.

With the retirement of Arthur Chance in 1971 I was appointed Orthopaedic Surgeon to the Adelaide and Dr Steevens'. Shortly afterwards both Dunlop and I started to use the Charnley replacement system. John Sugars chose to use the Ling Lee (now Exeter) prosthesis. By now knee replacement was also underway—the early hinge replacements being succeeded by the Geomedic and later the total condylar surface type prostheses.

The Irish Orthopaedic Club had been in existence for many years. It met twice every year and provided a forum where orthopaedic surgeons from all over Ireland would meet to present papers, discuss cases and meet socially afterwards. This was an invaluable institution and provided an excellent forum for discussing both clinical problems and medical politics. The members of the Irish Orthopaedic Club were drawn from both North and South and the chairmanship alternated as did the locations of the meetings. The Club was a most valued institution and is perpetuated today as the Irish Orthopaedic Association. With the development of formal training and the recognition of differences between the National Health Service in the UK and that in the Republic, it was felt inappropriate that the Club should spend a lot of time discussing matters which would not be of particular interest to one group or the other. Accordingly, about 1972, the Institute of Orthopaedic Surgeons was established at a meeting in Dublin. It was intended that it would represent the concerns and aspirations of orthopaedic surgeons in the Republic as a group. At the time, formal training programmes were being established in the UK, having already been developed in the US for a very long time. Higher training in orthopaedic surgery was developing. The Institute of Orthopaedic Surgeons was to be responsible for the development of training programmes and the rotation of trainees through suitable posts within the Irish orthopaedic system.

Perhaps as a result of the establishment of the Institute, the orthopaedic surgeons in Dr Steevens' and the Adelaide, together with Michael Pegum, who had been appointed to the Meath, and Derek Robinson, whose work there was primarily involved with trauma, formed an orthopaedic sub-group within the Federation.

This sub-group was to be responsible for the development of the Federated Hospitals' orthopaedic unit and felt it should plan for the future. In a document detailing how orthopaedics should develop in the Federation and Dublin the sub-group extrapolated the population growth based on the 1971 Census figures and determined the requirements for orthopaedic surgeons and orthopaedic beds in the year 2000. These were based on a *Report on Orthopaedic Services* compiled by the British Orthopaedic Association for the NHS.

With this in mind, the establishment of new orthopaedic posts was considered. In 1978 Frank Dowling was appointed jointly to Dr Steevens' and Our Lady's in Crumlin. His adult interest was to be spinal surgery and the development of a spinal unit and his interest in paediatric orthopaedics would enable him to fill the post in Our Lady's Hospital in Crumlin created by the retirement of Gerard Brady.

On the retirements of Jack Cherry from Dr Steevens' and Naas, and Brian Regan from Crumlin, Frank Dowling was joined by Mr E. Fogarty in a similar appointment thus establishing a two-man spinal unit in Dr Steevens'. John McElwain was appointed to Dr Steevens' with an attachment to Naas where he supervised the management of trauma, previously carried out by Mr Cherry.

Following the retirement of Boyd Dunlop and John Sugars, Hugh Smyth, who had an interest in upper limb surgery, and Gary Fenelon whose interest was in hip revision surgery and trauma, also joined the group. Both these posts were created in conjunction with St James's in order to enable expansion and development of the A&E department there.

In this way, by the early 1980s the orthopaedic consultant establishment within the Federated Hospitals had expanded from four to seven. All of these surgeons had an attachment to Dr Steevens' and a partial attachment to other hospitals; however, their elective adult orthopaedic commitment was in every case in Dr Steevens'. Unlike their early predecessors, their practice was devoted entirely to elective and traumatic orthopaedics.

Such an expansion of consultant staff was, of course, accompanied by some increase in the number of junior staff attached to them. These numbers never seemed to reach the desired level. However, the Orthopaedic Sub-group brought together the staff in Dr Steevens', the Meath and the Adelaide. As part of the educational programme a clinical meeting for trainees was held every Tuesday. The trainees and the junior staff within the orthopaedic unit were free to attend lectures and other parts of the educational programme provided by Cappagh.

Once a month the orthopaedic sub-group met to hold a business meeting. Discussions at these meetings revolved around the development of the unit. In the early 1980s the Central Council of the Federated Hospitals decided that it would be appropriate for all the orthopaedic services to be established in Dr Steevens'. To this end all the orthopaedic surgeons and staff were assigned to Dr Steevens', although John Sugars and Derek Robinson did not actually move when this arrangement was formally established. I retained my attachment and clinical duties in the Adelaide and of course already had an attachment to Dr Steevens'. So by 1983 an orthopaedic unit was established in Dr Steevens' with seven surgeons providing a comprehensive elective orthopaedic and trauma adult service. Children's services were still provided in Crumlin by Frank Dowling and Mr Fogarty. An additional service was also provided to the National Children's Hospital in Harcourt Street by myself and Hugh Smyth.

Another appointment was made about this time—David Moore was appointed between Dr Steevens' and Our Lady's in Crumlin. His adult specialty was spinal surgery so the spinal unit at this point was staffed by three well-trained and experienced spinal surgeons.

In order to accommodate the orthopaedic service in Dr Steevens' two new sterile air theatres were built and a new physiotherapy department was provided. In addition, a completely new A&E department was built with a drive-in ambulance entrance opposite Heuston Station.

A Comhairle report on orthopaedics had advised that there should be two major orthopaedic units in Dublin. One was to be sited at Cappagh and the other within the Federated Hospital group. In pursuit of this end the Federated Hospitals' orthopaedic sub-group decided that it should continue to develop and build the orthopaedic unit in Dr Steevens'. By this time the development of Tallaght Hospital had commenced and the question was whether the orthopaedic unit would move to Tallaght when it was initially built or whether it would move there as part of second phase development. It was decided the unit should continue to develop in Dr Steevens' and if it so happened that a move to Tallaght was delayed the major unit on the south side of the city could be continued in Dr Steevens'.

In the event the closure of Dr Steevens' was forced upon it by the Department of Health in 1987 and the orthopaedic services were then moved to the Adelaide where a completely new theatre suite had to be built to accommodate them. This move also meant that the expenditure on the development of orthopaedic facilities in Dr Steevens' over the previous seven to ten years had been a complete waste of money.

The actual move back to the Adelaide was accompanied by considerable negotiation about the number of beds which would be made available there. At a very protracted meeting of the Medical Committee of the Federated Hospitals it was finally decided that the beds in the Adelaide should be divided equally between the general surgeons and the orthopaedic surgeons. This meant that there were about 35 beds available for each specialty but the number of surgeons working from the orthopaedic beds was seven whereas the general surgical beds were to be utilised by only three general surgeons, at least initially. This did appear to be anomalous.

The move to Tallaght was now imminent and long, frequent and protracted discussions took place with regard to the number of beds to be made available for orthopaedics in Tallaght. The orthopaedic sub-group was of the view that in order to accommodate seven surgeons a minimum of 70 beds would be required. The possibility that the Federated Hospitals' orthopaedic unit might move as a whole to Cappagh was explored and indeed the impression was gained that such a move would be welcomed by the staff in Cappagh. Loyalty, however, prevailed over wisdom. The Cappagh option was turned down and the move to Tallaght took place when the hospital opened in 1998. Since then further expansion has occurred and although there are only 30 beds available in Tallaght and a limited number of theatre sessions provided, the total number of orthopaedic surgeons availing of the facilities now is ten. It remains difficult to see how an adequate service can continue to be provided in such circumstances.

On the positive side, however, compared with the situation in 1961 there is now a soundly developed cohesive orthopaedic unit in Tallaght which also supplies services to Naas, Our Lady's and to St James's. Super-specialties within the specialty have developed and now are well established including spinal, joint replacement, foot and upper limb services. It is to be hoped that further expansion of the unit will be possible in order that these services may develop their full potential.

28. Otorhinolaryngology

Eric Fenelon

The surgical profession in Ireland and especially in Dublin had, over the years, always thought of otolaryngology as the Cinderella of surgery, mainly directed towards removal of tonsils and adenoids for recurrent throat infections. How wrong they were!

From the early part of the 20th century, almost all the individual hospitals in Dublin had a consultant on the staff dealing with ENT problems. Originally, the consultant in most cases also took responsibility for the treatment of eye conditions, but around the late 1800s or early 1900s the two separated and each hospital would appoint individual consultants to each discipline. The group comprising the hospitals associated with Trinity College Dublin, later to become the Federated Dublin Voluntary Hospitals, had one consultant in each of the individual hospitals, though there were a few dual appointments.

In Sir Patrick Dun's R. R. (Bobby) Woods succeeded his father, Sir Robert Woods, a former President of the Royal College of Surgeons. Bobby was technically a first rate operator and was one of the early surgeons in Dublin to carry out the operation of laryngo-oesophagectomy which he did with considerable success. He was subsequently appointed also to St Luke's where he performed many of these operations. He was joined by Walter Doyle Kelly, who succeeded him on his death as solo ENT surgeon in Dun's until the Federated Hospitals moved to Tallaght.

At the turn of the century Horace Law was the ENT surgeon at the Adelaide and was succeeded by Sydney Furlong in 1939. Furlong had returned from the 1914–18 war where he had served as a pilot in the Royal Flying Corps and for his services was awarded an OBE. Initially he gave anaesthetics but, following Law's death in 1939, he was appointed ENT surgeon to the Adelaide. He was a very pleasant man and a good surgeon, but although his operating lists did not contain a large variety of conditions, his ear surgery was meticulous. He was also a very keen mechanical technician who often made his own instruments. Following his appointment to the Adelaide he was subsequently also appointed as ENT surgeon to the Meath.

I succeeded Sydney Furlong in the Adelaide in 1957 having originally been appointed as assistant general surgeon to the hospital in 1950. During the intervening period I gradually developed my interest in ear, nose and throat surgery. Sydney Furlong continued at the Meath and was, in turn, succeeded by Frank O'Loughran. The Adelaide had a retiring age of 65 years, though the Meath did not until the introduction of the common contract for hospital consultants in 1981. This established a retiring age for all consultants and also, very happily, a pension following retirement!

In Baggot Street, T. O. Graham, colloquially known as 'Togo', held sway and was joined there by Tom Wilson, a charming man who was known and respected in many parts of the world. A man of many talents he was an accomplished painter, author and musician. He was one of the Commissioners for Irish Lights and wrote a fine book describing the lighthouses around Ireland all of which he had visited in his capacity as Commissioner on the annual cruise of inspection. He was President of the College of Surgeons in 1958–60. He was also appointed ENT surgeon to Dr Steevens' and the National Children's. I succeeded Tom in Steevens' and, on his death, Walter Doyle Kelly succeeded him in the National Children's Hospital. We both remained in these posts until the move to Tallaght.

Tom Wilson's son, Thomas, also qualified as an ENT surgeon and was assigned by the Federated Hospitals to Mercer's and to Baggot Street, succeeding his father. Like his father, Thomas is an accomplished artist and his depictions of the seven hospitals illustrated the cover of the annual report of the Federation in 1975 (and are reused as chapter decorations in the second section of this book). He also has a fine voice and not unnaturally an interest in the physiology and pathology of voice production. He later resigned his post with the Federation to pursue and develop these interests further.

In about 1912 a number of small eye hospitals amalgamated and built the imposing Royal Victoria Eye and Ear Hospital in Adelaide Road, to which I was also appointed in the 1970s, along with Oliver McCullen, who was already a consultant in St Vincent's.

It is therefore apparent that, with all the multiple appointments, a great deal of one's time was spent travelling from hospital to hospital. There was also in the ENT profession, I am very glad to say, a strong camaraderie—this enhanced by the fact that there was more than enough work for everyone in the Federated Hospitals, and therefore no real competition.

In the earlier days one's junior staff was just a shared house surgeon, but by the 1970s the junior staff had increased considerably with not only a house surgeon, but also registrars and senior registrars, by which time higher training in all the specialties was being very actively encouraged by the

Royal Colleges on a much more formal basis then previously.

On the move of the Federated Hospitals to Tallaght the ENT department, now considerably enhanced, was expanded to include head and neck surgery. Two further consultant appointments were made to the new hospital in Tallaght. Don McShane, who moved with the Adelaide, has been joined by Brendan Conlon and John Kinsella, both of whom have joint appointments between Tallaght and St James's. Together they provide both a general adult and a paediatric ENT service with special interest in otology and head and neck surgery.

The Irish Otolaryngological Society, which was formed in 1961 by Tom Wilson and David Craig, a leading Belfast ENT surgeon, and included all the ENT surgeons of both Northern Ireland and the Republic, became, in about the year 2000, the Irish Otolaryngological Head and Neck Society. It was formed by all the Irish ENT surgeons with the notable exception of Togo Graham who felt it would downgrade the Royal Academy of Medicine ENT section, of which he was a keen member. Fortunately it did not do so but enhanced the ENT profession considerably and both societies are flourishing to date.

From a historical point of view, it is interesting that previously consultant surgeons bought and owned their own surgical instruments, but subsequent to the change, government (Department of Health) funding provided grants to individual hospitals to buy essential equipment. This resulted in a very welcome upgrading of ENT instrumentation in most hospitals and certainly in the new hospital in Tallaght.

29. Pathology

Dermot Hourihane

I was appointed as Reader in Pathology in TCD in the summer of 1966; the post carried an honorary consultant appointment to the Federated Dublin Voluntary Hospitals. The professor of pathology at the time had recently been appointed to the chair, W. T .E McCaughey, known as Elliott. My predecessor was Joan Mullaney (née McCarthy) who made a unilateral declaration of independence from TCD and was in the Meath laboratory reading the histology slides for that hospital, and then there were the hospital pathologists, Nick Jaswon in Steevens' and Harcourt Street and Niall Gallagher in Baggot Street and Dun's. The previous pathologist to Baggot Street was Celsus McCrea, who always said he had been dismissed by Judge Kingsmill Moore, on what grounds I never ascertained!, and who finished as pathologist in Daisy Hill in Newry. Betty Wallace was the pathologist in the Adelaide and there were several trainee pathologists based in the school of pathology, employed either by FDVH or TCD.

The Central Council of FDVH had decided to establish specialist laboratories in accordance with the professional developments in the western world, in order to have consultant haematologists, microbiologists and biochemists as well as consultant histopathologists. This development gave rise to a certain amount of competition and even antagonism in the individual hospitals who did not wish to lose services such as haematology and microbiology if they were to be centred in another hospital. In the end histopathology continued, as it had been for many years, to be based in the Trinity school of pathology, microbiology was centred in the Adelaide with Betty Wallace in charge, haematology was based in the Meath with Ian Temperley in charge and biochemistry was in Dun's with Paddy Leonard in charge. Some years later a separate immunology laboratory was established in Mercer's with Alex Whelan as the chief technologist; the first medical consultant for that laboratory was John Greally. Another later development was the establishment of a cytology laboratory in Baggot Street under Niall Gallagher.

The system of collection and dispatch of specimens and reports was immensely complicated as this was before computerisation, and vans driven by charming ladies who were generally widows, as I remember, moved the specimens from the hospital laboratory to the specialist laboratory in, say, the Adelaide or in Trinity, and reports were delivered back to the hospital of origin. As the traffic in Dublin grew progressively heavier, we eventually changed to motor bicycles which was an advance.

Elliott McCaughey was the chairman of the consultant pathologists' committee in the FDVH, and in about 1968 he complained in writing to the Central Council that he did not have enough authority to ensure centralisation as had been decided by the Central Council. A committee was set up under Minchin Clarke who was a lay governor of Dr Steevens' and subsequently became chairman of the Central Council. The committee included Robert Jacob and Douglas Mellon. This group recommended the appointment of a principal pathologist to take a place on the finance committee of the FDVH, with a clear recognition that Central Council needed to back the principal pathologist if it supported his/her proposals as he/she was not a member of the Central Council.

The system was somewhat unstable at this time as the FitzGerald Report was published in 1968 and recommended that the Federation be split in two, one half to go to St Kevin's (now St James's) and the second half to go to St Vincent's. Our professors of surgery and medicine, George Fegan and Peter Gatenby, were both members of the FitzGerald committee, but the consultants in the FDVH vigorously opposed its recommendation, most notably at a meeting of all the consultants held in Sir Patrick Dun's which was addressed by Brandon Stephens from the Meath and Stanley McCollum from the Adelaide and the National Children's Hospital. The point was emphasised that we would only remain powerful if we remained united in one hospital and that we should not be divided—an interesting attitude considering what subsequently occurred.

Another destabilising factor was the proposal from the Minister for Education Donogh O'Malley to merge TCD and UCD into a single university. This was vigorously, even fanatically, opposed by the vast majority of academic staff in each institution, and was finally dropped after years of debate.

Specialisation in pathology had arrived in the US and in Britain, but was slow to come to Ireland; it was particularly slow in our hospitals as they were individually too small to justify four different specialist consultants in the recognised disciplines; in addition, as we have seen, by having the specialist laboratories in different locations an immensely complicated system of collection and delivery was necessary.

During the 1970s it gradually became clear that the Meath, Adelaide and the National Children's Hospital were not going to move to St James's, but would go elsewhere although I have never been sure how that decision was arrived at and I have always regretted it.

The autopsies on my arrival were all conducted in the individual hospitals, usually by the local hospital pathologist, but in the case of the Meath and Adelaide, by staff from the school of pathology in Trinity. In the mid-1970s the hospitals agreed to allow the bodies to be transferred to what was then St James's for the conduct of the autopsy and brought back to the individual hospital for removal by the relatives. This was the system until the staff from the school of pathology moved to the Central Pathology Laboratory in St James's in 1980; the four hospitals (Dun's, Steevens', Baggot Street and Mercer's) were closed during the 1980s and all their services were then supplied from St James's.

The most difficult period, when it was almost impossible to supply a first-class service, had then developed in that the Meath, Adelaide and the National Children's Hospital remained in their original locations, and the service for the patients in those hospitals was supplied by the laboratory in St James's. This came to an end in 1998 when those hospitals closed and moved to Tallaght, with their own laboratory service.

Although the conditions were not ideal, the school of pathology was a very pleasant place to work, and there was an excellent atmosphere. We always had trainees, who mostly stayed within the laboratory disciplines, including Ken du Plessis, who became a haematologist in South Africa, Joan Gearty, now a histopathologist in Birmingham, Cintra Maharaj, who married a histopathologist and emigrated to Canada with him, and Jack Harbison who became our first whole-time forensic (state) pathologist. Dr John Dinn, an American graduate, also joined the staff and developed a histo-chemistry service for the study of neuromuscular disorders. He was unfortunately to die but the service he established has developed and continues.

There were several changes of personnel during the period up to 1980: Nick Jaswon resigned and moved to work in the National Health Service in the North of England, Elliott McCaughey left about 1970 and I replaced him in 1973, Joan Mullaney moved to be the histopathologist at the Eye and Ear Hospital, Betty Wallace went to a post in Brighton and was replaced by Conor Keane, Paddy Leonard left to work for a company in the United States, replaced by Clayton Love, and Eamonn Sweeney joined histopathology in the 1970s.

It was certainly a brave experiment by the Central Council in that for 15 years they had a specialist pathology service working towards unity of the

FDVH while the individual hospitals were very reluctant to contemplate or move towards unity, and in fact never did. The pathology service was a force towards unity as was the academic structure.

The forces against change within the hospitals were very strong so that if an individual consultant refused to give up beds to help form a unit of a recommended size then it usually did not happen, and there were several examples of this during those 15 years. Specialisation was not encouraged in the clinical field as the belief or wish in each individual hospital was to supply a comprehensive service as best they could. Such things as breast surgery, endocrine surgery, gastroenterology, cardiac and vascular surgery were very hard to develop in the small hospitals and even when they did develop, as did cardiac surgery in Baggot Street, they were subsumed into larger units eventually. Although the hospitals were very pleasant to work in and we have numerous pleasant memories of those years, the essential developments in specialisation, which were led by pathology and which spread into what was general medicine and general surgery at a later time, could only be achieved in a large hospital, which is why we have finished up in St James's and Tallaght.

30. Paediatrics

M. R. H. Taylor

Introduction

Although somewhat constrained by planning blight, the years leading up to the move of the National Children's Hospital to Tallaght in 1998 were full of innovation.

The reduction in the average duration of stay

In 1972 the mean duration of stay in the National Children's Hospital was approximately 14 days. This was a legacy from the days when little convalescent care could be given at home, the general level of education of parents in health matters was considerably lower, social services were very limited and poverty was common. Once the question 'Why does this child need to be in hospital?' started to be asked the duration of stay started to fall and over a number of years reached its current level of around 3.5 days.

The expansion of the x-ray department with the aid of funds from St Ultan's Hospital

The x-ray department in the National Children's Hospital in 1972 consisted of a wood and glass hut in the front hall which the radiologist, Sholto Douglas, used as a reporting room and a single general x-ray room located above the hospital kitchen (which was in the basement). The x-ray department was severely limited in the investigations which it could carry out and in the main this amounted to plain x-rays, barium studies of the intestinal tract, and intravenous pyelography. The department was expanded by the addition of ultrasound on the arrival of Dr Horton who replaced Sholto Douglas. After the arrival of Eric Colhoun and the closure of St Ultan's money was provided by St Ultan's to add a second improved x-ray room which was used for contrast studies including bronchography. An area for ultrasound examination was also added which greatly assisted in the investigation of children, especially those with abdominal and urinary tract problems. Isotope studies and computed tomography studies still had to be performed in other hospitals (mainly the Meath) and these studies required transfer of the patient to another hospital until the hospital moved to Tallaght in June 1998. Isotope studies and computed tomography were available from shortly after that hospital opened and magnetic resonance imaging (MRI) became available on site after a few years.

The provision of the intensive care unit

Planning of the intensive care unit was undertaken in the early 1970s. An area on the surgical landing was converted to provide one two-bedded and one single-bedded room plus a nursing station. A blood gas analyser was provided in the nursing area. A ventilator was bought for the unit but the anaesthetists declined to use it because of the inability to provide on site anaesthetic junior hospital doctor cover at night.

The provision of cubicles to reduce cross infection

Following outbreaks of gastroenteritis in the early 1970s measures were introduced to prevent the spread of infectious diseases, especially gastroenteritis, within the hospital. A major factor in this was the provision of single cubicles (which, in many cases could be used as parent-and-child rooms). The main cubicled area in the hospital was the Wicklow Clinic; cubicles were provided in the Wellington ward, on what had been part of the private area on the surgical landing. With funding provided by the Ladies' Guild a suite of about seven parent-and-child rooms were built and named the Steen Unit. They were officially named by Mrs Steen, who unveiled a commemorative plaque.

The provision of mother and child rooms to allow parents to sleep in hospital with their children

At one time, visiting in the National Children's Hospital was limited to one hour per day (including parents other than breast feeding mothers, of whom there were few). The hospital was considered to be in loco parentis. This was the norm in Ireland and the United Kingdom at the time. However, it was obvious that it was very traumatic for children to be separated from their parents and so gradually it became accepted that 'Parents are not visitors' and so visiting times should not apply to them. It also became accepted that parents might not only be a presence beside the child but should do all the caring that they would normally do at home and also aid the nursing staff in providing treatment. A study was undertaken which showed that when parents (who were in almost all instances mothers) lived in the hospital with their children the children went home 30 per cent earlier than those whose parents did not live in.

Sibling visiting

After considerable discussion regarding the potential for cross infection both from and to siblings it was decided on the instigation of Matron Mrs Ann Taylor to allow sibling visiting unless there was a specific reason not to permit it. In the past the main concern had been that siblings might be incubating an infectious disease which could then spread to patients or visitors. Sibling visiting proved a success and only in a few instances was it necessary to exclude siblings when parents requested that they visit. In most cases, when sibling visiting would have been inappropriate parents did not request it.

The expansion of the medical records department

The medical records department was expanded to deal with the increasing number of patients' charts. The department had been immediately inside the 'back' door from Clonmel Street which was the outpatients' entrance. (At one time the door had been bolted shut at a set time in the day and all patients who had come in before that time would be seen that day. There was no appointment system.) The medical records department was moved to an expanded area largely underneath the new parent-and-child cubicles. This space proved to be inadequate even with the microfilming of part or all of 'dormant' charts and so the 'stick house' which had been used for storing kindling wood in the days of open fires, and had later become the respiratory laboratory, was used for medical records storage. The medical records department in Harcourt Street worked well and missing charts were a rarity.

The arrival of an A&E consultant (Mary McKay) and the translocation and expansion of the A&E department

There was a dramatic improvement in the A&E service provided by the National Children's Hospital following Mary McKay's appointment as consultant in A&E and the expansion of the department. The department moved from the outpatients' area to the side of the corridor to the Wicklow Clinic and now had two rooms; in addition an ambulance access route for trolleys was provided through the archway and the garden. Prior to Mary McKay's arrival the A&E service was provided by non consultant hospital doctors with the medical or surgical consultant on duty providing consultant cover. Dr McKay provided a focus and an intellectual and knowledge resource for the development of the service. Her energy, interest and application to her work were prodigious; it was regrettable that these qualities were not appreciated and emulated by the hospital board which failed to back her adequately to maintain her position even though a later court judgment was that she had been treated 'appallingly' both by the hospital and Comhairle. Seven years after the move to Tallaght Dr McKay moved to Temple Street, a sad loss to the hospital and a poor reflection on both the National Children's Hospital and AMNCH.

The provision of an ultrasound service by Dr Colhoun

Eric Colhoun replaced Dr Horton who returned to the USA after a short time as consultant radiologist. On the closure of St Ultan's money was provided by St Ultan's for development of the imaging services in the National Children's Hospital. The hospital was then equipped with a general x-ray room, a fluoroscopy room and an ultrasound room. In 1972 there had only been a single general x-ray room above the kitchen. Dr Colhoun's enormous enthusiasm, energy and ability to deal superbly with the most frightened and difficult of patients lifted the department to new heights. In addition to this, his quality of image interpretation is superb. He is in the top echelon of paediatric radiologists. Dr Colhoun provided a personal ultrasound service which in particular revolutionised the care of children with urinary tract infections and abdominal symptoms in our hospital.

The expansion of the operating theatre suite with provision of a recovery area

A major restructuring of the operating theatre area was undertaken. This involved expanding the operating theatre space, providing a recovery area, changing rooms, a clean-up area for instruments and relocation of the autoclave. Access was also provided to the new parent-and-child ward known as the Steen Ward though with the loss of one parent-and-child cubicle.

The provision of a canteen

A canteen was provided by taking in the hospital boardroom and converting the doctors' dining room to a boardroom. The house governor's office was moved to what had been the sisters' sitting room. The nurses' dining room was then opened through to the old boardroom. The end of the old board room nearest to the front hall was partitioned off and used to provide a new porter's desk/reception desk and switchboard. The old porter's desk was removed from the front hail. A canteen was provided in the space left by the remainder of the old boardroom and the nurses' dining room.

Home treatment for coagulation disorders

Professor Temperley introduced home treatment for coagulation disorders in his modernisation of the treatment of these disorders in Ireland. This allowed parents of children with coagulation disorders to manage their children at home to a far greater extent than had been possible in the past. The children were managed on lines approaching those of children with diabetes so that parents maintained suitable coagulation levels in their children by injecting coagulation factor preparations at home and attending the hospital as required to check progress instead of attending hospital for every injection. This revolutionised management of these conditions. Unfortunately, at a later date some of the coagulation factor preparations used were found to contain the acquired immune deficiency (AIDS) virus with fatal consequences for the infected patients.

It can be seen from the above that things did not stand still in the years before 1998. Significant developments took place so that when the NCH moved to its new site, together with the Adelaide and Meath, it was in a singularly good position to provide a very good paediatric service for the people of Tallaght.

31. Physiotherapy

Kay Keating*

Origins of the Dublin School of Physiotherapy

The first school of physiotherapy in Ireland was founded in 1905 at 86 Lower Leeson Street. It was known initially as the Irish School of Massage, later as the Irish School of Massage and Medical Electricity and finally, in 1942, as the Dublin School of Physiotherapy. In 1914 the school moved to 12 Hume Street and in 1973 to its present location in St James's Hospital.

The founder and first principal was a trained nurse—Amelia Hogg, who died in 1940. In the early years she was assisted by Louisa Despard, who died in 1935. Miss Despard was interested in electrical treatment about which she wrote a textbook and held a six week course in Leeson Street in 1908.

Miss Hogg was the driving force in the development of the school for the first 20 years. She strove for its recognition and acceptance. She also maintained close links with similar institutions in Britain. The Society of Trained Masseuses was founded in England in 1894 by four nurses trained fully in the art of massage, the object being to prevent their skills falling into disrepute.

The first Dublin School examinations were held in 1908 and were organised by the Nurses' Co-operative of which Miss Hogg was a member. Two of the members of the Incorporated Society of Trained Masseuses travelled to Dublin to examine the students. Examinations in medical gymnastics were held in Dublin for the first time in 1918, otherwise students had to travel to London or Manchester to be examined.

Another powerful force associated with the Dublin School was Agnes Amy Leonora Allen. She began her training under Miss Hogg in 1912 and gained her certificate from the Incorporated Society of Trained Masseuses in 1914. When Miss Hogg retired in 1922 Miss Allen became principal of the school, a post which she held until 1969. In the early 1960s she was joined as co-principal by Henrietta Lucy Micks who had trained in 1920.

* With additional material from Sandy Wagstaff and extracts from FDVH Central Council Minutes.

Miss Micks subsequently qualified as a teacher of electrotherapy, massage and medical gymnastics. She was easily identifiable round Dublin on account of her bright copper hair and her red sports car which she drove at high speed.

The Mater School of Physiotherapy and diplomas

In 1955 a second physiotherapy training centre opened in Dublin; it was attached to the Mater. At the time, medical and associated educational courses were organised along denominational lines and there were Catholic hospitals and Protestant hospitals whose teaching tended to be associated with either UCD or TCD respectively. The 'ban' which made it difficult for Roman Catholics to attend Trinity of course contributed to this.

The first principal of the school, Sister Kevin Reynolds, and Dermot Roden, the medical director, concluded an agreement with the National University of Ireland (NUI) under which students who had satisfied the Chartered Society of Physiotherapists examiners were awarded a Diploma in Physiotherapy from NUI.

This of course stimulated Trinity and the Dublin School and in 1957 Trinity introduced a similar diploma for students from the school. Both schools therefore had university diploma status, but it was not until 1983 that both diploma courses were upgraded to degree standard.

The involvement of the Federated Hospitals

In 1961, when the Federated Hospitals Act was passed, physiotherapy training was being provided in the Dublin School of Physiotherapy in association with Trinity and in the Mater in association with UCD.

Although not directly involved with the administration of the Dublin School the Federated Hospitals had a considerable interest in its activities because the physiotherapy services in the constituent hospitals were dependant on the school's students and indeed the teachers who provided them. In similar fashion, the Mater School provided physiotherapy services for both the Mater and St Vincent's. In each hospital the students were supervised by senior staff, qualified members of the Chartered Society of Physiotherapist.

The Central Council of Federation, possibly because its influence over the activities of the individual hospitals was limited (despite the Act), was able to and indeed did take an active interest in the continuation of the Dublin School of Physiotherapy which was a rare area of common ground between the individual hospitals. It is noted in Central Council minutes in

1963 that the school at that time was in some administrative difficulty. Representatives of Central Council and TCD met with the school proprietors—Miss Allen and Miss Micks—to discuss the situation and future of the school.

In 1964 Vernon Harty, a member of Central Council, discussed the situation with the Chartered Society in London. It would appear that they were less than happy about the standards of the Dublin School. Following this visit Central Council agreed in principle that the Federation should offer to operate the school.

Negotiations between the Federation, Trinity, the Dublin School and the Department of Health were protracted. Funds were sought from the Department and a bid offered for a house for the school in Leeson Park. This was not successful due to lack of funds—there was a shortfall of some £3–4,000.

In 1968 the Department recommended that a new principal teacher be appointed and that the school be based in Trinity. In July 1969 the Chartered Society questioned the standard of training in the Dublin School and indicated that it would be unable to approve acceptance of students by the school for 1970 unless improvements took place. In October Miss Micks said that she did not propose to enrol students for future years. In April 1970 Central Council made enquiries from the Dublin Health Authority about the possibility of siting the school in the hospital then called St Kevin's. Discussions were already underway about its future with Trinity.

There were more delays but in November 1971 agreement was reached between the Dublin School of Physiotherapy, the Federation, and Trinity that the three bodies would amalgamate and move to St James's (previously St Kevin's) in 1972. The school in Hume Street closed and Professor Jessop, of Trinity medical school, and the Federation administrator, Nevin Dowling, after a search recommended that Jack Stockton be appointed as the new principal. He had been in charge of the Naval School in Haslar in Portsmouth and had headed the Physiotherapy School in Pretoria. He was working as a teacher at St Thomas's at the time of his appointment to the Dublin School of Physiotherapy. He was ably assisted by Miss Manifold, who moved with the school from Hume Street, and by Noreen Foley who had also been appointed as a teacher. Finally, the school moved to prefab accommodation on the St James's site and the Federation took over the responsibility for its administration and financing. In 1974 Paul Wagstaff joined the staff, moving from the London Hospital. His move was smoothed by Vernon Harty. In 1980 Jack Stockton retired and was replaced by Paul Wagstaff as head of the school. It was at this stage that negotiations began between the

two schools and their respective universities to establish a four-year honours degree programme.

Diplomas and degrees

In 1979, due to a shortage of teachers, the MEd course in Trinity established an additional option in paramedical studies for physiotherapists and
others who wished to train as teachers in their respective fields. The Federation was instrumental in this development.

To replace the diploma courses four-year honours degree courses were
established in Trinity (BSc) with the Dublin School, and in UCD (B. Physiotherapy) with the Mater School. These started in 1983. Northern Ireland
already had a degree programme running. Together with the two programmes in Dublin these were the first such courses established in the UK
and Ireland. This move was fully supported by the Federation. When the
degree programme started the Dublin School became part of the medical
faculty in TCD. The Federation ceased its involvement in physiotherapy
administration, although Desmond Dempsey—Nevin Dowling's successor—maintained strong links with the physiotherapists sitting on the Education Committee of the Irish Society of Chartered Physiotherapists for a
number of years.

The Irish Society of Chartered Physiotherapists

Up to 1983 physiotherapists in Ireland had been members of the British
Chartered Society of Physiotherapists. It became apparent by then that in
order to regulate and negotiate for the profession efficiently in Ireland a
separate organisation was needed. Thus, with the blessing of the Chartered
Society, the Irish Society of Chartered Physiotherapists came into being.

Today, physiotherapy training and practice in Ireland maintain standards which are of the highest quality. There are now schools in Trinity,
UCD, the Royal College of Surgeons in Ireland and in Limerick University. It is a tribute to Miss Hogg, Miss Allen, their colleagues and their
successors that the profession is in such a healthy state. There is no doubt
either that the members of the Federated Hospitals Central Council who
were involved with the Dublin School in the 1960s would also be proud of
the results of their efforts to maintain and help to develop the practice of
physiotherapy in Dublin and the country as a whole.

32. Plastic surgery and oral and maxillo-facial surgery

J. B. Prendiville, D. L. Lawlor and F. Brady

*The evolution of plastic surgery in Dr Steevens' Hospital, Dublin**

J. B. Prendiville

In 1710 Dr Richard Steevens, on his deathbed, initiated the whole concept of the voluntary hospital system, which, in time, established itself as the prime hospital system throughout Britain, its colonies and Europe. He left his estate to be used, after his sister's death, to establish a voluntary hospital in Dublin for 'such patients as were curable'. Its implementation was slow. The Trustees met in March 1717 and the building commenced in 1720 but patients were not admitted until 1733.

In the meantime, the Charitable Infirmary in Dublin was opened, in a previously existing house, in 1718 by six Dublin surgeons. The Westminster Society was established with its hospital opening its doors in 1720, and Guy's Hospital opened in 1724—all on the principles laid down by Dr Steevens.

In the board room of Dr Steevens' Hospital there is a fascinating gentleman's library of the early 18th century of some 3,000 volumes, with 21 incunabula, all beautifully encased and fully indexed. No books have been added to or taken from the library since its establishment in 1733 by a Dr Worth. He was a governor of the hospital and donated his collection. There are books of plastic surgical interest such as by Ambrose Pare and Tagliacozzi, and a very comprehensive collection of the more famous medical books published before that time.

* This is a shortened version of the eleventh of a series of histories of plastic surgery centres adapted, when necessary, (by A. F. Wallace and C. W. Chapman) from records forming part of the archives of the British Association of Plastic Surgeons. *British Journal of Plastic Surgery* (198 8), 4 1, 200–205 © 1988 The Trustees of British Association of Plastic Surgeons.

Plastic surgery

Abraham Colles repaired cleft lips in Steevens' in 1800 using silver pins and screws, with figure-of-eight thread to hold the lip together. Maurice Collis in 1868 described a method of creating a 'cupid's bow' on cleft lips although this had been attempted previously by Richard Butcher working in Mercer's Hospital, Dublin. A large series of Indian rhinoplasties was carried out in the middle of the 19th century and recorded, in particular, by John Hamilton (1864) with photographs of wood engravings.

In the present century William Doolin, who trained with Victor Veau in Paris and Kilner in Oxford, set up a one-man service in Temple Street Hospital where he did most outstanding work in the cleft palate field and in burns. Similarly, A. B. Clery took a considerable interest in plastic surgery in the Richmond Hospital in the late 1940s and during and after the Second World War, but there is no record of his having undergone any formal training. I attempted to persuade Clery to establish a unit in the Richmond Hospital, but although we were close friends he declined to set up a plastic surgery unit. Such work as he did in plastic surgery was very good and I remember, in particular, a reconstruction in 1947 of an amputated lower jaw and lip with bilateral superficial temporal scalp flaps as described by Esser, and more recently by McGregor. At about the same time Tommy Kilner was appointed to the Meath Hospital where he came every three months, in particular to operate on hypospadiacs for Mr T. J. Lane.

Having been a trainee for one year (1951) in Wythenshawe Hospital, Manchester and for three years in Chepstow and the United Cardiff Hospitals (1952, 1954 and 1954), I returned to Dublin in 1955 to the plastic surgery unit where I was given beds, by 'grace and favour', from Arthur Chance. In January 1957 I was appointed by the governors to the hospital staff and on the retirement of Chance was promoted to the rank of senior surgeon, with all the attendant rights and privileges.

The unit in Steevens' evolved. I persuaded the Board to appoint Niall Hogan as oral surgeon and subsequently I received the Derby winnings of the horse Ragusa from Mr and Mrs L. R. Mullion for the construction and equipping of the maxillo-facial unit. Major soft tissue trauma, burns, clefts and head and neck cancer were diverted almost completely from the general surgeons and in a relatively short space of time. A hand clinic was established in the 1960s.

In 1962 I was assigned a senior registrar in plastic surgery by the Board, and the Department of Health agreed to the finance. The first occupant of this position was a Mr Khan who returned to Pakistan in later years. The next senior registrar was Gearoid Lynch(1964–6) who was appointed subsequently to the professorial department of the Richmond Hospital. Gerry Edwards followed Lynch (1966–8). Matt McHugh was senior registrar from 1970 to 1979. McHugh was given leave of absence to work with David Matthews at Great Ormond Street, at the hand unit in Derby and at Canniesburn during his years in training, On McHugh's appointment as consultant, Denis Lawlor was appointed senior registrar (1979–84). He was given a year's leave of absence to work with Bernard O'Brien in Melbourne, training in microsurgery.

With the development of the Federated Hospitals the appointment of consultants has been made centrally since the 1960s. In January 1971 the Central Council of the Federation, at my request, appointed Gerry Edwards and Seamus Ó Riain as consultants, with me as Director, to the plastic unit. Matt McHugh was appointed consultant plastic surgeon in 1979, Denis Lawlor in January 1985.

Initially there were 43 adult beds, which were increased subsequently to 46 on the closure of the venereology department, with a proviso that 5 beds would be made available for general surgical emergencies during the hospital 'on-call' rota. There were an additional 15 children's beds and cots which were devoted almost exclusively to plastic surgery, there being no other demand for them in the hospital. In 1980 an intensive care unit for burns was constructed with theatre, dressing rooms, therapy bath and 5 beds for major burns. In all there are 61–6 beds in use in the unit.

The plastic and maxillo-facial surgery unit

With the appointment of Dr Hogan as maxillo-facial surgeon 8 beds were designated for this specialty, which operated in conjunction with the plastic service as the plastic and maxillo-facial unit. Dr Geoff Kronn assisted Hogan although his appointment to the hospital was that of dental surgeon. A senior registrar and shared SHO were subsequently assigned to oral surgery. With the construction of the plastic and maxillo-facial department (from the Mullions' gift) the two specialties were associated even more intimately, with the office, speech therapy department, laboratory and dental departments all together in the unit. Hogan was assigned an SHO in conjunction with the plastic unit and Mr Forde was appointed dental technician and prosthetic appliance maker. Mr Vincent Morris was appointed cleft palate orthodontist, initially for three sessions but subsequently for five with an assistant from the Dental Hospital, where he worked also.

Miss Nora Dawson was appointed in conjunction with Harcourt Street Children's Hospital, providing the first speech therapy service in Dublin, in 1958.

The cleft palate clinic

The clinic was established during the 1960s with the speech therapist, audiologist and orthodontist combining on the one afternoon for assessments to minimise travel for patients coming long distances from throughout Ireland. In 1977 the need for a second maxillo-facial surgeon was agreed after many years of negotiations and Frank Brady was appointed. With Dr Hogan's retirement in 1983, Mr H. Barry replaced him. There is an active casualty department and an orthopaedic unit of 79 beds with five consultants. Currently the staff of the unit consists of five plastic surgeons, two oral surgeons, one orthodontist, ear, nose and throat attendance at the cleft palate clinic, a conservative dentist, a speech therapist, an audiologist and a paediatrician as well as trainees and rotating junior hospital staff. Steevens' is to be phased out in favour of the new hospitals with the plastic and maxillo-facial unit moving to St James's, with over 1,000 beds, and the orthopaedic unit to a new hospital at Tallaght on the south side of Dublin.

Plastic surgery in the Federated Hospitals (Dr Steevens'/St James's)
1980 to the present

D. L. Lawlor

I returned from the O'Brien Institute in Melbourne in 1981 to complete my senior registrar training. I introduced microsurgery to the specialty and this allowed for micro replantation and microvascular reconstruction with free tissue transfer. This increased expertise allowed for more major surgical resections and reconstruction. Limbs that would otherwise have had to be amputated following major trauma could now be salvaged.

I was appointed as a consultant in 1984. Following three months training in cosmetic surgery in London I took up my post in April 1985 and was assigned not only to Dr Steevens' but also to the Mater and James Connolly Memorial Hospitals.

Plastic surgery suffered a major blow with the abrupt closure of Dr Steevens' in October 1987. In Dr Steevens' there were ample beds to allow for elective surgery and trauma to co-exist. Indeed the waiting time for elective surgery was in months. The specialty was transferred to St James's Hospital in January 1988. Because facilities at St James's were not yet completed I arranged for the unit to be transferred to James Connolly Memorial Hospital with the maxillo-facial department for the months of November/December 1987.

The plastic surgery unit had been earmarked to be transferred to St James's in 1993 and it was no surprise that facilities were inadequate in Hospital 5 in January 1988. We shared a ward of 31 beds with the maxillo-facial surgeons and these also included paediatric beds. This was to be a temporary arrangement until 1992 when the new St James's was to open. Unfortunately, the temporary situation became permanent. As time went on, and with the huge increase in trauma, elective plastic surgery suffered. Waiting lists spiralled, going from a few months in Dr Steevens' to years in St James's for some cases. However, one area that did benefit from the transfer to St James's was the management of burns patients. A custom-built burns unit of 20 beds opened prior to 1992. It was reduced to 13 beds to allow for a visitor facility within the unit.

The activity of the unit was greatly compromised in the period following the transfer to St James's. This resulted in the loss of recognition for specialist senior registrar training which was not restored until October 1994 when Margaret O'Donnell was appointed and took up her post. She went to the Royal Adelaide in Australia in 1997 to complete her training and on her return took up a consultant post at St Vincent's and at St James's as consultant to the burns unit. Patricia Eadie, who did most of her training in the United Kingdom, also trained at the O'Brien Institute in Melbourne before taking up her appointment in St James's in 1994. David Orr was trained in the United Kingdom and at the Royal Adelaide and was appointed as a consultant in 1998. Gerry Edwards retired from the plastic surgery department in 1999 and sadly died shortly afterwards after a brief illness. Matt McHugh retired from the department in 2003 and two new consultants were appointed in 2004, Eamonn Beausang and David O'Donovan. They both completed their training in the United Kingdom and North America.

A new laser unit opened in Hospital 7 in 1994 following the donation of laser equipment by Mrs Norma Smurfit. Laser treatment has revolutionised such conditions as port wine stains and through her generosity a large number of patients have benefited enormously.

Since the beginning the unit has been managed by Nurse Mary Kilmurray who also worked in the plastic unit at Dr Steevens'. Sister Kathleen Nolan transferred with us from Dr Steevens' and was our theatre sister in St James's until she retired in 2004. She has now been replaced by Sister Catriona McKenna.

The clinical photographer Neasa Doyle transferred with us from Dr Steevens' and is responsible to this day for the audio-visual and photographic department.

Presently there are four senior specialist registrar posts in St James's in plastic surgery. Margaret O'Donnell is on two years' leave of absence from the burns unit and is replaced by locum consultant Catriona Lawlor from Canada.

*The development of the maxillo-facial unit before and after
its transfer to St James's*

Frank Brady

With the development of the plastic surgery unit under Brendan Prendiville, the board of Dr Steevens' appointed Niall Hogan as oral surgeon to the hospital. Mr Prendiville subsequently received the winnings of the 1963 Derby winner Ragusa from Mr and Mrs Mullion, and donated the money to the hospital for the construction and equipment of the first maxillo-facial unit in the country.

With Niall Hogan's appointment, 8 beds were designated to the evolving surgical specialty of maxillo-facial surgery. The plastic and maxillo-facial unit continued to develop in tandem. Geoff Kronn was appointed as dental surgeon to the hospital on a part-time basis to assist Niall Hogan. With the increasing referral workload, it was realised that the maxillo-facial unit needed more staff, and I was appointed in 1971 to the post of SHO. This appointment was shared with the plastic surgery service.

Further appointments to the unit included part-time attachment of Vincent Morris, orthodontist and senior lecturer at the Dublin Dental Hospital, to the cleft palate clinic. Joint cleft palate clinics between plastic surgery, maxillo-facial surgery and orthodontics were established. Mr Forde was appointed as maxillo-facial technician to the newly formed laboratory. Niall Hogan encouraged me to obtain full surgical and specialist training in the rapidly developing specialty of oral and maxillo-facial surgery (OMFS), and I went abroad to obtain this training.

I was initially attached to the maxillo-facial unit in Westminster/Roehampton in London and subsequently at the University of California, Los Angeles, where I held the post of senior registrar of the associate professor. I returned to join Niall Hogan and the plastic and maxillo-facial surgical team in 1979 as consultant maxillo-facial surgeon to Dr Steevens', with attachments to the Richmond and St Vincent's. At this time, maxillo-facial surgery was developing as a separate, though closely allied, specialty to plastic surgery. Close co-operation between the two disciplines continued.

The maxillo-facial unit was subsequently recognised by the Department of Health as the national unit. David Ryan was appointed as first senior registrar in OMFS and Dermot Fitzpatrick was appointed as maxillo-facial technician and was assisted by Moira Ryan in the increasingly busy maxillo-facial laboratory. Hugh Barry, oral surgeon at the Dublin Dental Hospital, was granted sessions at Dr Steevens' to assist the maxillo-facial team. In addition to the management of facial bone trauma, the area of facial bone reconstruction—orthognathic surgery—developed in conjunction with the orthodontic team.

With the closure of Dr Steevens', the maxillo-facial unit was transferred to the new St James's. OMFS subsequently became recognised by Comhairle na nÓspidéal and the Irish Medical Council as a distinct surgical specialty. With the retirement of Vincent Morris, D. Eamonn McKiernan was appointed to St James's as consultant orthodontist, with a specific remit for cleft palate orthodontic and the orthodontic management of orthognathic surgery. Cliff Beirne and later Leo Stassen were appointed consultants in maxillo-facial surgery at St James's, bringing the complement of maxillo-facial surgeons to three. Aisling O'Mahony was recently appointed as maxillo-facial prosthodontist, with a specific interest in cleft prosthodontics. There are now four full-time technicians in the laboratory.

The national unit continues to develop and expand. Strong professional links continue to be made between the maxillo-facial unit and the plastic surgery unit in St James's, and there are regular combined craniofacial and cleft clinics between the two units, including Our Lady's, where David Orr, plastic surgeon, and Michael Earley, plastic surgeon, are significantly involved. It is interesting to note that the first orthognathic surgical case (facial bone osteotomy) was performed in 1981; up to 150 similar cases are now performed annually.

Bibliography

Butcher, R. G. *Essays and Reports*. Dublin: Fannin 1865.

Collis, M. *Quarterly Journal of Medical Science* Dublin 1868.

Doolin, W. 'Congenital clefts of lip and palate' *Irish Journal of Medical Science* 1938 p. 708.

Evans, D. and Howard, L . G. R. *Romance of the Voluntary Hospital Movement* Dublin: Hutchinson *n.d.*

Kirkpatrick, T. P. C. *The History of Steevens' Hospital* Dublin: University Press 1924.

33. Radiology

David McInerney and Gerry Hurley

At the time of Roentgen's discovery of x-rays in 1895, the hospitals which were to constitute the Federated Dublin Voluntary Hospitals were at the forefront of medical practice in Dublin. The first clinical x-ray in Dublin is likely to have been taken in one of these hospitals, perhaps by Dr W. S. Haughton who installed the first x-ray apparatus in Sir Patrick Dun's in February, 1896, or by Lane Joynt in the Meath Hospital, but optimal development was hindered by the small size of the individual institutions and the division of the radiologists' time between different hospitals.

By the 1960s the largest radiology department within the FDVH was at the Meath where Sholto Douglas is thought to have performed the first peripheral angiogram in Dublin in the early 1950s using a cassette box constructed of wood to his own design. Urological radiology was much advanced under the influence of T. J. D. Lane who had founded the urology service following his return from the Mayo Clinic in the late 1940s. As in all the other Federated Hospitals radiology commenced in the basement, the only place in old hospitals where extra space could be found. In truth, radiology departments never escaped from the basements of these old hospitals before their relocation to new premises.

Assisting Sholto Douglas in the Meath Hospital was Joan McCarthy, whose main commitment was to the National Children's Hospital in Harcourt Street, the oldest continuously functioning children's hospital in Britain or Ireland. In the 1970s, as health investment in Ireland finally picked, up a succession of new radiologists were appointed to these hospitals. G. D. Hurley, who had been a consultant in Nottingham was the first and he was followed by David McInerney returning from Adelaide, South Australia, Samuel Hamilton returning from Vancouver and Eric Colhoun who had completed his training in Cardiff. Following the closure of that portion of the Federation that relocated to St James's, these departments were joined by Noel O'Connell and by John Gately.

Radiologists from Federation Hospitals had been intimately involved in setting up the Faculty of Radiologists in 1961 and subsequently many trainees commenced their training in these hospitals as radiology registrars.

Adequate equipping of the older hospitals was difficult to achieve as the Department of Health preferred to devote its capital to fully equipping newly built hospitals. Consequently it came to pass that the new hospital in Tallaght had at its opening the most up to date radiology department in Ireland when the Meath, the Adelaide and the National Children's Hospital moved out. This new department had the first fully functioning filmless PACS archiving and communication system in the country.

The Royal City of Dublin Hospital in Baggot Street was to the fore in developing cardiac and thoracic radiology throughout the 1950s and 1960s, with the collaboration of the late Keith Shaw, a pioneer in thoracic surgery in Ireland, Gerry Gearty in cardiology and Noel O'Connell in radiology. One of the first cardiac radiology suites in Ireland was installed there.

Noel O'Connell, who went on to become Dean of the Faculty of Radiologists from 1976 to 1978, developed chest radiology extensively. Throughout his professional career Dr O'Connell made a substantial and ongoing commitment to the development of radiology education.

In Sir Patrick Dun's a considerable gastroenterology radiology practice was developed by H. J. R. Henderson, Dr O'Connell and Dr P. Freyne in association with Professor Donald Weir.

Mercer's was the smallest of the Federated Hospitals and was attended by James McNulty. Dr McNulty had a distinguished academic record in the USA and managed to continue his academic output despite the limitations of his facilities in Dublin. He went on to publish *Radiology of the Liver* in the 1970s, while a radiologist in the Federation, and this has remained a popular reference book since.

Dr Steevens' had a considerable orthopaedic and trauma practice. The first purpose-built A&E department was constructed there under the influence of J. B. Prendiville. James McNulty, P. Lorregan and D. McInerney attended Dr Steevens'. This hospital was the oldest structure within the Federation and was purchased, after its closure, by the Health Board and restored to its original early 18th-century splendour.

The Adelaide in Peter Street was attended by H. J. R. Henderson and D. McInerney. General and vascular surgery was of particular interest in the Adelaide and Dr Henderson performed peripheral angiograms at an early stage using an unusual method. In order to ensure that the single cassettes which he used could be exposed at the proper moment following injection of contrast medium which was injected using a translumbar needle a Geiger counter was placed adjacent to the patient's knees. This was connected to a gramophone sound box which was provided by a Dublin electrical company. When the injected contrast medium containing the isotope reached the patient's knees it activated the Geiger counter which became loudly audible in the angiogram room through the gramophone. At this point the single 17 x 14 inch cassette was exposed. This distinctive method led to surprisingly good results for the time.

It was clear by the late 1970s that physical limitation would prevent the Federated Hospitals from ever becoming significant players in radiology. For this reason the Federation radiologists welcomed the move to substantial new premises in the new hospitals at St James's and Tallaght though they still look back with some regret on the distinctive features of the old hospitals where so many elements of traditional medical practice had been retained up to the very end.

34. Renal medicine

Brian Keogh

While Richard Bright in the 19th century left an indelible mark on our understanding of glomerulonephritis and proteinura (the latter terms formerly lumped together as Bright's Disease), this condition is now the commonest cause of renal failure in the western world. At the same time as Bright was attempting to associate glomerulonephritis with proteinura, Jonathan Osborne graduated MB in Dublin University in 1818 and lectured at Trinity in materia medica. He lectured at Park Street Medical School in 1825 and subsequently at the University School of Physic. During his early career he became interested in the examination of urine; his first publication on that subject being a sketch on the physiology and pathology of the urine.

Together with William Charles Wells of St Thomas's Hospital, London and John Blackall of Exeter, his name was indeed linked with that of Richard Bright, who demonstrated in his reports of medical cases in 1827 the association of dropsy with renal disease and the distinction between cardiac and renal dropsy. Jonathan Osborne's book *On the Dropsies connected with Perspiration and Coagulable Urine* was published in 1835. He noted the condition in the introduction to his treatise 'which I do not hesitate to call renal dropsy and acknowledge the pioneer work of Bright'.

On first reading Bright's communication he stated: 'I was quite unprepared to admit its correctness and I have become a convert to his opinion only by virtue of a long series of observations, many of which were instituted in the cause of overthrowing it'. It is interesting that these observations were made in Sir Patrick Dun's.

The frontispiece of his book is a colour presentation of a sectioned kidney in advanced disease: 'The yellow/grey granular mass impermeable to injection is seen filling up the cortical portion of the kidney while the tubular portion has become contracted, insulated and more or less indistinct towards their papillary extremities'. The above history is beautifully outlined in J. D. H. Widdess' *History of the Royal College of Physicians of Ireland 1654–1963*.

It can be appreciated that although the first renal physician in the Federated Hospitals was Jonathan Osborne (1794–1864) the role of the renal physician only became established in a more formalised way in the 1960s, particularly in the Federated Hospitals and the Trinity medical school where Professor Gatenby showed the importance of the specialties within the discipline of medicine: namely gastroenterology, cardiology, endocrinology and nephrology.

At the Meath, which preceded St James's as a home of the clinical medical school, Eddie Bourke developed renal medicine following his appointment in 1969 as a lecturer in medicine and nephrology. He stimulated considerable research at the time, particularly in conjunction with the biochemistry department of Trinity College Dublin.

It must be remembered that during that period the centre for dialysis was, in fact, Jervis Street which considered itself the national renal unit, both for dialysis and transplantation. In the 1970s, Jervis Street was certainly very much supported by the Department of Health and the question of centralising dialysis there was part of the formal agenda. In 1974 Eddie Bourke ordered the first dialysis machines for the Meath, which brought about considerable controversy, as there was no funding whatever for these machines. Much consternation occurred with this development, particularly within the now growing specialty of renal medicine in Dublin. Eddie Bourke resigned in 1977 and I replaced him as consultant renal physician and expanded the services over the following years. This indeed was a very difficult experience, given the lack of support from the Department of Health. Fortunately, dialysis machines were acquired by a number of charitable donations. The unit was well supported thanks to the foresight of John Colfer and his administration at the time. It is interesting in retrospect how, in fact, the unit survived by providing a service for the Eastern Health Board fulfilling the needs for dialysis on the south side.

There was continuous expansion of dialysis throughout the 1960s and 1970s to cope with the increased demand. In the late 1970s the Meath Hospital continued to expand and to provide dialysis for the south side of Dublin. An important development was introduced at the Meath in 1979— continuous ambulatory peritoneal dialysis (CAPD). This form of treatment is complementary to haemodialysis. The renal unit at the Meath was the first to introduce this new therapy in these islands. This therapy is now widely accepted both in Europe and in the USA as an important form of complementary treatment for patients with end stage renal disease. Some 60 patients yearly are treated by this particular technique; it has been most successful in improving the quality of life of patients, with, in particular, a very low infection rate and excellent patient survival. This achievement is accepted internationally.

While the expansion of the unit continued, space was a major problem and in 1987 a modern renal unit was built for the Meath as an extension of West Wing II. This development was opened in 1987 by the Minister for Health at the time, Rory O'Hanlon. The building cost approximately £500,000. A grant of £300,000 was given by the Department of Health and the rest was contributed privately by Mr Louis Cohen who made a major donation towards the cost of the new building in memory of his brother Israel who died in the hospital in 1977. The Meath Hospital Board also made a major contribution to this development.

With the new building in place, it is interesting that the renal unit continued to expand with the numbers increasing by approximately 14 per cent per year.

In 1998 the unit moved to Tallaght, to a new site where there were 14 stations, which included two isolation rooms. At the time of the development of Tallaght this was generally considered to be a major increase but regrettably it was not large enough to cope with the problems now faced, in the year 2005. The unit is now full and over 90 patients are on long term dialysis and still 70 patients continue on CAPD. The unit continues to expand and the present plan is for the expansion into a stand alone station unit to cater for the growing population in the Tallaght area. Given that there are now over 550,000 people in the area, it is critical that the unit expand to meet future needs.

The renal unit at Tallaght has very close links with the hospitals at Naas, Tullamore, Mullingar and Kilkenny. It will have a very considerable role in the future in providing the necessary dialysis for the expanding population of patients with end stage renal disease. It is envisaged that over the next five to ten years, the requirements for dialysis will increase by 10–14 per cent per annum; hence the need to plan for the future.

In discussing the role of the renal unit in Tallaght we must reflect back on the remarkable work carried out by Jonathan Osborne in Sir Patrick Dun's in the 19th century. It is fitting that the renal unit in Tallaght should be named after him. While the philosophy of Jonathan Osborne continues at Tallaght Hospital, clinical research will remain an integral part of the development of the unit in the future. A further increase in consultant numbers together with proposed private/public partnership of dialysis expansion will provide a major stimulus to our future development.

35. *Urology*

Michael Butler

Urology is the oldest branch of surgery, and dates back to prehistoric times. The incentive for the development of this venerable surgical craft was the high incidence of bladder stones and outlet obstruction. The oldest recorded bladder calculus is dated from 4800 BC. In the 5th century BC Hippocrates wrote a treatise on bladder stones, and described accurately the operation of lithotomy. He cautioned 'not to cut for stone without the requisite skills, training and experience in the procedure'. It is interesting to note that his concerns are reflected today in the context of modern surgical practice based on a foundation of formal structured training programmes. The warning against surgical procedures carried out by the untrained and untutored is equally relevant today. The concept of a properly trained surgeon underpins much of the activity that we now take for granted in our modern hospital setting.

Two conditions led to the development of urology surgery—urinary obstructions and bladder stones. In the case of stone disease those afflicted sought relief from pain from any quarter that held out any prospect of success. The condition at that time was so prevalent that it was inevitable that invention of a surgical procedure would provoke ingenuity on the part of surgeons involved in its management. Cutting for stone through the perineum was practised from prehistoric times by ancient Hindus, Arabs, Greeks and Romans. The most famous lithotomist in Europe was Jacques Beaulieu, better known as the Frère Jacques. He was born in Burgundy in 1650. He wandered around Europe as an indigent lithotomist, and when he died in 1714 he was credited with 3,500 stone operations. The surgery was associated with a high morbidity and mortality and this inevitably led to an attempt to remove stones endoscopically by fragmentation. Surgeons applied themselves with increasing ingenuity and sophistication to this problem.

Sir Philip Crampton, a surgeon at the Meath, made a major contribution by inventing a vacuum bottle to extract the stone fragments. The concept of evacuation of the stone fragments was fundamental, but prior to the introduction of rubber it was not possible to devise an effective evacuator. It fell to Bigelow of Boston to introduce a working glass evacuator activated by a powerful rubber bulb in 1870 and the problem was solved.

The operation of lithotomy was placed on a sound scientific footing by the great French surgeon Calot who studied the surgical anatomy of the perineum in cadavers, and applied his findings to improving the surgical technique of lithotomy. Sir William Dease introduced the operation to Dublin, and achieved excellent results with a mortality of four patients from 88 operations. William Dease was appointed to the Meath in 1793, and was the first surgeon to have a specialist interest in urological conditions there. It is interesting to observe his zeal to collect and publish his analysed results; this is the first instance of surgical audit, which was to become such an important feature of the department of urology at the Meath.

The work of two distinguished Irish surgeons in the management of prostatic enlargement is well documented. The contributions of Peter Freyer and Terence Millin have been well described. Freyer, following on the work of Eugene Fuller, in New York performed his transvesical prostatectomy in 1901. Freyer was blessed with superb surgical skills which enabled him to successfully undertake prostatectomy on all comers. This was of singular importance as five of six patients with prostatic disease were afflicted with significant co-morbidity that rendered them high-risk patients. Freyer popularised the transvesical method and justified the procedure by regular publication of convincing results.[1] Despite the advantages of the transvesical approach it is an awkward procedure with limited visualisation of the prostate cavity after enucleation of the gland. Control of bleeding can be difficult.

Terence Millin, born in County Down and Trinity educated, popularised the retropubic approach to the prostate.[2] The major advantage of the technique is excellent visualisation of the prostatic cavity, which expedited control of bleeding. The technique of retropubic prostatectomy, known as a Millin prostatectomy, rapidly achieved popularity. It is an operation that is easy to learn and easy to do. It came at an appropriate time after the Second World War when so many young surgeons were discharged into civilian life after six long years devoted to military surgery. The surgical environment of the time was ready made for an elegant and relatively simple procedure that could be attained with a limited amount of training.

Despite these important advances in open prostatectomy accomplished with lower mortality rates, it was apparent that better results with less morbidity were being obtained in the United States by transurethral endoscopic procedures. Mortality rates of less than 1 per cent were regularly achieved in dedicated institutions such as the Mayo Clinic in the 1930s. The Meath urological department owes its existence to the achievement of these extraordinary results.

T. J. D. Lane was appointed to the Meath in 1928 and had a diverse medical career as pathologist, radiologist, and surgeon. Early in his surgical career he developed a particular interest in urological problems, and was greatly impressed by the published results of prostatic surgery emanating from the United States.

Following close study of the results from the USA he clearly comprehended the importance of sub specialisation. He outlined his advocacy of specialisation on the occasion of the authorisation by the Minister for Health of plans for the development of a specialised urological department at the Meath. In a letter to Dermot O'Flynn, (later his assistant) dated 25 October 1951, he referred to his paper on specialisation indicating 'I have been preaching the doctrine for years'. He highlighted the consequence of lack of specialisation in urology. He went on to say that 'less than 20 years ago the mortality for the operation of prostatectomy at the Meath was 20 per cent—a truly terrible figure'. This figure compared reasonably well with the London general hospitals, but was twice as high as the figure reported from the specialised unit at St Peter's in that city (where Millin was established). It seemed right and proper then, that the Irish patient should be given the advantages of specialisation. Lane observed that specialisation demanded for its development and progress plenty of material i.e. patients.

A specialised unit which wins access to hundreds of cases of commoner diseases and to dozens or half dozens of the rarer ones per year gives those who work in it a unique opportunity. While perfection cannot be attained, the very numbers permit a closer approach to it to be reached. The daily or weekly or fortnightly performance of the same or similar task tends, if performed in the proper spirit, to lead to its improved and better performance. The limitation of effort obviously enables more to be learned about a focussed field, both as regards the nature of the diseases within it and the best way to deal with them. Safety measures, impossible to introduce or not worth the while introducing when dealing with only a dozen cases, must be introduced when dealing with a gross, and when introduced yield valuable dividends. Specialised units without a sufficient number of patients are certain to be inefficient and quite possibly dangerous. There is no room for parochialism and provincialism in a matter as vital as this. The question is a national one, highlighted because of the smallness of our population. The matter is a national one affecting not only the patient in the South or the West or any other point of the compass, but patients in certain categories throughout the country. The only patients not seriously affected today are the well-to-do, who thanks to Aer Lingus are within an hour or two or a little more of the big specialised centres in England, Scotland, France and Holland. Poor and less well off are entirely dependent on local services and talent, and it is to them above all that the proper development of specialised services is of first rate and vital importance. This was emphasised as long ago as 1933 in a communication on the subject of specialisation in Ireland read to the Biological Club.

Lane had very strong support for his specialised urological department from many of his colleagues at the Meath Hospital and amongst his surgical friends and colleagues in Dublin and the provinces. He freely acknowledges that it would have been hard to develop the urological department at the Meath had it not been for the fullest support from the Medical Board and the joint committee.

His optimistic expectation for the development of the new genitourinary unit, was dashed by the 'Knights' Escapade' at the Meath.[3] The attempt by the Knights of Columbanus to take over control of the hospital affected all its functions and every member of the staff. In this regard Lane may have been particularly vulnerable. He was a Roman Catholic in a Church of Ireland hospital who stood firm in his support of his Protestant medical colleagues. The consequence of his loyalty to his friends and colleagues was a decision by the new 'stacked' Board to divert funds away from the proposed urological department and redirect them towards a new nurses' home. A letter of 25 November 1950 from Lane to O'Flynn indicates Lane's pessimism. He wrote: 'I know you have been following the Meath Hospital case. I'm afraid all chance of a genitourinary department for me has now gone, and with it the hope I had of having you as my assistant.' However, Lane was a dogged character. He was highly respected and had many international friends. He was able to galvanise their help.

Two distinguished British urologists, David Band of Edinburgh and Walter Galbraith of Glasgow, undertook to write a letter to the Irish government in support of the new genitourinary unit. Galbraith was president of the British Association of Urological Surgeons, and Band was editor of the *British Journal of Urology*. They addressed their unprecedented letter of support to the chairman of the Select Committee Meath Hospital Bill, Dáil Éireann, and to Noel Browne, Minister for Health, the Taoiseach John A. Costello, and to Éamon de Valera, the leader of the opposition. The letter was carefully worded and sensitively written to emphasise the importance of the proposed unit for the country. It highlighted Lane's international reputation, and the standing of the Meath in the worldwide context of urology. The letter concluded that 'any restriction imposed on the development of his urological department would be a disaster to the advancement of urological specialist practice in the English-speaking world'. Concurrently, other attempts to resolve the Meath debacle were being undertaken. In a letter of 10 January 1951 Lane wrote to O'Flynn, Galbraith and Band, 'the last few days have produced a considerable gleam of hope. The Archbishop [John Charles McQuaid] has come down on the side of fair play and justice, and two of my Protestant colleagues who have had three interviews with him have been enormously impressed by his outlook and promptness in moving to our help.'. On 25 January 1951 Dolly Lane kept O'Flynn abreast of further developments. She wrote: 'The Meath Hospital Bill came before the select committee yesterday, and they made good progress in dealing with some 70 amendments. It should be ready for its third reading about Feb 14th, and with luck the *present crowd* should be out by the first of April.'

As anticipated, the Meath Hospital Bill passed through the Oireachtas in March 1951, and was finally signed into law by the President of Ireland on 14 March 1951. With this final settlement of the issue between the Knights and the Meath, the development of the urology department progressed surprisingly quickly. A meeting between Lane and the Minister for Health took place on 8 October 1951 at which the Minister agreed to the demolition of the west wing of the hospital and construction of a genitourinary department of 80 beds. The Minister offered £125,000 for the project, and all associated work to bring it to a successful conclusion. The newly constituted Medical Board agreed the appointment of a urological assistant. Dermot O'Flynn's name was proffered to the Board, and approved by the Minister for Health. Lane then made a formal approach to the Hospitals Commission for an appropriate salary to expedite the new appointment. O'Flynn was officially appointed to the unit in January 1952 and in May of the same year Victor Lane was appointed as a second urological assistant.

These two appointments enabled Tom Lane to concentrate on the important task of planning in detail the proposed unit. The architects Robinson Keefe and Devane were appointed to oversee the design of the new unit. Tom Lane formed a close working relationship with Andrew Devane, and they spent long hours, more often outside of regular office hours, planning the details of the new department. Devane was a hands-on architect, and spent time in the hospital during working hours in an attempt to understand the functional needs of a surgical department. The result was a custom built urological department which was unique in these islands. The contract to build the unit was given to L. M. Byrne and Company, builders. The configuration of the unit was based around 76 beds on 3 landings, with 3 operating theatres and the outpatients on the ground floor. James

Ryan TD and T. F. O'Higgins TD were Health Ministers during the period of planning and construction. The foundation stone was laid by Dr Ryan on 27 January 1954.

Tom Lane was a genuinely humble and self-effacing man, despite a ferocious determination to succeed. Characteristically, the first patients admitted for surgery were children with hypospadias. Professor T. P. Kilner, Nuffield Professor of Plastic Surgery at Oxford, and Eric Peate, both longstanding friends of T. J. D., who had carried out corrective surgery for many years at the unit, were invited to perform the first surgical procedures at the new unit, a unique and generous gesture bestowed on them by Tom Lane.

During Lane's visit to the Mayo Clinic in May 1938 the great American surgeon Gershon Thompson advised that the path to reduced mortality and an important step in developing a urological department was to rely on a team of nurse specialists, looking after patients by day and night. He held that this was fundamental to obtaining world-class results. On his return from Rochester, training this coterie of nurses was one of Tom Lane's first tasks. Sister Betty Cunningham was the first nurse specialist appointed and she had a profound impact on the quality of nursing care at the unit. This is reflected in the superb results achieved for transurethral resection. By the end of 1939 Lane reported on 120 cases with 3 deaths—a mortality of 2½ per cent. Practitioners countrywide appreciated the impact of specialisation, and the urological workload developed so rapidly that within one year the number of specialist genitourinary nurses was increased to 6.

The success of specialised nursing initiated by the Lane/Cunningham team has continued to the present time. The baton has been passed on through the efforts of Sisters Maureen Fallon, Catherine McDaid and Kate Fitzpatrick in the theatres, and through the efforts of Sisters Maura Dunne and Frances Healy in the outpatients, and Sisters Marie Cooney, Annie McNeil, Mary Mangan, Anne Carey, Imelda Joyce and Christine McManus on the wards. These outstanding sisters have had the support over the years of many dedicated nurses too numerous to mention. The unit has also had the support of successive matrons both at the Meath and at Tallaght, from Miss Magee and Betty O'Dwyer.

The tradition of specialised nursing in the department was reaffirmed when in 2002, most appropriately, the current members of the nursing staff at the urological department founded the Irish Urological Nurses' Association which has met on two occasions at Tallaght. The Association embraces nurses engaged in urology in hospitals both north and south of the border. The establishment of the new association is a source of pride to all members of the urological department. The important contribution of nursing at the unit has always been acknowledged. Happily, the tradition has endured through the transfer to Tallaght. The special partnership between urologists and nurses in the unit is perhaps best summed up in the tribute paid to T. J. D. in *The Irish Times* on his death in 1967 by Sister Ann McNeil who was Sister in charge of St Andrew's (one of the wards in the department) for over a decade.

> Mr Lane was an idealist in his profession, untiring in his concern and devotion to his patients and was not influenced by wealth or position. To his staff he was a friend and advisor in times of illness and distress and always someone we respected and admired. At times we may have been hesitant to adapt ourselves to his rigid methods of perfection, but soon we realised the depth of his dedication and it inspired us to copy his example. This city has lost a great surgeon, the patients who have been under his care an irreplaceable doctor, and the nurses 'the loyalty' of their strongest advocate.

T. J. D. Lane retired in the mid 1960s. The workload during this early period had increased enormously. Dermot O'Flynn and Victor Lane were committed not only to the Meath unit, but also had onerous duties in St Kevin's which was shortly to become a major teaching hospital aligned to TCD medical school. There were over 50 urological beds available at St Kevin's. Patients admitted there were transferred for surgery to the Meath. St Kevin's, which was shortly to be renamed St James's, constituted a substantial commitment. Additionally, when the National Rehabilitation Centre was opened at Rochestown Avenue in the early 1960s, Dermot O'Flynn was appointed to provide management of urological problems at the new unit. Expert urological service is of prime importance in the outcome for patients with spinal cord injuries and in children with spina bifida. O'Flynn's many important contributions to spinal cord injuries at Rochestown were acknowledged internationally through his many publications on this difficult and important subject. The genitourinary department provided a paediatric urological service to the National Children's Hospital through the appointment of Victor Lane and later by John Thornhill.

As clearly anticipated by Tom Lane as early as 1932, the volume of patients and urological conditions rendered the genitourinary department fertile ground for the training of young surgeons. The Meath is a founding member of the senior registrar training scheme in urology. The higher surgical training scheme commenced in 1970 and because of the exceptional caseload the unit was given two training posts. While there are four registrar posts currently at the unit, two specialist registrar trainees continue to be recognised by the Higher Surgical Training Committee.

The increased commitment at the Meath, St James's and the Rehabilitation Centre, combined with an increase in time needed to train young surgeons, led to a gradual expansion in consultant staff. In 1974 I was appointed to the staff with duties at the Meath, St James's and the Rehabilitation Centre. This appointment led to further diversification in the workload with new interests in female urology, prosthetic and reconstructive surgery. St James's expanded rapidly in 1979 and a fourth urologist was appointed. Bernard Fallon, who was trained in the US at the University of Iowa, took up an appointment for about 18 months. He returned to the US and was replaced in 1980 by John Fitzpatrick who subsequently left to take up the appointment of Professor of Surgery at UCD in 1986. This was a unique achievement as no previous fulltime urologist had ever been appointed to a full surgical chair. This position is usually occupied by a general surgeon.

The years between 1983 and 1990 were a watershed period for stone disease. The Meath was always a major contributor to the management of this disease. The unit was at the forefront of percutaneous endoscopic surgery, and was involved at an early stage in the progressively developing modern management of ureteric stones by ureteroscopic techniques. In 1986 the Meath acquired the first extracorporeal lithotripter in the country. The machine was financed by the Department of Health and through private donations. The urology department received generous contributions from the AIB and the Jefferson Smurfit Foundation. Concurrent with the upsurge in interest in stone disease, the Irish Stone Foundation was established by Dermot O'Flynn. Initially its main objective was to support research into the cause of stone disease in Ireland but it also played a major role in fundraising for the new lithotripter. Over the years its brief has expanded into support of research in all branches of urology. As a result, research flourished at the unit. Studies were undertaken both in clinical and basic sciences. Many of these studies led to higher degrees, and were important contributors to career pathways for trainees aspiring to a consultancy in urology. The Stone Foundation provided and continues to provide funding to enable young trainees to take one or two years out of clinical duties to work fulltime in a research laboratory. This support is a continuation of a tradition of original research at the genitourinary department and a determination to contribute to the advancement of urological surgery in all its aspects .

Dermot O'Flynn retired in 1986 and John Fitzpatrick took up his new post at the Mater in the same year. Victor Lane retired a few years later. Their replacements, Ted McDermott, Ronnie Grainger and John Thornhill, were all appointed between 1986 and 1990. All new appointees were products of the higher surgical training scheme, and worked as registrars at the Meath. They brought new skills and interests to the unit. McDermott and Grainger each spent a postgraduate fellowship year in Ann Arbor with Edward McGuire studying the problems of female urology, while John Thornhill went to the University of Indiana and studied with John Donohue. Donohue's department at Indiana made fundamental contributions to the management of testicular cancer. Through the skills acquired in Indiana by John Thornhill and brought back to Tallaght the unit is now recognised as a referral centre for the treatment of testis cancer and in particular in the area of surgery for advanced tumours.

Many urology patients admitted for surgery are elderly and frail, and require particular anaesthetic expertise. Over 42 years, anaesthesia at the unit has been provided by a number of superb teams, with members including the late Bertie Wilson, John Cusson, Fergus Quilty and Dr McGrath. More recently an excellent service was provided by Una O'Callaghan, Joe Galvin, Kevin O'Sullivan, B. Brennan and Patricia Delaney. A newer generation of anaesthetists who commenced their consultant careers at the Meath have transferred to the new hospital at Tallaght. The unit is particularly well served by the outstanding team of Mary Stritch, Gerry Fitzpatrick, Con Cooney, Paul Doherty, Catriona O'Sullivan, Sally-Ann Colgan and Marie Donnelly. Apart from service commitments they have made other contributions to the welfare of urological patients. In association with the late Brian Mayne a grading system to assess operative risk was devised some ten odd years ago. It predated ASA scores which are currently in use. Provision of solid data to assess surgical outcomes against risk was a typical innovation of T. J. D. Lane and Dermot O'Flynn. It led to the eventual development of a punch card based data retrieval system which functioned perfectly up to present times. This has only recently been supplanted by a computerised system.

Intense specialisation has led to both co-operation and a reliance on other disciplines, most especially radiology. The genitourinary department has always maintained close co-operation with the department of radiology. Sholto Douglas and Joan McCarthy were held in high regard for their outstanding radiological opinion, but the interaction between x-ray and GU moved onto a different level with the arrival of radiologists with interventional skills. Urological problems lend themselves particularly well to diagnostic and therapeutic interventional radiological solutions. Gerry Hurley, in particular, and more recently William Torregianni, have taken a special interest in providing such a service for the unit. Skilled services

fundamental to a first-class urological service are at the disposal of the surgeons. More importantly the skills of the interventionalist are readily and
cheerfully made available both within and outside regular working hours.
The ease of access to such a service has made an enormous impact on the
effectiveness of the urological department. The radiologists have been supported over the years by all members of the radiology department whom
we would like to acknowledge.

References

[1] Sir Peter Freyer *Clinical Lectures on Enlargement of the Prostate* New York: War
Wood and Co. 1920.
[1] Barry O'Donnell *Terence Millin: A Remarkable Irish Surgeon* Dublin: A. & A.
Farmar 2002.
[3] See P. B. B. Gatenby *Dublin's Meath Hospital* Dublin: Town House 1996.

36. Vascular surgery

Gregor Shanik

The birth of vascular surgery as we know it today occurred in the 1950s. It was pioneered by the great among the vascular surgeons, Dr deBakey in the United States, Dr Kunlin in France and Dr Dos Santos, the father of modern angiography, in Portugal. Irish vascular surgeons, including Professors McGowan, FitzGerald and Kinnear, were the pioneers of peripheral vascular surgery in Ireland. Professor Nigel Kinnear in the late 1950s started the practice of peripheral vascular surgery at the Adelaide. He was one of the first to perform porto-caval shunts for cirrhosis and performed many successful aorto-iliac endarterectomies, bypass grafts for aneurysm and aorto occlusive vascular disease.

Almost simultaneously, Professor William McGowan at the Richmond, William Hederman at the Mater and Professor Patrick FitzGerald at St Vincent's were beginning to sub-specialise in the practice of peripheral vascular surgery. It was the beginning of a new dawn in treatment of peripheral vascular disease with the advent of the Fogarty balloon embolectomy catheter, Dacron grafts for aneurysm and peripheral bypass surgery and the use of reversed vein bypasses for femoro-popliteal occlusive disease. Cardiac surgery as we know it today was in its infancy at that time and pioneers such as Keith Shaw in Baggot Street and Professor Eoin O'Malley at the Mater were busy in the animal laboratories perfecting coronary artery valve techniques which would soon revolutionise the treatment of heart disease.

Professor George Fegan began his research into venous disease and the treatment of varicose veins and venous ulceration in the late 1950s at Sir Patrick Dun's. He was responsible for a revolution in the treatment of varicose veins and venous ulceration using injection sclerotherapy with compression. He was, and is today, recognised as one of the founding fathers of compression injection sclerotherapy and the technique has been used worldwide since his original treatise on the subject in the *British Journal of Surgery* in the early 1960s.

He also carried out numerous in-depth research projects including autologous valve transplantation which was initiated by Robert Quill, consultant surgeon to the Federation and St James's.

Household names within the Federation such as Michael Pegum, Bill Beesley and James Milliken, to name but a few, were part of the research team at Sir Patrick Dun's and many papers emanated from this group and were read at such prestigious societies as the Surgical Research Society of Great Britain and Ireland.

The practice of vascular surgery in the Adelaide, Meath, Sir Patrick Dun's and Baggot Street continued until the retirement of Professor Nigel Kinnear in the mid 1970s. J. C. Milliken took up the mantle of vascular surgeon at Sir Patrick Dun's and Baggot Street in the 1960s. He was one of the second generation of vascular surgeons in Ireland and continued his practice of venous surgery, peripheral vascular surgery and aneurysm surgery at both hospitals. He pioneered many new techniques such as gas endarterectomy of the superficial femoral arteries and carotid artery surgery which remained controversial at that time.

With the closure of five of the Federated Hospitals and their move, along with the Trinity medical school, to St James's a change occurred within the development of peripheral vascular surgery. I was appointed to Trinity working at St James's and the Federated Hospitals as a vascular surgeon. This was the beginning of a department of vascular surgery centred at St James's. With the closure of Sir Patrick Dun's and Baggot Street the vast majority of the venous centre was moved to St James's under the direction of J. C. Milliken. In the mid 1980s Dermot Moore was appointed as a third vascular surgeon and he continued to perform vascular surgery at Baggot Street until its closure.

A non-invasive vascular laboratory was opened in order to triage patients with peripheral vascular and carotid disease without resorting to invasive angiography. This was run by Wiley Kingston who was succeeded by Mary Paula Colgan who today oversees the running of two vascular laboratories and the centre of venous disease. Newly acquired techniques were implemented such as tibial bypass and the routine performance of both aneurysm and carotid surgery. Martin Feeley was appointed as a vascular surgeon in the late 1980s to the Adelaide and Meath. This was necessitated by the rapid increase in the number of elderly patients requiring surgery for the prevention of stroke, ruptured aneurysm and critical ischaemia of the lower limbs.

Vascular surgery changed direction in the early 1990s with the introduction of minimally invasive techniques closely allied to interventional radiology. Today, almost 50 per cent, if not more, of all operations in vascular surgery are performed using endovascular techniques and a new endovascular theatre has been opened at St James's to cope with the increasing demand. The procedures carried out include stenting for carotid artery stenosis, repair of ruptured aneurysms using stent grafts introduced from the groin and sub-intimal angioplasty of the femoral and tibial vessels using guidewire techniques.

The field of endovascular intervention is rapidly expanding in the same way as coronary artery angioplasty and the number of open operations will gradually diminish because of it.

The future of vascular surgery originally commenced by the pioneers in the Federated Hospitals is now secure in the sister hospitals of St James's and the AMNCH group. Currently five vascular surgeons between the two hospitals deliver a service to the Midlands, Kildare, Tallaght and Dublin city centre. With the advent of surgeons specializing solely in the field of peripheral vascular surgery such as Martin Feeley, Dermot Moore, Prakash Madhavan and Sean Tierney, the future of vascular surgery remains bright.

Postscript

David FitzPatrick

It is hoped that the reader will have built up, from the various accounts provided in this book, a concept of the voluntary tradition of the Federated Dublin Voluntary Hospitals and how they have melded their individual cultures when joining together in the two new institutions and since 1961 have contributed to the development of various specialties in Dublin, Ireland and indeed further afield.

Inevitably some details and accounts of developments in some specialised areas have been omitted for which I must apologise, as I must also do for any errors or other omissions—*mea culpa*.

We must now look to the future—the voluntary tradition, to which I make no apology for referring again, is I believe in safe hands in each of the new hospitals in which the Federated ones have been reincarnated. I often think that while there undoubtedly are continuing problems with regard to planning, development, staffing and finance they are no greater now than those which would have assailed the base hospitals had they remained on their sites in central Dublin. The difficulties now are different and probably less as the new hospitals are less affected by structural and design problems. It should be emphasised and I hope has become apparent that falling over backwards to accommodate the Department of Health and Children is not always the best policy and that verbal commitments from the Department are often worth only the paper they are not written upon, or less!

It is a tribute to all involved in AMNCH and St James's that everyone now identifies with the new institutions and few if any look back with regret at the 'Elysian fields' whence they emerged. The base hospitals have not totally disappeared and funds from all of them have been used in the new developments. Most of those from Steevens', Dun's, Baggot Street and Mercer's have been applied to projects in St James's but, as its name implies, AMNCH retains the support of its three parent bodies through the Meath Hospital Foundation, the National Children's Hospital Company and the Adelaide Hospital Society. These three also retain influence by nominating members of the AMNCH hospital board.

It is not possible to conclude without mention of St Loman's Hospital which was incorporated into the new AMNCH hospital shortly after it opened. This book has been devoted to the hospitals which formed the Federation and as such the broad development of psychiatric services has not been addressed, though indeed discussion of the provision of psychiatric services within the Federation is one of the deficiencies in the book which I regret.

If this collection of papers has enabled the reader to recognise the difficulties involved in the transfer of the base hospitals and the medical contributions made by their staffs in the past 45 years, during times of extreme financial constraint, then my purpose will have been well served.

Why did Edward Worth (1678–1733) leave his books to Dr Steevens' Hospital?

W. J. Mc Cormack

The collection comprising the Edward Worth library is made up of some 4,500 volumes, the earliest dating from 1475. Most are sumptuously bound in decorated leather or vellum. Approximately one third of the collection is made up of medical and related scientific works, with classics, history, literature, philosophy, reference, and travel accounting for much of the remainder. Though the collection contains a small number of books which Worth inherited from his father (the Revd John Worth, 1648–88, sometime dean of Saint Patrick's Cathedral), the greatest number of books were bought by Edward Worth himself. Born in Dublin, educated in Oxford and the Netherlands, holding degrees from three universities, Worth remains an enigma—and not least of the puzzle lies in why he left his magnificent library to Dr Steevens' hospital in the first place.

The hospital was founded by Griselda Steevens, using money left to her by her brother Richard for that purpose. Commenced in 1717 it finally opened its doors to patients in 1733, a few months after Edward Worth's death. Some two hundred and seventy-odd years later, the room designed to house the collection remains the only part of Thomas Burgh's structure which continues to fulfil its originally intended function. Electrical, fire-retardant and security systems apart, it continues largely unaltered since the completion of work. Visitors often express delight and surprise at the Library's cosiness as well as its eighteenth-century severe elegance. Touching detail about the craftsmen employed in building the book-shelves has survived, while larger questions about their purpose and location remain to puzzle us.[1] The presence in 1733 of 4,500 valuable books in an unfinished hospital building is almost as inexplicable as their happy survival.

Materials for a solution to the puzzle are scant or at least scattered beyond immediate view. What's more (or less), the Worth family is little known, beyond the holding of this ecclesiastical office or that legal one. Edward

Worth's last will and testament, of which we have only some copied portions, was emphatic on intention—but largely silent on motivation. Why was Worth's collection of magnificently preserved books assigned to the hospital planned by Richard Steevens and accomplished by his sister? The expedition with which they were—literally—carted from Worth's town house to the first floor of the new building on the Liffey banks indicates that no risk of any other outcome was tolerated. Once vellum and incunabula, sprinkled calf and gold-embossment were safe under Griselda Steevens' unblinking gaze, the boxes remained undisturbed for a number of years. A surviving example of these original boxes—we believe—has been identified in the last few months, and retrieved from the cellars of the hospital.

A newspaper announcement of the removal from Werburgh Street to the hospital suggests that Worth's library was not wholly a secret in Georgian Dublin.[2] In Trinity College and in Marsh's Library (built 1701, regulated by statute 1707) envious eyebrows must have been raised. It is true that Burgh's great library building for the College was not completed until 1732—two years after Burgh's death—and thus unavailable to Worth when he first composed his will in November 1723. But less than ten years later, it stood pristine and spaciously welcoming. The contrast with the muddy building site up-river could hardly have been more obvious.

Throughout the little known of Edward Worth's career in Ireland, links with the Steevens family constitute a rare instance of positive association. The body established by Griselda Steevens in 1717 to secure a site for the hospital and initiate works included Worth among the fifteen trustees. When, in 1729/30, the Irish parliament legislated to authorise the establishment of Steevens' Hospital, Worth's name again appeared as a foundational governor. Despite an uncle who served as a junior baron of exchequer—and he had died in 1721—Worth had little direct political experience. It was not he, but a namesake and nephew, who had sat in the Commons for New Ross in the parliaments of 1715-27.[3] In the absence of fuller evidence, it seems reasonable therefore to suppose that this appointment was not a political job, but that he was nominated as a governor at Griselda Steevens' behest. The preparation of a bill for the purposes of establishing the hospital broadly coincides with the time at which Worth was modifying his will by codicil (November 1729), modifications which refine and reinforce his determination to leave books to the hospital by specifying more clearly what books were destined to go there.

Nevertheless, friendship with the Steevens family can hardly provide a complete rationale of the decision. If, as the late Vincent Kinane concluded, Worth was seriously ill throughout much of his last decade, he cannot have been assured that the hospital would be ready at the moment of his will's execution. And indeed, it wasn't—though only by a matter of a few months. Long engagement in Miss Steevens' project did not necessarily imply a commitment of the books to her public role, any more than friendship precluded the bequeathing of the books privately.

In this nexus, with the emergent medical profession at its centre, the College of Physicians is conspicuously unmentioned. After his return from the Netherlands in 1701 or 1702, Worth had submitted his name for election to the college; once elected, he then refused to serve as President and indeed was repeatedly fined for dereliction of duty as a Fellow. Early in the 18th century, the Physicians had no collegiate real estate of their own; they met in the home of Sir Patrick Dun's widow—much to her annoyance—and had particular difficulty in housing the books which constituted the nucleus of their library. One way or another, when making his original will, Worth had been unlikely to offer up his fine bindings to the care of a body with which he had feuded and which had little experience in the business of minding books.[4]

If experience was to be the yard-stick, then Trinity College had more than a century's advantage over any rival. The new Library stood proud of the flood-prone quad, raised upon a colonnade into which delivery carts were to be drawn by horses. When the gaffer at Dr Steevens' Hospital took delivery of Worth's books, he committed them to the first floor (north-east corner), where no chamber was yet prepared but where they would be impervious to damp or a surge on the nearby Camac as it debouched into the tidal Liffey. In imitation of the raised long room in the college, or simply following common sense, those in charge of completing the hospital wards provided a first-rate, if extremely isolated, environment for the books. To the east, the new hospital faced into woodland; to the south lay its extensive grounds in which eventually St Patrick's Hospital would stand by the decree of another enigmatic Dubliner; well westward stood the Royal Hospital, home to the veterans of war and conquest, while the Liffey threatened to slop its natural banks on to Griselda's northern doorstep.

Would not the 20 incunabula be safer in Trinity, where scholars might more readily have access to them, not to mention Aldine printings, rare Calderon piracies, and lavish bindings? Worth cannot have been unaware of the financial implications of his bequest, for he had spent very large sums of money in assembling a collection made all the more valuable through commissioned bindings and by the simple fact of its being an individual connoisseur's achievement. In measuring the benefit to Dr Steevens' Hospital, as opposed to Trinity College, one should not neglect the possibility that the donor intended to provide a capital asset, a bulwark against hard times, for an institution embarking on the largely untried provision of surgical and medical treatment to the curable poor in Dublin. Trinity, by vulgar comparison, lay swaddled in ermine.

There is no reason to believe Worth a social reformer *avant la lettre* or even a philanthropist, though Griselda Steevens undoubtedly earned the latter title. Worth's full-length portrait, once more unrivalled by images of other worthies, now dominates his library, showing him accoutred in red robes of the day, sitting nervously forward. When he had returned from acquiring medical qualifications in the Low Countries, he had petitioned not only the College of Physicians, but also Trinity College, for professional certification. No less a person than the University Chancellor, James Butler, the 2nd duke of Ormonde, approved the award of an MD degree in 1702. This high level of patronage may reflect at once an element of opposition within the college and a relationship between Worth's family and the duke. William Worth, the collector's uncle, had held an appointment on the Ormonde estates from which he had been dismissed on the familiar grounds of absorbing portions of an income supposedly nurtured for his employer. The duke, in turn, had been impeached for treason in 1715 as part of the great assault on Toryism. By 1723 he was living in exile and official disgrace, having been replaced at the top of the University of Dublin by the Prince of Wales (later George II).

Accepting the genealogy upon which T. P. C. Kirkpatrick (in 1924) and James Kelly (in 2004) are broadly agreed, we find the Worth family to have been a rum lot politically.[5] As dean of Cork, the Revd Edward Worth (died 1669) devised ecclesiastical arrangements acceptable to Henry Cromwell during the Commonwealth, yet managed to acquire a bishopric at the Restoration. His son, William (the 3rd baron of exchequer referred to already), had something of a reputation as a Tory while falling out with the arch-Tory, Ormonde. The bishop's other son, John (father of the book collector), seems to have owned some books of a very specifically Catholic and Jesuit kind, despite being dean of St Patrick's Cathedral at the time of his death (1688).[6] Though very little can be established about Edward the Collector's private views, suspicions of atheism, foppism, and Toryism cling to this product of the new Dutch medical schools.

Perhaps the most remarkable evasion accomplished by Worth in disposing of his books was that of by-passing the public library established by Narcissus Marsh (1638–1713) in 1701. Protected by an act of the Irish parliament in 1707, what became known simply as Marsh's Library stood (indeed still stands) beside the cathedral of which Worth's father had been dean. With the Huguenot refugee Elias Bouhéreau as its first librarian, Marsh's was the meeting point of several important collections of books within which Worth's no less remarkable collection could have found a secure and established home. However, links between Marsh's and the cathedral, likewise links between Marsh's and Trinity College, may not have enhanced its attractions in the testator's eyes.

Opposition to the legislation promoted by William King, archbishop of Dublin, for the legal protection of Marsh's Library cannot have escaped the memory of the distinguished Dubliners seeking a similar act to establish Dr Steevens's Hospital in 1729, especially with respect to Worth's intention to leave his books to the emergent institution.[7] The prolonged effort of commencing (in 1717), sustaining and completing (in 1733) the building up-river doubtless reflected delays and frustrations of various kinds, but it also provided a long period of reflection in which Edward Worth was able to assess, and re-assess, the advisability of leaving his books to the hospital. Indeed, during the period, and especially in the years after his uncle's death in 1721, the number of books grew impressively. Between the first signing of his will, and the making of a codicil, Worth would have witnessed progress of Burgh's two buildings—the library in Trinity College and the hospital for Griselda Steevens. From July 1717 onwards, he had been a trustee in relation to the latter project. Personal involvement in the origins of Dr Steevens' Hospital should be acknowledged as a major factor in the decision to leave the books to it, whatever the merits and reputation of Dublin's other libraries and professional/learned societies.

Commentary on the style of building which resulted in Dr Steevens' Hospital provides a parallel for discussion of Worth's motivation in choosing it as a home for his legacy. The role of Thomas Burgh is obvious, providing a guarantee (so to speak) of concern for an environment in which books would be conserved.[8] Ironically, conditions in the Worth Library turned out to be far superior to those in the Long Room where 'great windows opening to the south' admitted highly damaging light and heat. Dutch influence has also been noted in the austerity of the Steevens building and even in the provisions for the library; here Worth's professional training in Leiden and Utrecht is relevant. But Dutch influence might be regarded as Williamite or Whiggish allegiance, in which context the 18th-century Worths strike ambiguous poses.

If one suspends considerations of Worth's motives for a moment, to revisit issues of intention, some welcome clarity may emerge. Worth did not intend a public library of the kind initiated for Ireland by Narcissus Marsh and later augmented by Richard Robinson in Armagh. His will stipulated that his books were to be available to the physician, surgeon and chaplain of Dr Steevens' Hospital. No doubt this decidedly exclusive statement was never intended literally to admit only three readers: at variance with it was another provision of the will whereby copies of the Worth Library's catalogue were to be placed in Marsh's Library and in the College Library, presumably for consultation by potential readers. But the exclusive statement does indicate that Worth saw his bequest to the hospital as constituting something more active than a mere capital asset.

That said, the condition of the books today does not suggest assiduous study of them by the salaried officers of Dr Steevens' foundation. In practice, if not in conscious principle, successive trios of approved readers would seem to have recognised that Worth chose and acquired items as a connoisseur rather than as a medical practitioner or humanistic scholar, and they left the books in the state they—successively—gained access to them. Only Bryan Robinson (a governor of the hospital under the Act, died 1754) introduced into the collection evidence of his own understanding of it.[9]

With mention of Robinson's name, one encounters the first possibility of an ideological purpose behind the establishment and maintenance of the Worth Library. A notable Dublin physician, Robinson devoted much time to the application of Newtonian science to the practice of medicine, specifically with reference to the problem of measuring the speed at which blood circulated in the human body. A copy of his *Dissertation on the Aether of Sir Isaac Newton* was deposited in the Worth Library in 1743, being one of the very few items added after the books were moved to the hospital. Robinson also edited Richard Helsham's *Lectures on Natural Philosophy* (1739) which served as a standard medical textbook in the Trinity medical schools for many years. Both men were followers of Isaac Newton (1642–1727).[10] Less immediately relevant to the issue of discerning an intellectual or ideological consistency behind the glass-fronted bookcases is the preservation of nine volumes of plays by the Spanish dramatist, Calderon de la Barca (1600–81) in rare and textually important pirated editions. These distinctly non-medical books bear the owner-signature of John Conduitt (1688–1737), a relative of Newton's by marriage and a major source of information on the great man's early life.

It is tempting to consider that Edward Worth envisaged his library as constituting a kind of ideological underpinning of the several important new institutions which had been built in the same area west of Dublin— the Royal Hospital at Kilmainham, the Royal Barracks (now the National Museum at Collins Barracks) across the river, and the magazine fort to the west in Phoenix Park. Certainly no other collection—apart from Marsh's, closer to town—existed to fulfil any such role. However, the eclectic subject matter of Worth's Library, the attention paid to the condition and appearance of books rather than simply their content, and the inclusion of early printing evidently for its own sake, would argue against any such purposefulness. More particularly, the absence of *Principia Mathematica* in its first (1687) edition might be thought damaging to any view of the collection as reflecting a determined Newtonian construction. There are, of course, other kinds of inflection to be discerned in the range of books making up the Worth Library—for example, the relatively low number of Irish printings, or the almost complete exclusion of manuscripts.

Finally, one can return to look once again at the physical lay-out of the accommodation made available for the books in the 1730s. Unlike Marsh's Library, the arrangement is not based on the Oxford collegiate model, nor on the new large-chamber built by Burgh in Trinity College, Dublin. With their glazed doors, the bookcases in Dr Steevens' Hospital line a room distinguished also by its fine fireplace and Corinthian columns at the north end. For centuries, this served as a boardroom for the hospital's governors; when not filling that role, it had an informal, even clubbish appearance. The number of books requiring shelf-space in the 1730s obliged the carpenters to devise an asymmetrical solution here or there, a free-standing press or two and, in one area, a somewhat desperate insertion of narrow shelves made from inferior timber. All in all, the Worth Library manifested the gentlemanly enthusiasm of a practising scientist whose known views or associations were not clear-cut. When Edward Worth died, the books he had collected were housed in the hospital of which he had agreed to be a governor, and despite a hiccough in our own time have been there ever since. The firm intention of the benefactor to bequeath his books to the hospital, and to have them preserved there, was clearly visible, and this intention was confirmed by Mr Justice Keane at the time of the High Court proceedings (concluded June 1993).[11] As to motivation, we must wait until Edward Worth finds his Boswell or his Borges.

References

[1] T. P. C. Kirkpatrick *The History of Doctor Steevens' Hospital, Dublin, 1720–1920* Dublin: printed at the University Press, 1924. pp. 62–3.

[2] See *Dublin Weekly Journal* 12 May 1733.

[3] Pending further enquiries, I do not fully accept the account given in Edith Mary Johnston Liik, *History of the Irish Parliament 1692–1800; Commons, Constituencies and Statutes* Belfast: Ulster Historical Association, 2002. vol 4 pp. 557–8.

[4] See J. D. H. Widdess, *A History of the Royal College of Physicians of Ireland 1654–1963* Edinbugh: Livingstone, 1963.

[5] See Kirkpatrick p 58; James Kelly, *Sir Edward Newenham MP, 1734–1814; Defender of the Protestant Constitution.* Dublin: Four Courts, 2004. p. 299. It should be noted that the details in Johnston Liik, and the general implication of Toby Barnard's entry on Edward Worth, bishop of Killaloe, in the new DNB, do not concur.

[6] About 170 books once the property of John Worth can be found in the Edward Worth Library; other books bearing his signature are preserved in the Library, TCD.

[7] See David Hayton, 'Opposition to the Statutory Establishment of Marsh's Library in 1707; a Case Study in Irish Ecclesiastical Politics in the Reign of Queen Anne' in Muriel McCarthy and Ann Simmons (eds), *The Making of Marsh's Library: Learning, Politics and Religion in Ireland, 1650–1750.* Dublin: Four Courts, 2004. pp. 163–86.

[8] For a succinct account, see Christine Casey, *Dublin [The Buildings of Ireland series].* New Haven, London: Yale University Press, 2005. pp. 681–4.

[9] In 1733, the first holders of these designated officers were Brian (or Bryan) Robinson (c. 1680–1754), physician; John Nichols (died 1767), surgeon; and Revd. Peter Cooke (c.1700–87), chaplain. Nichols held office until 1756, Cooke until 1787. The office of physician changed hands more often, with Robinson succeeded in 1734 by Richard Helsham (1683–1738) only to return for two subsequent periods. It appears that two men may have jointly held the post of physician in the early years.

Index

abortion referendum, 69
Abraham, Johnson, 79
Abrahamson, Professor Leonard, 112
Adams, Robert, 126
Adelaide and Meath Hospital, Dublin
  Incorporating the National Children's
  Hospital (AMNCH), 1, 3, 15, 26, 29, 32, 60,
  82, 91, 144, 153, 173, 179–80, 181, 216, 222,
  301, 303
  A&E, 3
  architecture, 56–7, 93
  board, structure of, 59, 99–100
  Charter, 44–51, 75–8, 94–7, 98–100, 100–4,
    170, 207
  formation of, 43–51
  management structures, 59, 67–8, 76–7,
    93–4, 104
  medical science faculty, 95–6
  nursing services, 241, 242, 243–4
  opened, 105
  plans for, 58–9, 59–60, 60–1, 169–70
  size of, 56, 57–8
  specialties
    anaesthesia, 155
    cardiology, 168
    clinical medicine, 175, 179–80
    dermatology, 194
    endocrinology, 195, 199–201
    gastroenterology, 205–7, 208
    geriatric care, 145, 146–50
    haematology, 227, 232
    microbiology, 181, 183, 186–7
    orthopaedics, 258, 259, 279
    otorhinolaryngology, 260, 261, 262
    paediatrics, 268, 270, 271
    pathology, 265, 266
    radiology, 284, 285
    renal medicine, 288
    surgery, 216
    urology, 294–5, 297
  teaching agreement, 61, 100
  transfers to, 124–5, 127, 217
  uniforms, 188
Adelaide Hospital, 2, 19, 20, 111, 116, 126, 127,
  136, 139, 178
  changes, 21

in FDVH, 14, 114, 211
financial pressures, 69–72, 74–6, 197–8
history of, 65–78
Kingston Group, 72–4
nursing, 242–3, 251–2
size of, 151
specialties, 172
  cardiac services, 160, 164
  cardiology, 166, 167–8
  dermatology, 188, 189, 190–4
  diabetes, 200, 201
  endocrinology, 195–6
  ENT and gynaecology, 82, 83
  gastroenterology, 204–6
  geriatric care, 145, 146, 147
  gynaecology, 218, 220–2
  haematology, 224
  infection control, 184
  intensive care, 157–8
  microbiology, 34, 181, 182, 183, 225
  neurology, 235–6, 236, 237, 238–9
  orthopaedics, 254, 256–7, 257–8, 259
  otorhinolaryngology, 260–1, 262
  pathology, 263, 264
  radiology, 284–5
  surgery, 212, 214, 215–16
  vascular surgery, 299, 300
transfer to Tallaght, 82, 86–7, 88, 92, 93–4,
  100–4, 169–70, 217, 227, 264–5, 271, 284
  protection of Charter, 44–51
  Protestant ethos, 70–1, 73–4, 77, 93–5, 98–
    104, 169–70
Adelaide Hospital Research Foundation, 193
Adelaide Hospital Society, 45, 46, 50, 51, 78, 96,
  303
Adelaide School of Nursing, 45, 96, 98, 100,
  242–3
Adrian Stokes Memorial Fellowship, 224
A&E services, 2–3, 144, 154, 215, 269–70, 284
Aer Lingus, 44
age-related health care, 145–50
AIB, 296
AIDS, 185, 187, 228, 229, 271
Alberti, Professor George, 196
All-Ireland Institute of Psychiatry, 147

Hogan, Liam, 36
Hogan, Lorcan, 32
Hogan, Niall, 80–1, 277, 278, 279, 281
Hogan, Peg, 245
Hogg, Amelia, 272, 275
Holles Street Hospital, 222
Holmes, Gordon, 235
Hone, Rosemary, 185
Hope, D. S., 85, 87
Horner, Nuala, 225
Horton, Dr, 267, 270
Hospital for Sick Children, Great Ormond St,
  121, 182, 243, 278
Hospitals Commission, 1, 2, 12, 112–13, 293
Hospitals Federation and Amalgamation Act,
  1961, 1, 14, 21, 42, 67, 79, 82, 91, 114, 130, 151,
  161, 254
  aims of, 25–6
Hospitals Sweepstakes, 111–12
Houlden, Valerie, 192, 195
Houlihan, Peter, 98
Hourihane, Professor Dermot, 34, 138–9, 140,
  184, 263, 265
Howie, Professor Ian, 15–16, 17, 18, 28–9, 33,
  221, 223
Howlin, Brendan, 17, 44, 58, 99, 100, 170
Hughes, Marian, 148
Hume, John, 66
Humphreys, Professor Hilary, 185
Hunt, Dame Agnes, 253
Hurley, Gerry D., 56–7, 157, 283, 297
Hutchinson, David A., 16
Hutchinson, Michael, 172, 236, 237, 239
Huxley, Miss, 246

IMPACT, 103–4
Incorporated Orthopaedic Hospital, 255
Incorporated Society of Trained Masseuses, 272
infection control, 183–4
Institute of Molecular Medicine, 18, 42, 179,
  204, 232
Institute of Nursing, 246
Institute of Orthopaedic Surgeons, 256
Institution for Sick Children, Pitt St, 120, 243,
  244
intensive care, 157–8
International Diabetes Federation, 196
Irish Association of Dermatologists, 188
Irish Blood Transfusion Service, 226
Irish Cardiac Society, 160, 161, 162
Irish Diabetes Federation, 200
Irish Epilepsy Association, 116, 236
Irish Gerontological Society, 148
Irish Haemophilia Society, 227, 229–30
Irish Health Research Board, 148

Irish Heart Foundation, 148, 163
Irish Journal of Medical Science, 109, 148
Irish Life Assurance Company, 44, 48, 72, 94,
  169
Irish Medical Association (IMA), 19, 118
Irish Medical Council, 282
Irish Medical Organisation (IMO), 207
Irish Neurological Association, 237
Irish Nurses' Organisation (INO), 104
Irish Orthopaedic Club, 256
Irish Otolaryngological Head and Neck Society,
  262
Irish Paediatric Association, 122
Irish School of Massage and Medical
  Electricity, 272
Irish Society of Chartered Physiotherapists, 275
Irish Society of Gastroenterology, 202, 207
Irish Stone Foundation, 296
Irish Times, 70, 72, 99, 116, 295
Irish Turf Club, 255
Irish Unrelated Bone Marrow Registry, 231
Irish Urological Nurses' Association, 294–5
Irish Volunteers, 11
Irwin, John, 164

Jackman, Frank, 56
Jackson, Fred, 226, 228
Jackson, Norman, 139, 189
Jacob, R. E., 115
Jacob, Robert, 264
James Connolly Memorial Hospital, 53, 67, 153,
  279, 280
Jasper, 236
Jaswon, Nick, 82, 224, 263, 265
Jefferson Smurfit Foundation, 296
Jermyn, Nicholas, 99, 205
Jervis Street Hospital, 13–14, 19, 109, 111, 115,
  154, 287
Jessop, Professor W. J. E., 14, 27, 130, 136, 171,
  181, 274
John Durkan Leukaemia Laboratory, 232
Johns Hopkins, Baltimore, 121, 236
Johnson, Alan, 196
Johnson, Charles, 243
Johnston, Sir Charles, 120
Johnston, Francis, 8
Jones, Sir Robert, 253
Journal of the Medical Association of Éire, 109
Joyce, Cyril, 227
Joyce, Sister Imelda, 294
Joyce, James, 196
Joynt, Lane, 283
Judge, Leona, 147
Judkins, 163
Julian, Desmond, 163